Orthodontics: Principles and Practice

Orthodontics: Principles and Practice

Edited by

Daljit S. Gill

BDS (Hons), BSc (Hons), MSc (Lond.), FDS RCS (Eng.),
MOrth RCS (Eng.), FDS (Orth) RCS (Eng.)
Consultant Orthodontist and Honorary Senior Lecturer, UCLH Eastman
Dental Hospital and UCL Eastman Dental Institute, London
Honorary Consultant, Great Ormond Street Hospital, London, UK

Farhad B. Naini

BDS (Lond.), MSc (Lond.), FDS RCS (Eng.), MOrth RCS (Eng.),
FDS (Orth) RCS (Eng.), GCAP (KCL), FHEA
Consultant Orthodontist, Kingston and St George's Hospitals, London
Honorary Senior Lecturer, Craniofacial Anatomy, Biology and Development,
St George's Medical School, University of London, London, UK

DentalUpdate

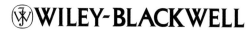

WILEY-BLACKWELL

A John Wiley & Sons, Ltd., Publication

This edition first published 2011 © 2011 Daljit S. Gill, Farhad B. Naini and Dental Update

Blackwell Publishing was acquired by John Wiley & Sons in February 2007. Blackwell's publishing program has been merged with Wiley's global Scientific, Technical and Medical business to form Wiley-Blackwell.

Registered office: John Wiley & Sons, Ltd, The Atrium, Southern Gate, Chichester, West Sussex, PO19 8SQ, UK

Editorial offices: 9600 Garsington Road, Oxford, OX4 2DQ, UK
The Atrium, Southern Gate, Chichester, West Sussex, PO19 8SQ, UK
2121 State Avenue, Ames, Iowa 50014-8300, USA

For details of our global editorial offices, for customer services and for information about how to apply for permission to reuse the copyright material in this book please see our website at www.wiley.com/wiley-blackwell.

The right of the author to be identified as the author of this work has been asserted in accordance with the UK Copyright, Designs and Patents Act 1988.

Designations used by companies to distinguish their products are often claimed as trademarks. All brand names and product names used in this book are trade names, service marks, trademarks or registered trademarks of their respective owners. The publisher is not associated with any product or vendor mentioned in this book. This publication is designed to provide accurate and authoritative information in regard to the subject matter covered. It is sold on the understanding that the publisher is not engaged in rendering professional services. If professional advice or other expert assistance is required, the services of a competent professional should be sought.

Library of Congress Cataloging-in-Publication Data
Orthodontics : principles and practice / edited by Daljit S. Gill, Farhad B. Naini.
      p. ; cm. -- (Dental update)
   Includes bibliographical references and index.
      ISBN-13: 978-1-4051-8747-3 (hardback : alk. paper)
   ISBN-10: 1-4051-8747-6 (hardback : alk. paper) 1. Orthodontics. I. Gill, Daljit S. II. Naini, Farhad B. III. Series: Dental update (Wiley-Blackwell)
   [DNLM: 1. Orthodontics--methods. 2. Orthodontic Appliances. 3. Tooth Diseases. WU 400]
   RK521.O778 2011
   617.6'43--dc23
                                                      2011019197

A catalogue record for this book is available from the British Library.

This book is published in the following electronic formats: ePDF 9781444346091; ePub 9781444346107; Mobi 9781444346114

Set in 9.5 on 12 pt Palatino by Toppan Best-set Premedia Limited
Printed and bound in Singapore by Markono Print Media Pte Ltd

1 2011

Contents

Contributors

David R. Bearn, PhD, MSc, BDS, MOrth RCS (Eng.), F (Orth) DS RCPS, FDS RCS (Edin.), FHEA, Professor of Orthodontics, University of Dundee, Scotland

Adrian Becker, BDS, LDS, DDO, Clinical Associate Professor Emeritus, Department of Orthodontics, Hebrew University Hadassah School of Dental Medicine founded by the Alpha Omega Fraternity, Jerusalem, Israel

Philip E. Benson, PhD, FDS (Orth), Reader and Honorary Consultant, School of Clinical Dentistry, University of Sheffield, Sheffield, UK

Daniel Burford, BDS, MSc, FDS, MSc MOrth, FDS (Orth), RCS (Eng.), Consultant Orthodontist, Medway NHS Foundation Trust, Gillingham, Kent, UK

Robert A.C. Chate, BDS, DOrth RCS (Eng.), DDOrth RCPS (Glasg.), MOrth RCS (Eng.), M Surg Dent RCS Ed, FDS RCS Ed., Consultant Orthodontist, Essex County Hospital, Colchester, UK

Stella Chaushu, DMD, MSc, Associate Professor and Chairperson, Department of Orthodontics, Hebrew University Hadassah School of Dental Medicine founded by the Alpha Omega Fraternity, Jerusalem, Israel

Lam L. Cheng, MDSc (Hons), BDSc (Hons), BDent St, MRACDS (Ortho), Morth RCS Edin, Honorary Associate Lecturer, Discipline of Orthodontics, Faculty of Dentistry, University of Sydney, Australia

Richard R.J. Cousley, BSc, BDS, MSc, FDS, MOrth, FDS (Orth) RCS, Consultant Orthodontist, Peterborough and Stamford Hospitals NHS Foundation Trust, Peterborough, UK

Susan J. Cunningham, PhD, BChD, FDS RCS, MSc, MOrth RCS, FHEA, Professor/ Honorary Consultant, Orthodontics, UCL Eastman Dental Institute, London, UK

M. Ali Darendeliler, BDS, PhD, DipOrth, CertifOrth, PrivDoc, Professor and Chair, Discipline of Orthodontics, Faculty of Dentistry, University of Sydney, and Head, Department of Orthodontics, Sydney Dental Hospital, Australia

Leandra Dopazo, DDS, MS, Clinical Assistant Professor, Department of Orthodontics, University of Florida, Gainesville, Florida, USA

Donald H. Enlow, PhD, Professor Emeritus, Department of Orthodontics, Case Western Reserve University, Cleveland, Ohio, USA

Nigel Fox, BChD, MSc, FDS RCPS, MOrth RCS (Eng.), Specialist Orthodontist, Select Orthodontics, Middlesbrough, UK

Daljit S. Gill, BDS (Hons), BSc (Hons), MSc (Lond.), FDS RCS (Eng.), MOrth RCS (Eng.), FDS (Orth) RCS (Eng.) Consultant Orthodontist and Honorary Senior Lecturer, UCLH Eastman Dental Hospital and UCL Eastman Dental Institute, London, and Honorary Consultant, Great Ormond Street Hospital, London, UK

Urban Hagg, DDS, Odont Dr (Lund.), FDS RCS (Edin.) (Hon), FHKAM, FCDSHK (Ortho), Chair and Professor in Orthodontics, Faculty of Dentistry, University of Hong Kong, Hong Kong, SAR, China

Mark G. Hans, DDS, MSD, Professor and Chairman, Department of Orthodontics, Case Western Reserve University, Cleveland, Ohio, USA

Nigel W.T. Harradine, BDS, FDS, MB BS, MSc, MOrth, Consultant Orthodontist Bristol Dental Hospital and School, Bristol, UK

Norman John Hay, BDS, FDS RCS (Eng.), MSc (Lond.), MOrth RCS (Eng.), FDS (Orth) RCS (Intercollegiate), Consultant Orthodontist, Great Ormond Street Hospital, London and Specialist in Orthodontics, Blandy House Dental Practice, Henley-on-Thames, London, UK

Sarah Hepburn, BSc, BDS, MFDS RCS (Eng.), MSc, MOrth, MSc Lingual, Principal of a Private Practice, Director of Harley Street Orthodontic Clinic, London, UK

Nigel Hunt, PhD, BDS, FDS RCPS, FDS RCS (Edin.), FDS RCS (Eng.), MOrth, FHEA, Chairman of Division of Craniofacial and Developmental Sciences, Head of Unit of Orthodontics, UCL Eastman Dental Institute, London, UK

Anthony Ireland, PhD, FDS MOrth (RCS Eng.), Consultant/Reader, Department of Child Dental Health, Bristol Dental Hospital and Consultant Orthodontist, Royal United Hospital, Bath UK

Shamique Ismail, BDS, FDS RCS, MSc, MOrth, RCS, FDS (Orth) RCS, Consultant Orthodontist, North West London Hospitals NHS Trust, UK

Ama Johal, BDS, MSc, PhD, FDS, MOrth, FDS (Orth) RCS, Senior Clinical Lecturer/Honorary Consultant Orthodontist, Barts & The London School of Medicine and Dentistry, Institute of Dentistry, Queen Mary University of London, London, UK

Robert Kirschen, BDS, MSc, MOrth, FDS RCS, Specialist in Orthodontics, Reigate Specialist Orthodontic Practice, Surrey, UK

Robert Lee, MDS, MOrth, FDS, Professor and Consultant Orthodontist, Barts & The London, Centre for Oral Growth & Development, Institute of Dentistry, London, UK

Kevin Lewis, BDS, LDSRCS, FDS RCS (Eng.), FFGDP (UK), Dental Director of Medical Protection, London, UK

Simon J. Littlewood, BDS, FDS (Orth), RCPS, MOrth RCS, MDSc, FDS RCS, Consultant Orthodontist, St Luke's Hospital, Bradford, UK

Gavin J. Mack, BDS, MSc, MFDS, MOrth, FDS (Orth), RCS, Consultant Orthodontist, King's College Hospital, London, UK

James McDonald, BDS, FDS RCS (Edin.), FDS, LDS, DOrth RCS (Eng.), Professor and Consultant Orthodontist, Dental Hospital, Edinburgh, UK

Niall J.P. McGuinness, PhD (QUB), DDS (U. Edin.), MScD (U.Wales), BA, BDentSc (U.Dubl.), FDS (Orth) RCPS (Glasg.), MOrth RCS (Edin.), Consultant Orthodontist and Honorary Senior Lecturer, Edinburgh Postgraduate Dental Institute, Edinburgh, UK

Grant T. McIntyre, BDS, FDS RCPS, MOrth RCS, PhD, FDS (Orth) RCPS, Consultant Orthodontist, Dundee Dental Hospital and School, Dundee, Scotland

Declan Millett, BDSc, DDS, FDS RCPS (Glasg.), DOrth RCS (Eng.), MOrth RCS (Eng.), Professor of Orthodontics, Cork University Dental School and Hospital, University College Cork, Ireland

Howard Moseley, BChD, MSc, FDS (Orth) RCPS, MOrth, FHEA, Consultant Orthodontist, Watford General Hospital, West Hertfordshire Hospitals NHS Trust and Consultant Orthodontist/Honorary Senior Lecturer, Eastman Dental Institute/University College Hospitals NHS Trust, London, UK

Peter A. Mossey, BDS, PhD, FDS RCS (Edin.), MOrth RCS (Eng.), FFD (Orth) RCSI, FDS RCPS (Glas.), FHEA, Professor of Craniofacial Development University of Dundee, Scotland

Alison Murray, BDS, MSc, FDS RCPS, MOrth RCS, Consultant Orthodontist, Derbyshire Royal Hospital, Derbyshire, UK

Farhad B. Naini, BDS (Lond.), MSc (Lond.), FDS RCS (Eng.), MOrth RCS (Eng.), FDS (Orth) RCS (Eng.), GCAP (KCL), FHEA, Consultant Orthodontist, Kingston and St George's Hospitals, London, and Honorary Senior Lecturer, Craniofacial Anatomy, Biology and Development, St George's Medical School, University of London, London, UK

Stephen L. Newell, BDS (Hons), MSc, FDS MOrth RCS (Eng.), Consultant Orthodontist, Medway NHS Foundation Trust, Gillingham, Kent, UK

Joseph Noar, MSc, BDS, FDS RCS, DOrth, MOrth RCS, FHEA, Consultant in Orthodontics and Honorary Senior Lecturer, Eastman Dental Hospital, University College London Hospitals NHS Trust, London, UK

Richard Parkhouse, BDS Hons (Lond.), FDS DOrth RCS (Eng.), FDS RCS (Edin.), Formerly Consultant Orthodontist, Glan Clwyd Hospital, Wales, UK

Jonathan Sandler, BDS (Hons) MSc, FDS RCPS, MOrth RCS, Consultant Orthodontist, Chesterfield Royal Hospital, Bakewell, UK

Jonathan R. Sandy, PhD, FDS, MOrth RCS (Eng.), FMedSci, Professor of Orthodontics, School of Oral & Dental Science, University of Bristol, Bristol, UK

Manish Valiathan, DDS, DOrth, MSD, DMD, Assistant Professor, Department of Orthodontics, Case Western Reserve University, Cleveland, Ohio, USA

Timothy T. Wheeler, DMD, PhD, Professor and Chair, Department of Orthodontics, University of Florida, USA

Dirk Wiechmann, DDS, Department of Orthodontics, Hanover Medical School, Hanover, Germany and Honorary Associate Professor, Faculty of Dentistry, University of Hong Kong, Hong Kong

Ricky W.K. Wong, BDS, MOrth, PhD, MOrth RCS (Edin.), MRACDS (Ortho), FRACDS, FHKAM, FCDSHK (Ortho), Associate Professor in Orthodontics, Postgraduate Programme Director in Orthodontics, Faculty of Dentistry, University of Hong Kong, Hong Kong, SAR, China

Preface

Orthodontics was the first established specialty within dentistry. The extensive and arduous training required to gain proficiency in orthodontic practice is precisely because of the significant and consequential responsibility of providing the highest level of care for patients.

It is important to dispel any myths at the outset – Orthodontics is not easy and misguided attempts to undertake orthodontic treatment without adequate understanding and training will inevitably result in problems for the patient and, at best, considerable confusion for the clinician.

Orthodontics: Principles & Practice has been designed to serve as an affordable, yet comprehensive reference for orthodontists in clinical practice and training, and dentists with a special interest in orthodontics. The text has been organized into four sections covering the entire spectrum of orthodontics, representing growth and development, diagnosis and treatment planning, the management of malocclusions and appliance techniques. In each of these sections the clinician will find chapters devoted to the critical core knowledge of each specific orthodontic problem or technique. Each chapter is logically arranged and evidence-based, describing the scientific and practical foundations of the subject area at hand.

The distinguished authors invited to prepare the chapters for this text are renowned experts in their respective fields; many have been leaders in developing the techniques and procedures that they describe. We appreciate the hard work and diligence of the contributing authors in preparing manuscripts for this textbook.

Our heartfelt thanks to the staff at Wiley-Blackwell, particularly Lucy Nash, Sophia Joyce, Lotika Singha and Anne Bassett, for believing in our mission and for working hard to bring this text to fruition. Special thanks to Professor Trevor Burke for supporting this project from the outset.

Experience, the mother of wisdom, may be defined as the action of putting our assimilated and reflective knowledge and practice to the test. It is our wish that the scientific and practical information in this book, together with credible clinical training, will provide the stepping stones towards sound clinical experience, and help develop the aptitudes, skills and judgement that may only be 'by industry achieved'.

We are donating the royalties for this book to *Changing Faces*, the leading UK charity that supports and represents people who have disfigurements to the face, hand or body from any cause, thereby complementing medical and surgical interventions by addressing the psychological and social challenges posed by such disfigurements.

DSG/FBN
2011

Dedication

To our families and our profession

Growth and Development

1

An introduction to human craniofacial growth and development

'Growth' is a general term implying simply that something changes in magnitude. It does not, however, presume to account for **how** it happens. For the clinician, such a loose meaning is often used quite properly. However, to try to understand 'how' it works, and what actually happens, the more descriptive and explanatory term 'development' is added. This connotes a maturational process involving progressive differentiation at the cellular and tissue levels, thereby focusing on the actual biological mechanism that accounts for growth.

'Growth and development' is an essential topic in many clinical disciplines and specialties, and the reason is important. Morphogenesis is a biological process having an underlying **control** system at the cellular and tissue levels. The clinician intervenes in the course of this control process at some appropriate stage and substitutes (augments, overpowers or replaces) some activities of the control mechanism with calculated clinical regulation. It is important to understand that the actual biological process of development itself is the same. That is, the histogenic functioning of the cells and tissues still

carry out their individual roles, but the **control signals** that selectively activate the composite of them are now clinically manipulated. It is the rate, timing, direction and magnitude of cellular divisions, and tissue differentiation that become altered when the clinician's signals modify or complement the body's own intrinsic growth signals. The subsequent course of development thus proceeds according to a programmed treatment plan by 'working with growth' (an old clinical tenet). Of course, if one does not understand the workings of the underlying biology, any real grasp of the actual basis for treatment design and results, and why, is an illusion. Importantly, craniofacial biology is independent of treatment intervention strategy. Therefore, although some clinicians may argue about the relative merits of different intervention strategies (e.g. extraction versus arch expansion), the biological rules of the game are the same.

Morphogenesis works constantly towards a state of composite, architectonic **balance** among all of the separate growing parts. This means that the various parts developmentally merge

Orthodontics: Principles and Practice, First Edition. Edited by Daljit S. Gill, Farhad B. Naini.
© 2011 Daljit S. Gill, Farhad B. Naini and Dental Update. Published 2011 by Blackwell Publishing Ltd.

into a functional whole, with each part complementing the others as they all grow and function together.

During development, balance is continuously transient and can never actually be achieved because growth itself constantly creates ongoing, normal regional imbalances. This requires other parts to constantly adapt (develop) as they all work toward composite equilibrium. It is such an imbalance itself that fires the signals which activate the interplay of histogenic responses. Balance, when achieved for a time, turns off the signals and regional growth activity ceases. The process recycles throughout childhood, into and through adulthood (with changing magnitude) and finally on to old age, sustaining a changing morphological equilibrium in response to ever-changing intrinsic and external conditions. For example, as a muscle continues to develop in mass and function, it will outpace the bone into which it inserts, both in size and in mechanical capacity. However, this imbalance signals the osteogenic, chondrogenic, neurogenic and fibrogenic tissues to immediately respond, and the whole bone with its connective tissues, vascular supply and innervation develops (undergoes modelling) to work continuously towards homeostasis.

By an understanding of how this process of progressive morphogenic and histogenic differentiation operates, the clinical specialist thus selectively augments the body's own intrinsic activating signals using controlled procedures to jump-start the modelling process in a way that achieves an intended treatment result. For example, in patients with maxillary transverse deficiency, rapid palatal expansion can be used to separate the right and left halves of the maxilla (displacement). This in turn initiates a period of increased remodelling activity in the midpalatal suture and dentoalveolus.

The genetic and functional **determinants** of a bone's development (i.e. the origin of the growth-regulating signals) reside in the composite of **soft tissues** that turn on or turn off, or speed up or slow down, the histogenic actions of the osteogenic connective tissues (periosteum, endosteum, sutures, periodontal ligament). Growth is not 'programmed' within the bone itself or its enclosing membranes. The 'blueprint' for the design, construction and growth of a bone thus lies in the muscles, tongue, lips, cheeks, integument, mucosae, connective tissues, nerves, blood vessels, airway, pharynx, the brain as an organ mass, tonsils, adenoids and so forth, all of which provide information signals that pace the histogenic tissues responsible for a bone's development.

A major problem with therapeutic modification of the growing face can be **relapse** (rebound subsequent to treatment). The potential for relapse exists when the functional, developmental or biomechanical aspects of growth among key parts are clinically altered to a physiologically imbalanced state. The possibility of instability exists because clinicians strive to bring about a state of aesthetic balance that at times produces physiological imbalance. Rebound is especially strong when the underlying conditions in the 'genic' tissues that led to the pretreatment dysplasia still exist and thus trigger the growth process to rebound in response to the clinically induced changes in morphology. The 'genic' tissues are attempting to restore physiological balance, thereby returning in a developmental direction towards the pretreatment state or some combination between. Physiological compensation is, in effect, a built-in protective mechanism that allows the final occlusion of the teeth to vary only a mere few millimetres, despite enormous variation in the human face (see Figure 1.1).

The evolutionary design of the human head is such that certain regional clinical situations naturally exist. For example, variations in headform design establish natural tendencies toward different kinds of malocclusions. The growth process, in response, develops some regional imbalances, the aggregate of which serves to make corrective adjustments. A Class I molar relationship with an aesthetically pleasing face is the common result in which the underlying

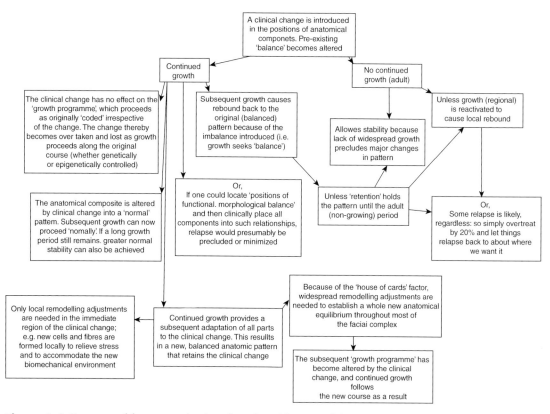

Figure 1.1 Summary of factors involved in clinical modification of the growth process.

factors that would otherwise have led to a more severe Class II or III malocclusion still exist but have been 'compensated for' by the growth process itself. The net effect is an overall, composite balance.

As pointed out above, clinical treatment can disturb a state of structural and functional equilibrium, and a natural rebound can follow. For example, a premature fusion of some cranial sutures can result in growth-retarded development of the nasomaxillary complex because the anterior endocranial fossae (a template for midfacial development) are foreshortened, as in the Crouzon or Apert syndrome. The altered nasomaxillary complex itself nonetheless has grown in a balanced state proportionate to its basicranial template, even though abnormal in comparison with a population norm for aesthetics

and function. Craniofacial surgery disturbs the former balance and some degree of natural rebound can be expected. The growth process attempts to restore the original state of equilibrium, since some extent of the original underlying conditions (e.g. the basicranium) can still exist that was not, or could not be, altered clinically. These are examples in which the biology of the growth process is essentially normal, either with treatment or without, but is producing abnormal results because of altered input control signals.

THE BIG PICTURE

No craniofacial component is developmentally self-contained and self-regulated. Growth of a component is not an isolated event unrelated to other parts. Growth is the composite change of all components. For example, it might be perceived that the developing palate is essentially responsible for its own intrinsic growth and anatomical positioning, and that an infant's palate is the same palate in the adult simply grown larger. The palate in later childhood, however, is not composed of the same tissue (with more simply added), and it does not occupy the same actual position. Many factors influence (impact) the growing palate from without, such as developmental rotations, displacements in conjunction with growth at sutures far removed, and multiple remodelling movements that relocate it to progressively new positions and adjust its size, shape and alignment continuously throughout the growth period.

Similarly, for the mandible, the multiple factors of middle cranial fossa expansion, anterior cranial fossa rotations, tooth eruption, pharyngeal growth, bilateral asymmetries, enlarging tongue, lips and cheeks, changing muscle actions, headform variations, an enlarging nasal airway, changing infant and childhood swallowing patterns, adenoids, head position associated with sleeping habits, body stance and an infinite spread of morphological and functional variations all have input in creating constantly changing states of structural balance.

As emphasised above, **development** is an architectonic process leading to an aggregate state of structural and functional equilibrium, with or without an imposed malocclusion or other morphologic dysplasia. Very little, if anything, can be exempted from the 'big picture' of factors affecting the operation of the growth control process and no region can be isolated. Meaningful insight into all of this underlies the basis for clinical diagnosis and treatment planning. Ideally, the target for clinical intervention should be the control process regulating the growth and development of the component out of balance. However, gaps in our understanding of these processes limit the clinician's ability to treat malocclusions in this manner. Since cause is unknown, clinicians target the effect of

the imbalance. Therefore, a thorough understanding of the process and pattern of facial growth serves as the foundation for craniofacial therapies.

A CORNERSTONE OF THE GROWTH PROCESS

A grasp of how facial growth operates begins with distinguishing between the two basic kinds of **growth movement**: remodelling and displacement (Figure 1.2). Each category of movement involves virtually all developing hard and soft tissues.

For the bony craniofacial complex, the process of growth **remodelling** is paced by the composite of soft tissues relating to each of the bones. The functions of remodelling are to: (1) progressively create the changing **size** of each whole bone; (2) sequentially **relocate** each of the component regions of the whole bone to allow for overall enlargement; (3) progressively **shape** the bone to accommodate its various functions; (4) provide progressive fine-tune **fitting** of all the separate bones to each other and to their contiguous, growing, functioning soft tissues; and (5) carry out continuous structural adjustments to **adapt** to the intrinsic and extrinsic changes in conditions. Although these remodelling functions relate to childhood growth, most also continue on into adulthood and old age in reduced degrees to provide the same ongoing functions. This is what is meant in freshman histology when it is stated that bones 'remodel throughout life', but without an explanation of the reasons. Added to this, now, is that all soft tissues *also* undergo equivalent changes and for all of the same reasons.

In Figures 1.3 and 1.4 note that many external (periosteal) surfaces are actually resorptive. Opposite surfaces are depository. This is required in order to sculpt the complex morphology of the facial bones.

As a bone enlarges, it is simultaneously carried away from other bones in direct articu-

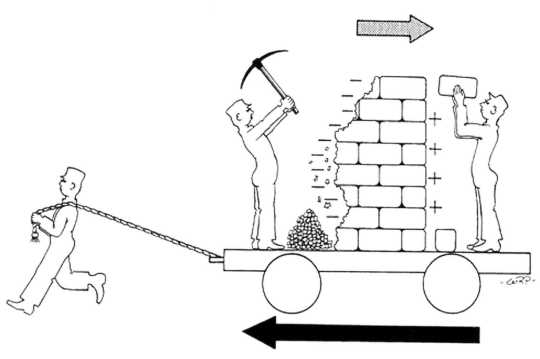

Figure 1.2 Diagrammatic depiction of displacement and remodelling – the two basic types of growth movement.

lation with it. This creates the 'space' between bones and allows bony enlargement to take place. The process is termed **displacement** (also called 'translation'). It is a physical movement of a whole bone and occurs while the bone simultaneously remodels by resorption and deposition. As the bone enlarges in a given direction within a bony interface, it is simultaneously displaced in the **opposite** direction (Figure 1.5). The relationships underscore why facial articulations (sutures and condyles) are important factors; they are often direct clinical targets.

The process of new bone deposition does not cause displacement by **pushing** against the articular contact surface of another bone. Rather, the bone is **carried** away by the expansive force of all the growing soft tissues surrounding and attached to it by anchoring fibres. As this takes place, new bone is added immediately (modelling), the whole bone enlarges

and the two separate bones thereby remain in contact. The nasomaxillary complex, for example, is in sutural contact with the floor of the cranium. The whole maxillary region, *in toto*, is **displaced** downwards and forwards away from the cranium by the expansive growth of the soft tissues in the midfacial region (Figure 1.6a). This then triggers new bone growth at the various sutural contact surfaces between the nasomaxillary composite and the cranial floor (Figure 1.6b). Displacement thus proceeds downwards and forwards an equivalent amount as maxillary remodelling simultaneously takes place in an opposite upward and backward direction (i.e. **towards** its contact with the cranial floor).

Similarly, the whole mandible (Figure 1.5) is **displaced** 'away' from its articulation in each glenoid fossa by the growth enlargement of the composite of soft tissues in the developing face. As this occurs, the condyle and ramus grow

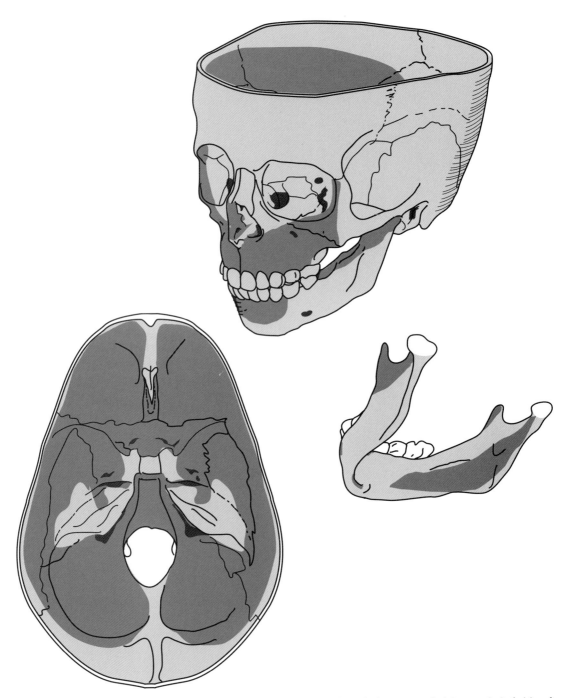

Figure 1.3 Summary diagram of the resorptive (darkly stippled) and depository (lightly stippled) fields of remodelling. (From Enlow DH, Kuroda T, Lewis AB. The morphological and morphogenetic basis for craniofacial form and pattern. Angle Orthod 1971;41:161. Reproduced with permission from the Angle Foundation.)

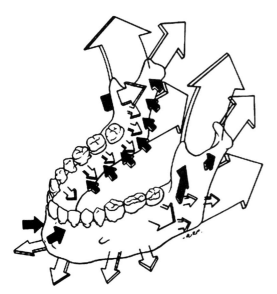

Figure 1.4 Black arrows are surface resorptive and white arrows are depository.

upwards and backwards (relocate) into the 'space' created by the displacement process. Note that the ramus also changes in both shape and size due to the remodelling process as it relocates posterosuperiorly. It becomes longer and wider to accommodate the increasing mass of masticatory muscles inserted onto it, the enlarged breadth of the pharyngeal space and the vertical lengthening of the nasomaxillary part of the growing face.

A beginning student is always confused because it is repeatedly heard and read that the face 'grows forwards and downwards'. It would seem reasonable, then, that the growth activity of the mandible and the maxilla would be in their anterior, forward-facing parts. However, it is mostly the displacement movement that is forwards and downwards, thereby complementing the predominantly posterosuperior vectors of remodelling. This is one fundamental reason, as mentioned above, that all joint contacts and bone ends are of basic significance in the growth picture. They are the points away from which displacement proceeds and, at the same time, the sites where remodelling

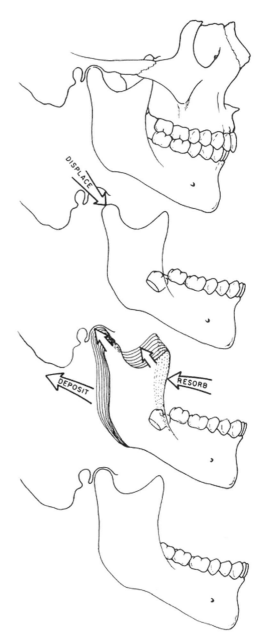

Figure 1.5 Illustrates the displacement of the mandible downwards and forwards with upward and backward remodelling.

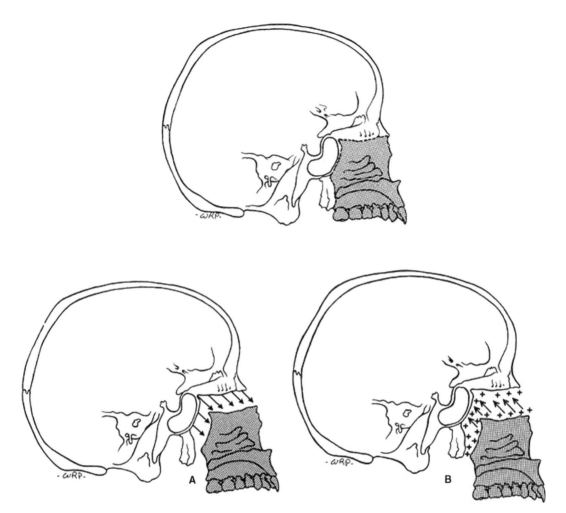

Figure 1.6 Illustrates the displacement of the nasomaxillary complex downward and forwards (A) with upward and backward (B) remodelling.

lengthens a given bone. Thus, they are key locations where clinical procedures can alter the growth process.

THE THREE PRINCIPAL REGIONS OF FACIAL AND NEUROCRANIAL DEVELOPMENT

The major but mutually interrelated form/function components involved in development are the brain with its associated sensory organs and basicranium, the facial and pharyngeal airway, and the oral complex. Although discussed below separately, they are, of course, developmentally inseparable. The fact that all three are interrelated becomes important when applying growth concepts to clinical situations since the developmental factors underlying most craniofacial dysplasias involve all three. In addition, very few clinical procedures address malocclusions at the level of the cranial base.

The brain and basicranium

The configuration of the neurocranium (and brain) determines a person's headform type which, in turn, sets up many of the proportionate and topographical features characterising facial type. A long and narrow basicranium (dolichocephalic) with its more elongate and open-angle configuration, for example, programmes the developmental process so that it characteristically leads to an anteroposteriorly and vertically elongated facial pattern and a more frequent built-in tendency for mandibular retrusion (Figure 1.7, top panel). A rounder basicranium (brachycephalic) is characterised by a proportionately wider but anteroposteriorly shorter configuration, a more closed basicranial flexure, and a vertically and protrusively shorter but wider midface (nasomaxillary complex). These features generally underlie a more orthognathic (or less retrognathic) profile or, in the extreme, a tendency for mandibular protrusion (Figure 1.7, bottom panel).

These characteristic features exist because the basicranium is the template that establishes the shape and perimeter of the facial growth fields. The mandible articulates by its condyles onto the ectocranial side of the middle endocranial fossae and the bicondylar dimension is thus determined by this part of the cranial floor. The nasomaxillary complex is suspended from the anterior endocranial fossae, and the width of the facial airway, the configuration of the palate and maxillary arch, and the placement of all these parts are thus established by it.

The airway

The facial and pharyngeal airway is a space determined by the multitude of separate parts comprising its enclosing walls. The configuration

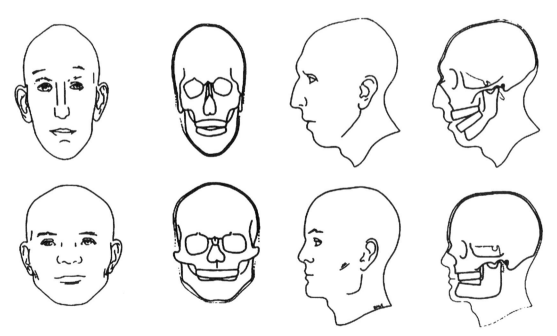

Figure 1.7 The underlying tendency for dolichocephaly towards Class II malocclusions with increased lower vertical facial height and brachycephaly towards Class III malocclusions with decreased lower vertical facial height. (From Enlow DH, Dale J. In: Ten Cate R. (ed.) Oral Histology, 4th edn. St. Louis: CV Mosby, 1994, with permission.)

and dimensions of the airway are thus a product of the composite growth and development of many hard and soft tissues along its pathway from nares to glottis.

Although determined by surrounding parts, those parts in turn are dependent on the airway for maintenance of their own functional and anatomical positions. If there develops any regional childhood variation along the course of the airway that significantly alters its configuration or size, growth then proceeds along a different course, leading to a variation in overall facial assembly that may exceed the bounds of normal pattern. The airway functions, in a real sense, as a keystone for the face. A keystone is that part of an arch which, if of proper shape and size, stabilises the positions of the remaining parts of the arch. In Figure 1.8 a few of the many 'arches' in a face can be recognised and the bony remodelling (+ and −) producing them. Horizontally and vertically, the arch form of the orbits, the nasal and oral sides of the palate, the maxillary arch, the sinuses, the zygomatic arches and so forth are all subject to airway configuration, size and integrity. Note that the airway is strategically pivotal to all of them.

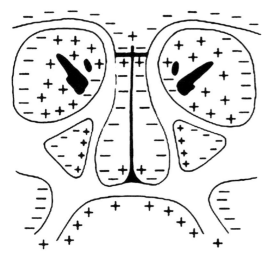

Figure 1.8 The depository (+) and resorptive (−) areas of the midface in coronal section.

Two easy personal tests can be performed illustrating the airway as a significant factor in programming the developmental course of the facial 'genic' tissues. This is useful in explanations of malocclusion aetiology for patients or their parents. First, starting with an open mouth, close the lips and jaws (note that your tongue will likely rise against the palate) and, momentarily, swallow. This evacuates the oral air into the pharynx, creating an oral vacuum. The effect is to stabilise the mandible and hold it in a closed position with minimal muscle effort. Now, open the jaws and lips, feeling a rush of air into the mouth. To hold the lower jaw in this 'mouth breathing' posture requires a different pattern of muscle activity, and the osteogenic, chondrogenic, periodontal, fibrogenic and other histogenic tissues thereby receive a correspondingly different pattern of signals. This causes different developmental responses to a different functional morphology adapted to the conditions. As emphasised before, the operation of the growth process itself functions normally. It is the nature of the **activating signals** that produces emerging deviations in the course of development that results in any morphological variation and perhaps malocclusion.

The second test is similar. Swallow with your teeth in occlusion and your lips touching. Next, swallow with your teeth and lips apart. Open-jawed swallows are possible, but can be difficult when one is accustomed to a closed mouth. Note the very different pattern of masticatory and hyoid muscle actions required. As with the mouth breathing test outlined above, altered signals are generated, and the genic tissues work toward a different balance combination, producing a variation in facial morphology. A factor often overlooked by clinicians is that these altered signals may result in different treatment responses to the same intervention. For example, patients' response to a removable orthopaedic appliance such as a bionator or twin block may vary dramatically based on their mode of breathing.

The oral region

In addition to the basicranial and airway factors described above affecting mandibular and maxillary shape, size and positioning, other basic considerations are involved. If a brain and basicranial asymmetry exists, this condition can either be passed on to cause a corresponding facial asymmetry, or compensated by the facial developmental process to either offset or reduce its magnitude. For the latter, remodelling adjustments produce an actual opposite asymmetry in the nasomaxillary complex and/or mandible that counteracts the basicranial condition. Advances in craniofacial imaging such as cone beam computed tomography have made it easier for clinicians to identify the site of facial asymmetry and plan treatment accordingly.

For the maxilla, if not developmentally compensated or only partially so, the maxillary arch can become deviated laterally, matching the lateral asymmetry of the anterior endocranial fossae. Or, vertically, one side can become lowered or elevated relative to the other, including the orbits, palate and maxillary arch. For the mandible, the middle endocranial fossae determine the placement of the temporomandibular joints and, if asymmetrical, one or the other will be lower or higher, forward or back. Whole mandible alignment necessarily follows if not fully or partially adjusted by remodelling during development.

Many other such compensatory adjustments by the remodelling process occur throughout growth and development in many ways. These involve the development of certain regional imbalances to offset others, resulting in a composite overall structural and functional equilibrium.

CRANIOFACIAL LEVELS

When the face is in balance, there exists a descending, cause-and-effect stratographic arrangement of structural **levels** in the design of the face. Beginning with the frontal lobes of the cerebrum,

the floor of the anterior endocranial fossae adapts in size and shape during their interrelated development. The ectocranial side of this floor is the roof of the nasal chambers, thus programming the perimeter of that key facial part of the airway. This configuration, in turn, is projected inferiorly to the next level, establishing the proportions and configuration of the nasal side of the palate. Then, the perimeter of the apical base of the maxillary dental arch is set by the oral side of the hard palate, all representing configurational projections from the anterior endocranial fossae. The next level following is maxillary intercanine width, and then mandibular intercanine width, all preprogrammed in configuration and in proportion to the basicranium.

The mandible has a component not represented in the maxilla, and that is its **ramus**. The anteroposterior size of the ramus develops by an amount approximating the horizontal span of the pharynx, which has a programmed anteroposterior dimension established by its ceiling, which is the ectocranial side of the middle endocranial fossae underlying the temporal lobes of the cerebrum. The ramus, thus, places the mandibular arch in occlusion with the maxillary arch following a pattern set up by the basicranium. Vertically, the developing ramus lowers the corpus by progressive amounts, adapting to the vertical growth of the middle cranial fossae (clivus) as well as the vertical expansion of the nasal airway and developing dentition.

The face, thus, is a stratified series of vertical levels all sharing a common developmental template. This makes possible a workable morphogenic system having a structural design allowing large numbers of separate parts to develop together in harmony and to carry out respective functions while it happens.

THE TWO BASIC CLINICAL TARGETS

There is one developmental concept that needs to be addressed with particular emphasis because of its great significance to the old clinical axiom 'working with growth'. While a factor such as the basicranium can prescribe and determine a 'growth field' in the contiguous facial complex, as described above, it is within the boundaries of that field that remodelling then engineers the **shape and size and functional fit** of all parts and develops them through time. However, it can be misunderstood if one presumes that all 'local growth' is regulated solely by a single local, intrinsic growth system. Remember, there are *two* kinds of growth activity: localised, regional **remodelling** ('genic' tissues); and the **displacement** movements of all the separate parts as they remodel. Thus, there are two corresponding histogenic recipients of clinical intervention.

To illustrate this fundamental concept, the incisor and premaxillary alveolar region of the maxilla develops into its adult shape and dimensions by the local remodelling process. But the principal source of the considerable extent of its downwards and forwards growth movement is by displacement, and *that* comes from biomechanical forces of growth enlargement occurring *outside* the premaxillary region itself. Thus, most of the growth movements responsible for the anatomical **placement** of this region, along with, passively, its teeth, are not controlled within its own tissues or any genetic blueprint therein, even though this might be a natural presumption. *Two* clinical targets thereby exist for orthodontists: local remodelling and, separately, the displacement of some whole part produced by the sum of developmental expansions occurring everywhere. There are certain clinical procedures that relate specifically to one or the other target and some that involve both. For example, rapid palatal expansion mimics displacement; incisor retraction primarily involves remodelling of the anterior portion of the alveolar arch, and functional appliance treatment involves both remodelling of the alveolar process and displacement of the mandible, triggering changes in the remodelling of the ramus.

These two basic growth movements are difficult to separate in clinical interventions since the majority of therapeutic procedures require the teeth to be used to deliver biomechanical forces to the surrounding tissues. This limits the clinician's ability to separate displacement from modelling using traditional cephalometric techniques. It is likely that the new three-dimensional imaging modalities currently available will help with this problem.

CHILD-TO-ADULT CHANGING PROPORTIONS

The three principal craniofacial growing parts (brain and basicranium, airway, oral region) each has its own separate timetable of development even though all are inseparably bound as an interrelated whole. Some body systems, such as the nervous and cardiovascular systems, develop earlier and faster compared with others, including the airway and oral regions. The reason is that airway growth is proportionate to growing body and lung size, and the oral region is linked to developmental stages involving the fifth and seventh cranial nerves and associated musculature, the suckling process, dental eruption stages and masticatory development.

The infant and young child are characterised by a wide-appearing face because of the precociously broad basicranial template, but the face otherwise is vertically short (Figure 1.9). This is because the nasal and oral regions are yet diminutive, matching the smallish body and pulmonary parts, and with masticatory development in a transitory state. The vertical height of the mandibular ramus is still relatively short because it is linked in developmental feedback with the shorter, later-maturing nasal and dental regions. Masticatory musculature is proportionately sized and shaped to progressively match increasing function and to interplay developmentally with the ramus.

During later childhood and into adolescence, vertical nasal enlargement keeps pace

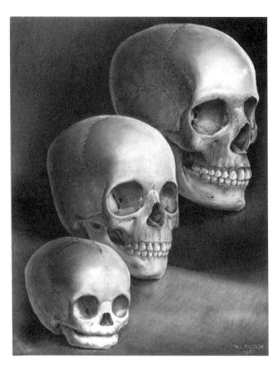

Figure 1.9 Infant, child and adult skulls showing the changes in both size and proportion that occur with growth and development. (Courtesy of William L. Brudon. From Enlow DH. The Human Face. New York: Harper & Row, 1968, with permission.)

with growing body and lung size, and dental and other oral components have approached adult sizes and configuration. The mandibular arch is lowered by increasing vertical ramus length. Overall, the early wide face has become altered in proportion by the later vertical changes. The end effect is particularly marked in the dolichocephalic long-headed and long-face patterns and less so in the brachycephalic headform type.

TOOTH MOVEMENT

To begin, a tooth is moved by either or both of two developmental means: by becoming actively moved in combination with its own remodelling periodontal connective tissue and alveolar socket; and by being carried along

passively as the entire maxilla or mandible is displaced anteroinferiorly during facial morphogenesis. Another basic and clinically significant concept is that **bone and connective tissues** (such as the periodontal connective tissue, periosteum, endosteum and submucosa, all of which participate directly and actively in a tooth's movement) have an intrinsic remodelling process that, when activated, move themselves as a growth function. When a tooth is moved, these other contiguous parts move with it by their own 'genic' remodelling process to sustain relationships. A tooth, however, *cannot move itself* in a comparable manner by its own remodelling. Teeth erupt 'fully grown' and are mobile, but not motile. A tooth is *moved* by biomechanical forces external to the tooth itself and there is an elaborate 'biology' in the composite process that produces a tooth's growth movements. A tooth must move (drift, erupt, etc.) during maxillary and mandibular growth in order to become properly placed in progressively changing anatomical positions. Whether the force producing the tooth's change in position is intrinsic or **clinically induced**, the biology is the same. As mentioned again because the point is important, it is the nature of the **activating signals** that is different, and this causes either the multiple array of genic tissues to alter the course of remodelling or the displacement process of a whole bone to become altered in direction or magnitude.

DRIFT

A worthy advance was made when it was realised that teeth undergo a process of **drift**. For many years this fundamental concept was limited to horizontal (mesial and distal) movements and the essential function was held to be a stabilisation of the dental palisade to compensate for interproximal attrition. Added to this, now, is that drift has a basic **growth** function. It serves to anatomically place the teeth in occlusion as the maxilla and mandible enlarge.

Such movements are significant considering that a jawbone lengthens considerably from prenatal to adult sizes. Also, the original drift concept was for horizontal movement. This is in addition to 'eruption' and should not be so termed. **Vertical drift** is a basic growth movement the clinician 'works with' because it can be modified by clinical intervention (i.e. orthodontic treatment).

Just as teeth undergo a drifting movement, the bone housing them also moves. Unlike a tooth, however, bone moves by the remodelling action of its enclosing osteogenic membranes, and this is also a direct target for clinical intervention. The intrinsic coordination of these bone–tooth movements is remarkable.

GROWTH ROTATIONS

Growth rotations occur throughout the craniofacial region and fall into two categories: remodelling rotations and displacement rotations. They are particularly important in orthodontics when they occur in the mandible. Small rotations occur in everyone during growth, however, when these are significant they can have a large impact on facial form. For example, a significant clockwise mandibular growth rotation can lead to a long face and an anticlockwise rotation to a short face deformity.

Growth rotations can also have a significant effect on determining the direction of tooth eruption.

FINAL THOUGHTS

It has been emphasised in the preceding pages that facial growth is a process requiring intimate morphogenic interrelationships among all of its component growing, changing and functioning soft and hard tissue parts. No part is developmentally independent and self-contained. This is a fundamental and very important principle of growth. As underscored earlier, the growth process works toward an ongoing state of composite functional and structural equilibrium. In clinical treatment, no key anatomical part can be fully segregated and altered without affecting 'balance' with other parts and their state of physiological equilibrium as well. In essence, orthodontic treatment seeks to maximise the effectiveness of anatomical compensations to achieve an aesthetically harmonious masticatory system.

Further Reading

Enlow D, Hans M. Essentials of Facial Growth, 2nd edn. Needham Press, Ann Arbor, MI, 2008.

Development of the dentition 2

INTRODUCTION

Occlusion, in the context of dentistry, has been simply defined as the 'contacts between teeth' albeit between the opposing arches.[1] The arrangement of the contacts between the upper and lower dentition when the teeth are in a position of maximal intercuspation is described as the **static occlusion**, and the pattern of the contacts that guide the movement of the mandible away from this position of maximal intercuspation is termed the **dynamic occlusion**.

Static occlusion can be described and classified through the assessment of incisor and molar relationships (Figures 2.1, 2.2) and the widely accepted static occlusal goals of orthodontic treatment are the six keys to occlusion described by Lawrence Andrews (Box 2.1).[2] Dynamic occlusion can be assessed clinically through the careful observation of the pattern of tooth contacts when the mandible is raised into centric occlusion and is then protruded anteriorly or moved laterally.

Normal occlusal development is intrinsically related to the development of the denti-

tion. The chronology of normal dental development is given in Table 2.1.

Although the teeth and the contacts between the upper and lower dentition provide a means of classifying and assessing the static and dynamic occlusion, a complete assessment of a patient's occlusion requires consideration of the periodontium, orofacial musculature, the temporomandibular joints and the underlying pattern of skeletal growth.

THE STAGES OF OCCLUSAL DEVELOPMENT

Primary Dentition (2.5 Years to 6 Years)

Intra-arch Alignment (Crowding/Spacing/Inclination of Incisors)

The fully developed primary dentition is established from the approximate age of 2.5 years. Ideally the arches are spaced, with the

Orthodontics: Principles and Practice, First Edition. Edited by Daljit S. Gill, Farhad B. Naini.
© 2011 Daljit S. Gill, Farhad B. Naini and Dental Update. Published 2011 by Blackwell Publishing Ltd.

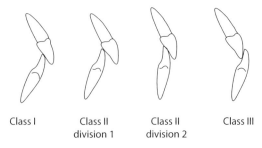

| Class I | Class II division 1 | Class II division 2 | Class III |

Figure 2.1 Incisor classification.

Class I: the lower incisor edges occlude with or are immediately below the cingulum plateau of the upper incisors.

Class II division 1: the lower incisor edges lie posterior to the cingulum plateau of the upper incisors, with the upper incisors being proclined or of an average inclination. The overjet is increased.

Class II division 2: the lower incisor edges lie posterior to the cingulum plateau of the upper incisors, with the upper incisors retroclined. The overjet is usually minimal but may be increased.

Class III: the lower incisor edges lie anterior to the cingulum plateau of the upper incisors, with the upper incisors. The overjet is reduced or reversed.

Box 2.1 The six keys of normal occlusion

1. Molar relationship:
   - The distal surface of the distobuccal cusp of the upper first permanent molar occludes with the mesial surface of the mesiobuccal cusp of the lower second permanent molar.
2. Crown angulation (mesiodistal tip):
   - The gingival portion of each crown is distal to the incisal portion and symmetrically varied with each tooth in the arch.
3. Crown inclination (labiolingual or buccolingual):
   - Incisor teeth with sufficient inclination to prevent overeruption
   - Upper canines and premolars have similar degree of lingual inclination, with increased lingual inclination for the molars
   - Lower posterior teeth from the canine to the molars have progressively increasing lingual inclination
4. No rotations of teeth
5. No spaces between teeth
6. Flat occlusal plane.

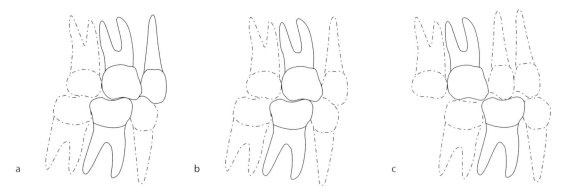

a   b   c

Figure 2.2a–c Molar classification.
(a) Class I: the mesiobuccal cusp of the maxillary first permanent molar lies in the buccal groove of the mandibular first permanent molar.
(b) Class II: the mesiobuccal cusp of the maxillary first permanent molar is mesial to the buccal groove of the mandibular first permanent molar.
(c) Class III: the mesiobuccal cusp of the maxillary first permanent molar is distal to the buccal groove of the mandibular first permanent molar.

Table 2.1 The chronology of dental development

		Calcification begins		Crown formation completed		Eruption begins		Root formation completed	
		Max	Mand	Max	Mand	Max	Mand	Max	Mand
Primary dentition	Central incisor	14 wks in utero	14 wks in utero	1.5 mths	1.5 mths	8–12 mths	6–10 mths	33 mths	33 mths
	Lateral incisor	15 wks in utero	15 wks in utero	2.5 mths	3 mths	9–13 mths	10–16 mths	33 mths	30 mths
	Canine	17 wks in utero	17 wks in utero	9 mths	8–9 mths	16–22 mths	17–23 mths	43 mths	43 mths
	First molar	15 wks in utero	15 wks in utero	6 mths	5–6 mths	13–19 mths	14–18 mths	37 mths	34 mths
	Second molar	19 wks in utero	18 wks in utero	11 mths	8–11 mths	25–33 mths	23–30 mths	47 mths	42 mths
Permanent dentition	Central incisor	3 mths	3 mths	3–4 yrs	3–4 yrs	6–8 yrs	6–7 yrs	8–10 yrs	7–9 yrs
	Lateral incisor	10 mths	4 mths	4–5 yrs	3–5 yrs	7–9 yrs	6–8 yrs	9–10 yrs	8–9 yrs
	Canine	5 mths	5 mths	4–5 yrs	4–5 yrs	10–12 yrs	9–11 yrs	11–13 yrs	11–13 yrs
	First premolar	18–24 mths	18–24 mths	6–7 yrs	5–6 yrs	9–11 yrs	9–11 yrs	11–13 yrs	11–13 yrs
	Second premolar	24–30 mths	24–30 mths	6–7 yrs	6–7 yrs	10–12 yrs	10–12 yrs	11–14 yrs	11–14 yrs
	First molar	6–8 mths in utero	6–8 mths in utero	2–4 yrs	2–4 yrs	6–7 yrs	6–7 yrs	9–11 yrs	8–10 yrs
	Second molar	30–36 mths	30–36 mths	6–8 yrs	6–8 yrs	12–13 yrs	11–12 yrs	13–16 yrs	11–16 yrs
	Third molar	7–9 yrs	8–10 yrs	12–13 yrs	12–13 yrs	17–19 yrs	17–19 yrs	19–20 yrs	20–21 yrs

Max, maxillary; mand, mandibular; wks, weeks; mths, months; yrs, years.

term 'primate space' or 'anthropoid space' being used to describe the space that is localized mesial to the upper primary canine and distal to the lower primary canine. Spacing in the primary dentition is desirable, with an excess of 6 mm of space in each arch being a favourable indication that the developing permanent dentition will be well aligned. An absence of space in the primary dentition has been associated with a 70% likelihood of crowding when the permanent dentition becomes established.[3] Within the upper and lower arches the primary teeth have a typically upright appearance.[4]

Inter-arch Relationship (Overjet/Overbite/Molar Relationship)

The incisor relationship in the primary dentition can be indicative of the likely arrangement when the permanent dentition develops if the overjet or reverse overjet is significant. Otherwise, minimal variations in overjet measurements have little predictive value, with a normal range of overjet being between 0 and 4 mm.

The overbite is relatively increased as the primary dentition erupts and typically this gradually reduces prior to the exfoliation of the incisors as a result of attrition and some forward growth of the mandible. Oral habits such as digit or pacifier sucking are common in this age group and if these persist anterior open bites develop.

The buccal occlusion in the primary dentition is often characterized by the mesiobuccal cusp of the upper second primary molar occluding in the buccal groove of the lower second primary molar, with the distal surfaces of both the upper and lower second primary molars being in the same vertical plane. This arrangement is due to the lower second primary molar being significantly larger than the upper second primary molar and is not necessarily predictive of a developing Angle's Class II molar relationship.

Functional Occlusion

Functional occlusion is difficult to assess in the primary dentition stage due to the changes that occur to the morphology of the teeth as a result of attrition and the underlying growth and development of the alveolar processes and the mandible and maxilla. In addition, young children can have a tendency to posture the mandible when asked to 'bite together' and this can complicate occlusal assessment.

While open bites that develop as a result of an ongoing oral habit will resolve if the habit is broken prior to the eruption of the permanent incisors, the lateral crossbites that can also develop as a consequence of the habit are more persistent and may be associated with a functional displacement of the mandible.

Transitional Dentition (6 Years to 12 Years)

Intra-arch Alignment (Crowding/Spacing/Inclination of Incisors)

An awareness of the typical changes that can occur during this transitional phase of dental development can enable a practitioner to reassure parents and patients that potentially unsightly appearances will improve spontaneously with further growth, and also enables appropriate referrals to be made for interceptive treatment (see Chapter 20) as required.

The lower permanent incisors develop in a lingual position relative to the primary incisors and as they erupt their alignment is typically irregular and they can appear mildly crowded. The lower incisors can then spontaneously align as space is created through three processes:

* A small increase in the transverse dimension between the canines of approximately 2 mm as permanent teeth erupt into a more lateral position within the arch.

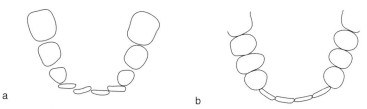

a   b

Figure 2.3 Relief of lower incisor crowding in the mixed dentition. (a) Mild (1–2 mm crowding of the lower permanent incisors in the early mixed dentition. (b) Lower incisor crowding is relieved through: (i) increase in intercanine width as the permanent canines erupt laterally in the arch; (ii) the permanent incisors move labially after eruption; (iii) the permanent canines use the primate spaces distal to the primary canines.

- The permanent incisors erupt into a more labial position ensuring a larger arc of a circle is available to accommodate the larger-sized teeth and the inclination of the incisors is more proclined. This can contribute 1–2 mm of space to relieve crowding.
- The primate space, localized distal to the lower primary canine, is utilized and the erupting incisors cause the canines to migrate distally in the arch, contributing to the increase in intercanine width and providing approximately 1 mm of space.[5]

These distinct mechanisms can increase the space available for the lingually positioned, mildly crowded permanent incisors, which are commonly seen in 8–9 year olds, to align spontaneously (Figure 2.3).

The upper primary incisors are typically spaced and the primate spaces are positioned mesial to the upper primary canines. This tends to ensure there is always sufficient space for the upper central incisors to erupt, and usually enough space to accommodate the lateral incisors. If crowding exists and space is limited for the lateral incisors, these teeth can be palatally excluded from the line of the arch.

A diastema is normal as the upper central incisors erupt and this may partially close with the eruption of the lateral incisors and tends to fully close as the permanent canines erupt. It has been suggested that a diastema of 2 mm or less is likely to close spontaneously as the dentition develops, whereas a diastema greater than 2 mm is likely to persist in the absence of clinical intervention.[6]

The upper lateral incisors can appear flared and distally tipped as the unerupted canines press on the distal aspect of the lateral incisor roots and this transitory, irregular arrangement has been termed the 'ugly duckling' stage of dental development.

From the age of 8–9 years the developing permanent canines should be palpable buccally. Other clinical indications to their position are the inclination of the lateral incisors and whether the primary canines are becoming increasingly mobile as a consequence of their roots being resorbed by the developing permanent canine. Concerns about the location of the developing canines after a clinical examination should be followed up with specialist advice and appropriate radiographic investigations.

Inter-arch Relationship (Overjet/Overbite/Buccal Segments)

A transitory open bite is common (17–18%) during the transition from the primary dentition to the permanent dentition.[7] This can be due to incomplete eruption of the incisors, and normal development will cause the open bite to resolve as the eruption process is completed. A persisting digit habit can act as mechanical interference to the eruption of the incisors and can lead to the development of an increased overjet and a persisting, typically asymmetrical open bite that will 'fit' around the offending digits when *in situ*. The eruption of the permanent incisors is an important stage of dental development to concentrate on eliminating persisting oral habits as the potential for spontaneous improvement in the open bites exists as the permanent incisors erupt.

The buccal segment relationships are represented by the occlusal relationships of the first permanent molars and described according to Angle's classification. The establishment of the molar relationship is guided by the occlusal relationship of the second primary molars and also influenced by the forward growth of the mandible and the mesial migration of the mandibular dentition, particularly the lower first molar migrating into the available leeway space (Figure 2.4).

Mild infraocclusion of primary molars is a common occurrence in the mixed dentition and is not necessarily a cause for concern. If the permanent successor is present a conservative approach can be adopted and the permanent tooth can be expected to erupt normally.[8] Intervention may be indicated if the adjacent permanent teeth significantly 'tip' into the

available space for the successor which can happen when the infraoccluded teeth slip below the contact points of the adjacent teeth.

Functional Occlusion

The functional occlusion in the mixed dentition can be disrupted by the ongoing processes of tooth exfoliation and eruption, which can cause disturbances in the intercuspal position and can cause transient displacements to be present.

The upper incisors can erupt in to a crossbite relationship with the lower incisors. If clinically appropriate, removable appliances can be used to 'push' the upper incisors over the bite and this can eliminate the functional displacement, prevent tooth wear and potential gingival recession, while improving dental aesthetics.

Similarly buccal crossbites may be associated with a functional displacement and expansion appliances can eliminate these displacements during this transitional stage of development, allowing the upper and lower arches to be coordinated and preventing the crossbite from becoming established in the permanent dentition.

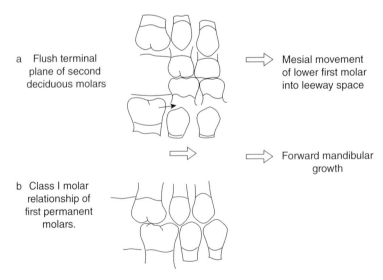

a   Flush terminal plane of second deciduous molars

Mesial movement of lower first molar into leeway space

Forward mandibular growth

b   Class I molar relationship of first permanent molars.

Figure 2.4 Establishing molar relationship in the mixed dentition.

Permanent Dentition (12 Years to 25 Years)

Intra-arch Alignment (Crowding/Spacing/Inclination of Incisors)

The permanent dentition stage begins with the exfoliation of the last primary tooth and the eruption of all the permanent teeth with the exception of the third molars. Ideally, the upper and lower arches are well aligned with no rotations or contact point displacements and tight interproximal contacts between all the teeth. Generalized crowding or spacing can be due to inherent tooth size–arch length discrepancies, and localized spacing, particularly in the region of diminutive upper lateral incisors, may be due to variations in the proportionate widths of the permanent teeth.

The variations in the inclination and angulation of the permanent dentition are more significant than the primary teeth, which are more vertically orientated within the alveolar processes. The crowns of molars and premolars tend to be slightly inclined towards the palate or tongue and the crowns of the canines tend to be slightly tipped in a mesial direction. The crowns of the incisors are slightly proclined in a labial direction, with the upper incisors being slightly angulated towards the midline. Variations in the inclination and angulation of the permanent dentition can occur in all three planes of space and can be representative of dental compensation for an underlying skeletal discrepancy.

Inter-arch Relationship (Overjet/Overbite/Buccal Segments)

In an ideal occlusion, a positive overjet and overbite exists, with the lower incisors lightly contacting the cingulum plateau of the upper incisors in the intercuspal position. A normal overbite can range between 10% and 50% of the height of the clinical crowns of the lower incisors and the overjet can range from 1 to 3 mm. The incisor relationship is classified according to the British Standards Institute classification and may be affected by the underlying skeletal pattern, the effects of the surrounding soft tissues or local factors such as digit habits.

The maxillary and mandibular first permanent molars are ideally in Angle's Class I occlusion, with the mesiobuccal cusp of the maxillary first molar contacting the buccal groove of the mandibular first molar, the premolars intercuspating fully and the maxillary canines occupying the embrasure space between the mandibular canines and first premolars.

The anteroposterior curve of the vertical height of the crowns of the teeth is called the curve of Spee in the lower arch and the compensating curve in the upper arch. The buccolingual curvature of the occlusal surfaces of the posterior dentition is termed the curve of Wilson.

Functional Occlusion

Ideally any slide from the position of initial contact on the retruded arc of closure to the position of maximal intercuspation is small (1–2 mm). In the intercuspal position there should be positive, evenly distributed contacts between all the posterior teeth with light contact between the incisors.

When the mandible is moved forwards from the position of maximal intercuspation, incisor guidance ideally results in an immediate disclusion of the posterior dentition. Similarly, lateral excursions of the lower jaw are guided by the canine or buccal dentition on the 'working' side, with an absence of contacts on the contralateral 'non-working' side.

Maturational changes throughout adulthood

Intra-arch Alignment (Crowding/Spacing/Inclination of Incisors)

Changes to occlusion can occur throughout adulthood at a relatively slow rate. There is a tendency towards development of crowding of the lower incisors, particularly in the late teens and early twenties, and proposed theories for this include the gradual mesial migration of the dentition and late mandibular growth.[9] Changes to the inclination and alignment of incisors with an associated increase in spacing can occur as teeth migrate labially as a consequence of periodontal disease.

Inter-arch Relationship (Overjet/Overbite/Buccal Segments)

Growth rotations of the maxilla and mandible persist throughout adulthood at a basal level and these typically occur at a rate that allows occlusal relationships to be maintained as a result of adaptatory changes in the position of the teeth and the supporting periodontium.[10,11]

Functional Occlusion

As attrition and tooth surface loss results in a reduction of the cusps and flattening of the morphology of the canines, a transition from a 'canine-guided' to a 'group function' occlusal scheme may occur.

FACIAL GROWTH AND THE DEVELOPMENT OF OCCLUSION

Underlying patterns of skeletal growth can affect the development of occlusion. If the skeletal discrepancy is mild or moderate, the inter-action between the underlying skeletal bases, the teeth and the surrounding soft tissues can allow dentoalveolar compensation to occur and for an occlusion to be maintained. If the skeletal discrepancy is severe the potential for dental compensation to occur at an alveolar level is exceeded and malocclusion may develop.

Transverse Skeletal Growth

Studies on facial growth have identified the transverse dimension as being the dimension that ceases growth at the earliest stage of development. This is reflected in the studies on arch form that indicate that the maximum intercanine width is attained on the eruption of the permanent canines and subsequently a gradual reduction in this dimension can be expected.

An underlying transverse skeletal discrepancy can result in a patient developing a buccal crossbite. Dentoalveolar compensation can occur in the transverse dimension to maintain an intercuspated occlusion and this is achieved by the lower posterior teeth being lingually inclined and the upper posterior teeth being buccally inclined.

Anteroposterior Skeletal Growth

Dentoalveolar compensation for skeletal Class II growth patterns can occur with labial tipping of the lower incisors and the palatal tipping of the upper incisors. Conversely, skeletal Class III growth patterns can result in the lowers incisors being retroclined and potentially crowded and the upper incisors being proclined and potentially spaced.

There is a tendency for mandibular growth to exceed that of maxillary growth as a child undergoes pubertal growth. The pubertal growth spurt in males lasts longer and occurs later than in females. The differential between maxillary and mandibular growth is favourable for patients with skeletal Class II patterns of facial growth and unfavourable for young patients with skeletal Class III patterns of facial growth.

Vertical Skeletal Growth

Mandibular growth rotations can occur in a clockwise or anticlockwise direction. When growth rotations are pronounced the development and maintenance of occlusion can be affected. Clockwise mandibular growth rotations are relatively less common and result in a downwards and backwards direction of mandibular growth, which can contribute to a reduction in overbite or even an anterior open bite. An anticlockwise growth rotation can lead to an upwards and forwards direction of mandibular growth and an increase in the depth of the overbite.

Irrespective of the direction of the mandibular growth rotation, crowding of the lower incisors may occur. A clockwise mandibular rotation presses the lower incisors into the musculature of the lower lip and an anticlockwise mandibular rotation forces the lower incisors against the palatal aspects of the upper incisors, both of which can cause progressive lower incisor crowding.[12]

Ethnic Variations and the Development of Occlusion

The concept of 'normal' occlusal development should be interpreted with an appreciation of the influence of a patient's ethnicity. The orthodontic literature describes varying incidences of malocclusions between different ethnic populations, an example being the increased tendency for midline diastemas to develop in African ethnic groups.[13]

Similarly, morphological variations in facial form between different ethnic groups have been investigated and reported, such as a relatively higher incidence of Class III skeletal patterns occurring within the Chinese population.[14]

An awareness of how ethnic variations can present at an occlusal level can allow practitioners to discuss with patients and parents the difference between malocclusion and variations in normal occlusion that reflect ethnicity.

SUMMARY

It is important that all practitioners have an awareness of the different stages of occlusal development. This is particularly important during the transitional, mixed dentition stage when the potential to undertake effective interceptive treatment exists.

A working knowledge of the average dental eruption dates is a minimum requirement. However, as dental age has been shown to correlate relatively poorly with chronological age,[15] it is important practitioners have an appreciation of the normal processes and stages of occlusal development. It is recommended that further investigations are indicated if the *sequence* of occlusal development is significantly disrupted or if there is a *discrepancy of more than 6 months* between the eruption dates of contralateral teeth within the same arch.

References

1. Davies S, Gray RMJ. What is occlusion? Br Dent J 2001;181:235–45.
2. Andrews LF. The six keys to normal occlusion. Am J Orthod Dentofacial Orthop 1972; 62:296–309.
3. Leighton BC. The value of prophecy in orthodontics. Trans Br Soc Study Orthod 1971;59:1–14.
4. Bishara S. Textbook of Orthodontics. WB Saunders, Harcourt Health Sciences, Philadelphia, PA, 2001.
5. Moorees CFA, Chadha JM. Available space for the incisors during dental development – a growth study based on physiologic age. Angle Orthod 1965;35:12–22.
6. Edwards JG. The diastema, the frenum, the frenectomy. Am J Orthod 1977;71:489–508.

7. Cozza P, Baccetti T, Franchi L, Mucedeto M, Polimeni A. Sucking habits and facial hyperdivergency as risk factors for anterior open bite in the mixed dentition. Am J Orthod Dentofacial Orthop 2005;128: 517–19.

8. Kurol J, Koch G. The effect of extraction of infraoccluded deciduous molars: A longitudinal study. Am J Orthod 1985;87:46–55.

9. Richardson ME. The aetiology of late lower arch crowding alternative to mesially directed forces: A review. Am J Orthod Dentofacial Orthop 1994;105:592–7.

10. Harris EF. A longitudinal study of arch size and form in untreated adults. Am J Orthod Dentofacial Orthop 1997;111:419–27.

11. Bishara SE, Treder JE, Jakobsen JR. Facial and Dental changes in adulthood. Am J Orthod Dentofacial Orthop 1997;111:401–9.

12. Bjork A. Prediction of mandibular growth rotation. Am J Orthod 1969;55:585–99.

13. Brunelle JA, Bhat M, Lipton JA. Prevalence and distribution of selected occlusal characteristics in the US population, 1988–1991. J Dent Res 1996;75:706–13.

14. Cooke MS, Wei SHY. A comparative study of southern Chinese and British Caucasian cephalometric standards. Angle Orthod 1989;59:131–8.

15. Hagg U, Taranger J. Maturation indicators and the pubertal growth spurt. Am J Orthod 1982;82:299–309.

Diagnosis and Treatment Planning 2

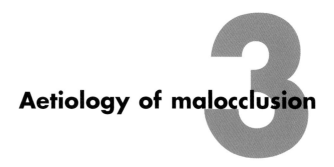

Aetiology of malocclusion

INTRODUCTION

Malocclusion may be defined as a significant deviation from what has been described as normal or 'ideal' occlusion.[1] Many components are involved in the development of the occlusion. The most important are:

- The size of the maxilla
- The size of the mandible, both ramus and body
- The factors which determine the relationship between the two skeletal bases, such as cranial base and environmental factors
- The arch form
- The size and morphology of the teeth
- The number of teeth present
- The soft tissue morphology and behaviour of lips, tongue and perioral musculature.

The study of twins has provided much useful information concerning the role of heredity and the environment in malocclusion. The method is based on the underlying principle that observed differences within a pair of monozygotic twins (whose genotype is identical) are due to environment and that differences within a pair of dizygotic twins (who share 50% of their total gene complement) are due to both environment and genotype. In this chapter we will investigate the environmental and genetic factors that play a part in contributing to commonly observed malocclusion traits.

CLASS I MALOCCLUSIONS

Vertical Skeletal Variation

Class I malocclusions are those that do not have an anteroposterior skeletal discrepancy and accounts for approximately 50% of all presenting malocclusions, but within this there may be vertical skeletal variation. The overall pattern of craniofacial development (short or long face) is established early and on average does not change with age. It is also acknowledged that facial maturity develops in females between 10 and 13 years and 2 years later for males. A number of studies[2–5] have shown high genetic

Orthodontics: Principles and Practice, First Edition. Edited by Daljit S. Gill, Farhad B. Naini.
© 2011 Daljit S. Gill, Farhad B. Naini and Dental Update. Published 2011 by Blackwell Publishing Ltd.

determination for total anterior facial height and for its lower component. Overall, vertical variables were found to have higher heritability than horizontal variables. Malocclusions are sometimes referred to as 'high angle' or 'low angle' malocclusions, which reflects the vertical skeletal and growth rotation patterns – a backward growth rotation being associated with an increased vertical dimension of the lower face (Figure 3.1), and a forward growth rotation associated with a reduced lower face height (often expressed in Class II division 2 malocclusion – see below).

Environmental factors such as lips, tongue and cheeks, muscle activity and certain functions (e.g. breathing and mastication) play an important part in occlusal development[6] and mouth breathing is an example of an environmental factor that alters the balance of muscle forces, producing a more vertical growth pattern and a narrow, V-shaped maxillary arch form with a deep palatal vault.[7] In circumstances where the lip morphology is unfavourable and lips are incompetent, the manifestation may be vertical maxillary excess with a 'gummy smile'.

Overbite and Tongue Position

An endogenous tongue thrust is a rare and still disputed phenomenon which is reserved for a persistent tongue thrust accompanied by an anterior open bite and associated circumoral muscle activity on swallowing. This is to be distinguished from the much more common forward tongue posture seen in incomplete overbites (Figure 3.2), particularly when there is a lower 'lip trap' in a Class II division 1 malocclusion (see below).

Crossbites

Crossbites can be buccal or lingual, unilateral or bilateral and with or without associated man-

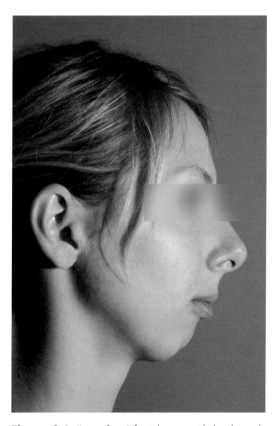

Figure 3.1 'Long face' facial type with backwards mandibular rotation possibly due to habitual mouth breathing, showing lip competence maintained with visible effort of mentalis muscle.

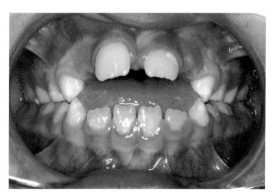

Figure 3.2 Anterior open bite and proclined upper incisors caused by persistent forward tongue posture, preventing normal vertical development of incisors.

dibular displacement. In terms of aetiology, genetic influences such as anteroposterior skeletal pattern and environmental influences such as digit sucking habits or mouth breathing may contribute. Crossbites in the absence of significant skeletal discrepancy are a good illustration of the environmental influence of lips, cheeks and tongue on the maxillary and mandibular arch widths and the equilibrium theory. Equilibrium theory proposes that the dentoalveolar portions of the jaws are in a neutral zone where the soft tissue forces of lips and tongue are in buccolingual balance.[8] This balance is upset by both digit sucking and mouth breathing, with the low tongue position and simultaneously increased buccal pressure on the maxillary arch from the cheeks resulting in maxillary narrowing and a broader lower arch. In unilateral crossbite with mandibular displacement, the maxillary narrowing is usually bilaterally symmetrical, and it is the mandibular deviation that creates the unilateral crossbite.

Asymmetry

While asymmetry may result from mandibular displacement as described above, structural mandibular asymmetry can result from early condylar trauma that causes unilateral deficiency in the growth of the mandibular ramus and therefore a displacement of the mandibular body to the affected side.

Crowding and Spacing

Crowding can be categorised into three distinctively different types according to aetiology. Primary crowding refers to tooth size and arch size discrepancy, with this ratio being more often increased (causing crowding) than reduced (which results in spacing), and this is genetically determined. Secondary crowding is caused by premature loss of primary molars, which is environmental in origin (Figure 3.3), while tertiary or 'late lower incisor crowding'

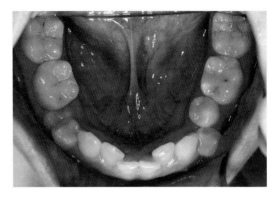

Figure 3.3 Secondary crowding in the lower arch following the early loss of primary molars. Note the crowding localised to the premolar region.

is a phenomenon that has both genetic and environmental contributions, the main determinant being differential jaw growth.

Hypodontia and Other Familial Dental Disturbances

The genetic background in tooth development is becoming progressively understood with the synthesis of tooth development biology and human studies focusing on inherited conditions that specifically interfere with tooth development.

Genes affecting early tooth development (e.g. *PAX9* and *MSX1*) are associated with familial hypodontia.[9] For example, patients with *PAX9* mutations typically lack at least six or more molars, but there is considerable intrafamilial variability in the particular teeth missing among affected members of such families. Genes expressed by odontoblasts (*COL1A1*, *COL1A2* and *DSPP*), and ameloblasts (*AMELX*, *ENAM*, *MMP20* and *KLK4*) during the crown formation stage, are associated with dentinogenesis imperfecta, dentin dysplasia and amelogenesis imperfecta. Late genes expressed during root formation (*ALPL* and *DLX3*) are associated with agenesis of dental cementum and taurodontism.

Brook[10] reported the prevalence of supernumerary teeth in British school children as 2.1% in the permanent dentition with a male: female ratio of 2:1. In Hong Kong, however, the prevalence is around 3% with a male: female ratio of 6.5:1.[11] The most frequently occurring type of supernumerary is a premaxillary conical midline tooth (mesiodens). These are more commonly present in parents and siblings of patients, although inheritance does not follow a simple mendelian pattern.[12–14]

Various studies in the past have indicated a genetic tendency for ectopic maxillary canines.[15] Peck et al.[16] concluded that palatally ectopic canines was an inherited trait, being one of the anomalies in a complex of genetically related dental disturbances, often occurring in combination with missing teeth, tooth size reduction, supernumerary teeth and other ectopically positioned teeth.

While the exact genetic nature of a range of abnormalities such as hypodontia, peg-shaped laterals, transpositions, supernumeraries and impactions is unknown, pedigree and twin studies reveal a familial association, and therefore they are likely to be connected with defects in these and other genes.

CLASS II DIVISION 1 MALOCCLUSIONS

Class II division 1 malocclusion has a prevalence of between 25% and 33% of all malocclusions in a typical Western population.[17] Extensive cephalometric studies have been carried out to determine the heritability of certain craniofacial parameters in Class II division 1 malocclusions.[18,19] These investigations have shown that the SNA angle (maxillary prominence) and SNB angle (mandibular prominence) are heritable, and in the Class II patient the mandible is significantly more retruded than in Class I patients, with the body of the mandible being smaller and overall mandibular length reduced.

Environmental factors can also contribute to the aetiology of Class II division 1 malocclusions. Bilateral condylar trauma can cause severe disruption to mandibular growth resulting in a Class II skeletal pattern and Class II division 1 malocclusion. Soft tissues can exert an influence on the dentoalveolar portions of the maxillary and mandibular arches, causing proclination of upper incisors and retroclination of lower incisors. Lip incompetence also encourages upper incisor proclination by virtue of the imbalance in labial and lingual pressures on the teeth. The need to achieve lip/tongue contact for an anterior oral seal during swallowing can encourage the lower lip to retrocline the lower incisors and the forward tongue position to procline the uppers, influencing the severity of the overjet (Figure 3.4). The presence

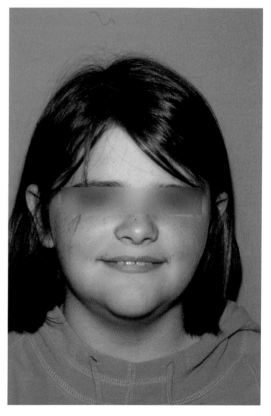

Figure 3.4 A 'lip trap', with the lower lip acting palatal to the upper incisors during function leading to proclination of the upper incisors.

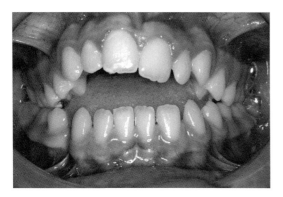

Figure 3.5 Anterior open bite due to a thumb sucking habit. Note the asymmetry of the open bite and the crossbite tendency posteriorly.

of a non-nutritive or thumb sucking habit beyond infancy can also result in proclination of the upper incisors and retroclination of the lower incisors. The increased overjet seen in these cases is often also associated with asymmetrical open bite (Figure 3.5). Cessation of the habit in the primary dentition is often followed by spontaneous reduction in severity of the malocclusion.

CLASS II DIVISION 2 MALOCCLUSIONS

Class II division 2 malocclusions occur in approximately 7–10% of a Western (largely Caucasian based) population.[17] This is a distinct clinical entity and is a more consistent collection of definable features occurring simultaneously, i.e. is more akin to a syndrome than the other malocclusion types. Class II division 2 malocclusion typically comprises the combination of deep overbite, retroclined incisors, Class II skeletal discrepancy, and high lip line with strap-like activity of the lower lip and an active mentalis muscle (Figure 3.6). This is often accompanied by particular dental features such as a poorly developed cingulum on the upper incisors and a characteristic crown-root angulation so that there is a poor incisal 'stop' for the lower incisor.

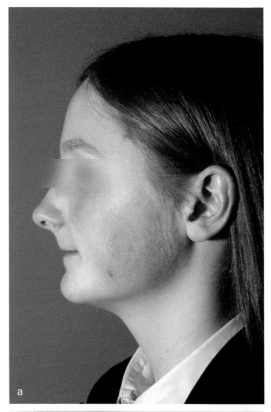

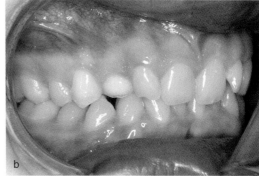

Figure 3.6 Typical features of Class II division 2 malocclusion with (a) thin hypertonic lips and (b) retroclined incisors with increased overbite.

Peck et al.[20] also describe characteristic smaller than average teeth when measured mesiodistally, reinforcing a similar observation made by Beresford,[21] and Robertson and Hilton[22] also found these teeth to be significantly 'thinner' in the labiolingual dimension. A further feature of the Class II division 2 is a tendency to a forward rotation of the mandible, which contributes to the deep bite, chin prominence and reduced lower face height. This last feature in turn has an influence on the position of the lower lip relative to the upper incisors, and an increase in masticatory muscle forces has been reported by Quinn and Yoshikawa.[23]

Familial occurrence of Class 2 division 2 has been documented in several published reports including twin and triplet studies[24,25] and in family pedigrees from Korkhaus (1930),[26] Rubbrecht (1930),[27] Trauner (1968)[28] and Peck et al. (1998).[20] In one study on monozygotic twin pairs,[25] 100% demonstrated concordance for the Class 2 Division 2 malocclusion, whilst almost 90% of the dizygotic twin pairs were discordant. This is strong evidence for genetics as the main aetiological factor in the development of Class 2 Division 2 malocclusions.

CLASS III MALOCCLUSIONS

Class III malocclusion represents a relatively small proportion (3–5%) of the total Caucasian population,[17] but there are ethnic variations. Class III malocclusions are most prevalent in Oriental populations, accounting up to 14% in a study of 9–15-year-old Chinese children.[29]

Two main subsets of Class III malocclusion can be recognised, one due to an apparent forward position of the mandible, and the other due to true mandibular prognathism. An apparent forward mandibular position may occur either due to a tooth causing interference on closure and mandibular displacement, or to foreshortening of the maxillary arch causing the normal mandible to project beyond the underdeveloped upper jaw. The second type, which is true mandibular prognathism, is brought about by either a large mandible or an acute cranial base angle with an anterior positioning of the glenoid fossa with protrusion of the mandible beyond a normal maxillary

arch.[30,31] Mandibular prognathism has been studied in familial and in twin studies,[32] and concordance in monozygotic twins is much higher than among dizygotic twins.

While there are these two main subset, the precise aetiology in a particular case is usually heterogeneous and both genetic and environmental factors may contribute. A series of autosomal genetic conditions can lead to Class III malocclusion due to mandibular prognathism or deficiency in the maxilla or the middle third of the face. The occlusal relationship is contributed to by the relative size of the maxillary and mandibular arches and the relative positions of the cranial base, the saddle angle and position of the temporomandibular articulation all of which are mainly under genetic control.

A wide range of environmental factors have also been suggested as contributory to the development of mandibular prognathism. Among these are enlarged tonsils,[33] nasal blockage,[34] congenital anatomical defects,[35] hormonal disturbances,[36] endocrine imbalances,[37] posture[38] and trauma/disease. It has also been reported that habitual head posture may influence the facial pattern and mandibular growth rotation and whether this is in a predominantly vertical or horizontal direction.

Soft tissues do not generally play a part in the aetiology of Class III malocclusion, and in fact there is a tendency for lip and tongue pressure to compensate for a skeletal Class III discrepancy by retroclining the lower incisors and proclining the uppers.

CLINICAL SIGNIFICANCE

Aetiological heterogeneity is a feature of most malocclusions, and it is important to appreciate the range of possibilities with respect to aetiology. The diagnosis of an individual malocclusion needs to be based on the observation of the clinical features, facilitated by cephalometric analysis of the facial and dental features when required.

Each malocclusion will occupy its own distinctive slot in the genetic/environmental spectrum and therefore the diagnostic goal is to determine the relative contribution of genetics and the environment. The greater the genetic component the worse the prognosis for a successful long-term outcome by means of orthodontic intervention. The difficulty, of course, is that it is seldom possible to determine the precise contribution from hereditary and environmental factors in a particular case. However, an understanding of possible causes enables a clinician to ascertain with a reasonable level of confidence whether the malocclusion is determined by genetic or environmental causes or a combination of both. Such knowledge and understanding is important not only in diagnosis and treatment planning but also in patient counselling and determination of the long-term prognosis for successful treatment and stability.

References

1. Andrews LF. The straight wire appliance. Br J Orthod 1979;6:125–43.
2. Horowitz SL, Osborne RG, DeGeorge FV. A cephalometric study of craniofacial forms in adult twins. Angle Orthod 1960; 30:1–5.
3. Manfredi C, Martina R, Grossi GB, Giuliani M. Heritability of 39 orthodontic cephalometric parameters on MZ, DZ twins and MN-paired singletons. Am J Orthod Dentofacial Orthop 1991;111:44–51.
4. Hunter WS. A study of the inheritance of craniofacial characteristics as seen in lateral cephalograms of 72 like-sexed twins. Eur Orthod Soc Report Cong 1965;41:59–70.
5. Dudas M, Sassouni V. The hereditary components of mandibular growth, a longitudinal twin study. Angle Orthod 1973;43: 314–22.
6. Solow B. Upper airway obstruction and facial development. In: Davidovitch Z (ed.) The Biological Mechanisms of Tooth Movement and Craniofacial Adaptation. The Ohio State University College of Dentistry, Columbus, OH, 1992:571–9.
7. Solow B, Kreiborg S. Soft tissue stretching: A possible control factor in craniofacial morphogenesis. Scand J Dent Res 1977;85: 505–7.
8. Proffit WR, Fields HW. Contemporary Orthodontics. CV Mosby Company, London, 1996.
9. Gerita A, Nieminen P, De Muynck S, Carels C. Exclusion of coding region mutations in MSX1, PAX9 and AXIn2 in eight patients with severe oligodontia phenotype. Orthod Craniofacial Res 2006;9:129–36.
10. Brook AH. Dental anomalies of number, form and size: their prevalence in British schoolchildren. J Int Assoc Dent Child 1974;5:37–53.
11. David PJ. Hypodontia and hyperdontia of permanent teeth in Hong Kong schoolchildren. Community Dent Oral Epidemiol 1987;15:218–20.
12. Brook AH. A unifying aetiological explanation for anomalies of human tooth number and size. Arch Oral Biol 1984;29:373–8.
13. Mercuri LG, O'Neill R. Multiple impacted and supernumerary teeth in sisters. Oral Surg Oral Med Oral Pathol 1980;50:293.
14. Mason C, Rule DC. Midline supernumeraries: a family affair. Dent Update 1995;22: 34–5.
15. Zilberman Y, Cohen B, Becker A. Familial trends in palatal canines, anomalous lateral incisors and related phenomena. Eur J Orthod 1990;12:135–9.
16. Peck S, Peck L, Kataja M. The palatally displaced canine as a dental anomaly of genetic origin. Angle Orthod 1994;64:249–56.
17. Jones ML, Oliver RG. Walther and Houston's Orthodontic Notes, 6th edn. Wright Publishers, Oxford, 2000.
18. Harris JE. A Multivariate Analysis of the Craniofacial Complex. School of Dentistry, University of Michigan, Ann Arbor, MI, 1963.

19. Harris JE. Genetic factors in the growth of the head: inheritance of the craniofacial complex and malocclusion. Dent Clin North Am 1975;19:151–60.
20. Peck S, Peck L, Kataja M. Class II Division 2 malocclusion: a heritable pattern. Angle Orthod 1998;68:9–17.
21. Beresford JS. Tooth size and class distinction. Dent Pract 1969;20:113–20.
22. Robertson NRE, Hilton R. Feature of the upper central incisors in Class II, Division 2. Angle Orthod 1965;35:51–3.
23. Quinn RS, Yoshikawa DK. A reassessment of force magnitude in orthodontics. Am J Orthod 1985;88:252–60.
24. Kloeppel W. Deckbiss bei Zwillingen. Fortschr Kieferorthop 1953;14:130–5.
25. Markovic MD. At the cross roads of orofacial genetics. Eur J Orthod 1992;14:469–81.
26. Korkhaus W. Investigations into the inheritance of orthodontic malformations. Dent Rec 1953;50:271–80.
27. Rubbrecht O. Les variations maxillo-facial sagittales et l'heredite mendelienne. Revue Belge Stomat 1930;27:1–24, 61–91, 119–53.
28. Trauner R. Leitfaden det praktischen Keiferorthopedie. Verlag Die Quintessenz, Berlin, 1968:20–1.
29. Lin JJ. Prevalence of malocclusion in Chinese children aged 9–15. Clin Dent Chin 1985;3:57–65.
30. Ellis E, McNamara JA. Components of adult class III malocclusion. J Oral Maxillofac Surg 1984;42:295–305.
31. Singh GD, McNamara JA, Lozanoff S. Morphometry of the cranial base in subjects with class III malocclusion. J Dent Res 1997;76:694–703.
32. Litton SF, Ackermann LV, Isaacson R, Shapiro BL. A genetic study of Class III malocclusion. Am J Orthod 1970;58:565–77.
33. Angle FH. Treatment of Malocclusion of the Teeth, 7th edn. SS White Manufacturing Company, Philadelphia, PA, 1907.
34. Davidov S, Geseva N, Donveca T, Dehova L. Incidence of prognathism in Bulgaria. Dent Abstr 1961;6:240.
35. Monteleone L, Duvigneaud JD. Prognathism. J Oral Surg 1963;21:190–5.
36. Pascoe J, Hayward JR, Costich ER. Mandibular prognathism, its etiology and a classification. J Oral Surg 1960;18:21–4.
37. Downs WG. Studies in the causes of dental anomalies. J Dent Res 1928;8:267–379.
38. Gold JK. A new approach to the treatment of mandibular prognathism. Am J Orthod 1949;35:893–912.

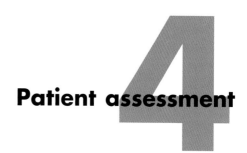

Patient assessment

INTRODUCTION

It is important to take a comprehensive history before undertaking an orthodontic examination. Orthodontic examination should begin as soon as the patient enters the surgery. The general stage of development, including stature/height and the presence of secondary sexual characteristics, should be noted. This information will allow one to determine the amount of growth that may be remaining.

EXTRAORAL ASSESSMENT

Assessment of Skeletal Pattern

The relative position of the maxilla and mandible, termed the skeletal pattern, has a large influence on the relationship of the maxillary and mandibular dentition. The skeletal pattern should be assessed in three dimensions:

- Anteroposterior (AP)
- Vertical
- Transverse.

Anteroposterior Dimension

The aim is to relate the AP position of the mandible to the maxilla and the relationship of these bones to the cranial base. Assessment of the position of each jaw relative to the cranial base gives an indication of which jaw may be contributing to a malocclusion. An assessment of the severity of the discrepancy will help to guide whether treatment can be provided with orthodontics alone or if a combination approach that also involves orthognathic surgery (see Chapter 25) is required. It is important to assess the patient in the natural head position, which is a standardised reproducible head orientation, as the tilt of the head can greatly influence the interpretation of the skeletal pattern. To achieve this, the patient should be sitting upright, relaxed, and looking straight ahead at a distant point at eye level and the teeth should be lightly in occlusion.

The most anterior part of the maxilla and the mandible can be palpated in the midline through the base of the lips (Figure 4.1). The relationship of the mandible relative to the maxilla can be classified as follows:

Orthodontics: Principles and Practice, First Edition. Edited by Daljit S. Gill, Farhad B. Naini.
© 2011 Daljit S. Gill, Farhad B. Naini and Dental Update. Published 2011 by Blackwell Publishing Ltd.

- Class I – when the mandible lies 2–3 mm posterior to the maxilla (Figure 4.2a). The profile is straight.
- Class II – when the mandible is retrusive relative to the maxilla (Figure 4.2b). The

profile is convex. The discrepancy should also be classified as mild, moderate or severe.
- Class III – when the maxilla is retrusive relative to the mandible (Figure 4.2c). The profile is concave. The discrepancy should also be classified as mild, moderate or severe.

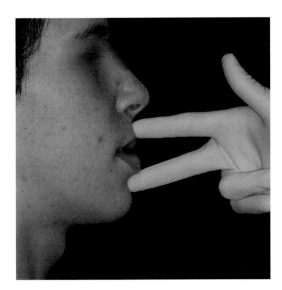

Figure 4.1 The anteroposterior relationship of the maxilla to the mandible can be assessed by palpating soft tissue A- and B-points. Ideally A-point should lie 2–3 mm ahead of B-point.

To determine the position of the mandible and maxilla relative to the cranial base, one imagines a vertical line drawn through soft tissue nasion in the natural head position. This line is termed the zero meridian[1,2] and represents the anterior limit of the cranial base. The anterior limit of the base of the upper lip (soft tissue A-point) should lie 2–3 mm ahead and the base of the lower lip (soft tissue B-point) 0–2 mm behind the zero meridian in Caucasians. When making this assessment, it is important to remember that ethnic variation exits in normal lower face protrusion. The face progressively becomes less protrusive as follows: African Caribbean > Asian > whites of northern European ancestry. The term used when both jaws are protrusive is bimaxillary protrusion, which is a common feature in African Caribbeans. As well as using the zero meridian as a guide, other clinical signs which *may* be present and are suggestive of maxillary retru-

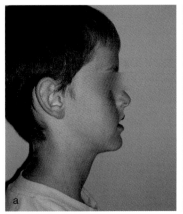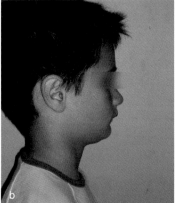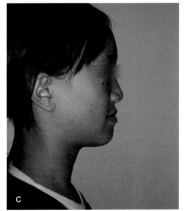

Figure 4.2 Profile photographs showing a (a) Class I, (b) Class II and (c) Class III skeletal pattern.

sion include paranasal flattening, an obtuse nasolabial angle, reduced incisor show at rest, prominent nasolabial folds (due to lack of skeletal support), a flat nasal bridge and lower scleral show.

Vertical Dimension

The vertical skeletal dimension can influence the degree of vertical incisor overlap, lip competency and overall facial aesthetics. There are two methods in which the vertical dimension should be assessed:

• Lower anterior face height (LAFH) proportion
• Frankfort-mandibular planes angle (FMPA).

Vertically in the frontal view, the face can be split into thirds. The LAFH (subnasale-menton) should be approximately equal to the middle face height (glabella-subnasale) for facial balance. However, if the middle face height is of incorrect dimension, the LAFH may be in proportion but also incorrect such that incisor overlap and lip competency are adversely affected. This is why some clinicians additionally measure the absolute LAFH. The normal absolute measurements for LAFH are given in Table 4.1. The LAFH can also be split into thirds and ideally the upper lip should represent one-third of the total height.

The FMPA is assessed in the profile view and gives an indication of the relationship between the LAFH and posterior face height (i.e. ramus height). It is considered to be normal

Table 4.1 Lower anterior face height measurement in young adults (age 16 years)[3]

	Male	Female
Caucasian	72 (6) mm	66 (4.5) mm
African Caribbean	74 (5.3) mm	67 (4.8) mm

Standard deviation is given in parenthesis.

when the line of the mandibular plane and Frankfort plane intersect in the occipital region. If the point of intersection is anterior to the occiput, the vertical dimension is usually increased and if it lies posterior to the occiput, it is reduced.

Transverse Dimension

The two components of the transverse dimension that should be assessed are:

• Facial symmetry
• Arch width.

It is quite common to find asymmetries in the face, but those that affect the mandible and maxilla are particularly important when planning orthodontic treatment.

The symmetry of facial structures can be assessed by constructing the facial midline between soft tissue nasion and the middle part of the upper lip at the vermillion border. The chin point should be coincident with this line. If there is an asymmetry of the chin point, it is also important to check for a compensatory cant in the maxillary occlusal plane. Asymmetries in the chin point can be produced by a lateral mandibular displacement on closing if there is an occlusal interference.

The relative width of the upper and lower arches affects the transverse relationship of the teeth. Often the maxilla is narrow, which results in a crossbite of the buccal segments if there has been inadequate dentoalveolar compensation (see Chapter 2). On intraoral palpation, the maxilla should be slightly wider than the mandible at the corresponding points. It is important to remember that the absolute transverse dimensions of the maxilla may be normal, but a *relative* transverse maxillary discrepancy, manifesting as a posterior crossbite, may exist due to incorrect AP positioning of the maxilla/mandible. The AP position can affect the transverse relationship as the dental arches get wider as one moves distally.

As well as the skeletal pattern, the facial soft tissues can influence tooth position. If there is an underlying skeletal discrepancy, the soft tissues may help to guide teeth into a more favourable position (dentoalveolar compensation) so that the occlusal relationship is improved. Soft tissue evaluation should involve examination of the lips, tongue, temporomandibular joints (TMJs) and assessment for habits.

The Lips

The following aspects of the lips should be examined:

- Lip fullness
- Lip tone
- Lower lip line
- Lip competency
- Method of achieving an anterior oral seal at rest/swallowing.

Lip fullness may be classified as protrusive, straight or retrusive. Where the lips lie in relationship to Ricketts' aesthetic line (E-line),[4] which runs between the tip of the nose and chin point, can help make this assessment. The upper lip should lie 4 mm behind this line. If the lower lip lies anterior to the line it is considered protrusive, if it lies 0–2 mm behind it is normal and if >2 mm posterior it is retrusive. If the nose is large, so that the E-line is displaced anteriorly, this may give a misleading result. Also, the lips tend to appear less protrusive during growth as the nose and chin point develop.

The nasolabial angle (NLA), formed by a tangent to the upper lip and columella of the nose, can give an indication of upper lip position. In Caucasians, the upper lip should slope slightly anteriorly (8–14°) to the vertical.[5] The NLA can be classified as normal (102 ± 8° males and females), acute (<90°) or obtuse (>90°). It may be increased, with a relatively normal upper lip position, if the columella of the nose slopes upwards excessively. There is ethnic variation, and it is normal for African Caribbeans to have an acute NLA.[3]

Lip fullness can influence the extraction/non-extraction decision during treatment planning. If the lips are retrusive, it may be preferable not to extract, depending on the amount of crowding, as this helps maintain incisor position and lip support. The opposite may be true if the lips are protrusive.

Concerning tonicity, the lips may be flaccid, where there is little muscular tone, have normal tone or be highly active. The term 'strap-like' lower lip is given to a highly active lower lip. Lip tonicity can influence the position of muscular balance, such that incisors tend to be more protrusive with reducing tonicity. If the lips are very active the incisors may be retroclined.

The lower lip line is the vertical relationship between the lower lip and maxillary incisors at rest. It is determined by the LAFH, AP mandibular position and the lower lip length. Ideally, the lower lip should lie adjacent to the middle third of the maxillary central incisor crown. In Class II division 1 malocclusion the lip line can be lower down, leading to proclination of the upper incisors (Figure 4.3a) and in Class II division 2 malocclusion it can be high (Figure 4.3b) leading to their retroclination. In Class II division 1, the stability of overjet correction is questionable if the lower lip does not cover at least the incisal third of the maxillary central incisors at rest.

The lips may be described as:

- Competent – a lip seal is produced with minimal muscular effort when the mandible is in the rest position.
- Potentially competent – the positioning of the upper incisors prevents a comfortable lip seal from being obtained.
- Incompetent – excessive muscular activity is required to produce a lip seal. Signs of excessive activity include puckering of the skin overlying the chin, due to mentalis contraction, and flattening of the labiomental fold when the lips are held together (Figure 4.4). If the interlabial distance at rest is >4 mm the lips can be considered incompetent. Patients

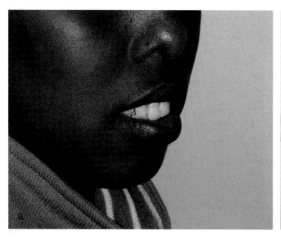 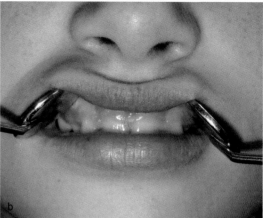

Figure 4.3 The lower lip line can influence incisor position. (a) A low lower lip line is associated with incisor proclination and poor stability of overjet correction and (b) A high lower lip line is associated with retroclined upper incisors.

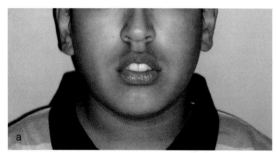 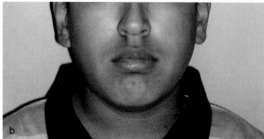

Figure 4.4a,b Excess muscular activity to close the lips is indicated by puckering of the chin due to mentalis contraction.

may learn to habitually keep the lips together with increased muscular effort and forward mandibular posturing.

Factors that influence lip competency include age ($\uparrow$ age $\rightarrow \downarrow$ lip separation), LAFH ($\uparrow$ LAFH $\rightarrow \uparrow$ lip separation), AP mandibular position ($\uparrow$ mandibular retrognathia $\rightarrow \uparrow$ lip separation), lip length (normal upper lip length in females = 20–22 mm and in males = 22–24 mm) and upper incisor position ($\uparrow$ protrusion $\rightarrow \uparrow$ lip separation).

The significance of lip competence lies in the stability of Class II division 1 malocclusion cor-

rection. If the lips fail to control upper incisor position following treatment there is a significant risk of relapse. An anterior oral seal at rest and during swallowing can be created by a number of mechanisms:

- Lip to lip contact ($\pm$ mandibular forward posturing)
- Tongue to lower lip contact
- Lower lip to palate contact
- Tongue to upper lip contact.

When a *lip to lip* seal can not be attained, an adaptive swallowing pattern must be produced

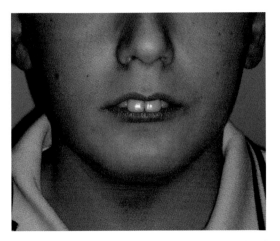

Figure 4.5 A lip trap, where the lower lip sits behind the upper incisors, can lead to upper incisor proclination and sometimes retroclination of the lower incisors.

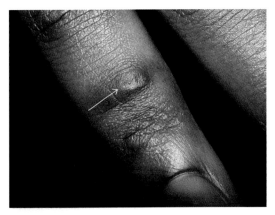

Figure 4.6 A vigorous digit sucking habit can leave a tell-tale callous on the digit where it rubs against the incisal edges.

to prevent expulsion of oral contents during swallowing. A *tongue to lower lip* seal (also termed an adaptive tongue thrust) is often found in Class II division 1 malocclusion and a clue to its existence is an overbite that is just incomplete. A *lower lip to palate* seal is also found in Class II division 1 malocclusion when the lower lip is caught behind the upper incisors (lower lip-trap, Figure 4.5). This often results in proclination of the upper and retroclination of the lower incisors. A *tongue to upper lip seal* is sometimes seen in Class III malocclusion.

Tongue

It is difficult to assess the size and position of the tongue unless it is grossly abnormal. During function, there may be an adaptive tongue thrust where the tongue is positioned anteriorly to help achieve a lip seal when the lips are incompetent. This adaptive mechanism often disappears following occlusal correction. Rarely, a patient may present with an endogenous tongue thrust where the tongue is thrust forwards forcibly during swallowing due to a

neuromuscular defect. Macroglossia is rarely seen and is difficult to diagnose unless it is moderate/severe. Signs of a tongue thrust and macroglossia include:

- Proclination of the upper and lower incisors
- Reverse curve of Spee in the lower arch
- Anterior open bite
- Presence of a lisp
- Presence of the tongue interposed between the incisors at rest
- Crenulations of the lateral border of the tongue.

Such findings should alert the clinician to the high risk of relapse if the AP incisor position is altered.

Habits

A clue to the presence of a vigorous digit sucking habit is the presence of a callous on the digit sucked in the area in contact with the incisors (Figure 4.6). Nail biting habits can potentiate orthodontically induced root resorption and are easily identified by examining the nails.

Temporomandibular Joint

It is important to note the presence of tenderness in the muscles of mastication, clicking or crepitus in the joints and the range of mandibular movements during orthodontic assessment. If pathology is found, there may be a history of parafunction or facial trauma.

INTRAORAL EXAMINATION

The aims of intraoral examination are to:

- Assess the mucosal/dental surfaces for pathology
- Determine the level of oral hygiene
- Establish whether dental development is normal
- Assess tooth position within and between the arches.

Assessment for Pathology

Every patient should have a full examination of the mucosal surfaces during routine assessment. Oral mucosal disease is uncommon in the majority of patients attending for orthodontic treatment, however, if left undetected it can be life-threatening in some circumstances. Dental pathology can have a significant influence on treatment planning. Of particular relevance is:

- Dental caries
- Dental hypoplasia and hypomineralisation
- Toothwear
- Sequelae of traumatic injuries to the dentition
- Gingivitis, periodontitis and gingival recession.

All teeth that have previously suffered trauma, and those with advanced caries or large restorations should undergo thermal or electrical vitality testing. Areas of significant enamel hypoplasia/hypomineralisation should

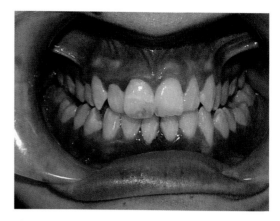

Figure 4.7 Areas of hypomineralisation and hypoplasia should be identified and documented using colour photography.

be documented, photographed and highlighted to the patient/parent(s) (Figure 4.7). Patients often become more aware of these defects during treatment as they begin to examine their teeth more closely, and this can lead them to incorrectly attribute the previously unrecognised enamel defects to orthodontic treatment. All patients should undergo the Basic Periodontal Examination (BPE) as part of their routine assessment. All dental disease *must* be controlled before contemplating orthodontic treatment and it is important that patients understand that they must continue to visit their general practitioner for routine dental maintenance during orthodontics.

Oral Hygiene

The level of oral hygiene can be assessed by examining for gingivitis, probing to elicit gingival bleeding, and with visual aids such as disclosing tablets/solution. The presence of a line of decalcification that follows the gingival margins of the teeth is indicative of plaque accumulation and a cariogenic diet. Poor hygiene during orthodontic treatment predisposes to decalcification, gingival hyperplasia, periodontal breakdown and removable appliance-related stomatitis.

Assessment of Dental Development

It is important to note the teeth present and the mobility of retained deciduous teeth. A mobile tooth often indicates eruption of the successor. The stage of dental development can be classified as follows:

- Deciduous dentition
- Early mixed dentition – marked by eruption of the permanent incisors and first molars
- Late mixed dentition – marked by eruption of all successional teeth, excluding the second premolars
- Permanent dentition.

The chronological age gives an indication of the teeth likely to be present within the mouth permitting for individual variation. Abnormalities in the sequence of eruption are more informative in detecting developmental disturbances. Asymmetries in dental development, particularly when ≥6 months, are also indicative of developmental disturbances and warrant radiographic assessment.

Developmental disturbances of tooth size are common. The maxillary lateral incisor is often diminutive or peg shaped. Microdontia can be associated with hypodontia. Macrodontia is less common and can occur as an isolated phenomenon or in association with supernumerary teeth. Tooth size discrepancies can impact on aesthetics, especially when the maxillary lateral incisor is affected, and can influence how well the arches occlude following comprehensive orthodontic treatment.

Assessment of Tooth Position

The segments of each arch should be assessed in turn: (1) labial segments, (2) canines and (3) buccal segments. It is important to quantify the amount of crowding or spacing within each segments and the inclination of the incisors and molars.

The inclination of the teeth is determined by a combination of skeletal and soft tissue factors. In Class II malocclusion, the lower incisors may be proclined (dentoalveolar compensation), if the soft tissues are favourable, to compensate for the AP skeletal discrepancy. Similarly in Class III malocclusion, the upper incisors may be proclined and the lowers retroclined. The existence of an abnormal frenal attachment should always be considered in the presence of a diastema.

Canine angulation may be classified as mesial, upright or distal. Mesially angulated canines may upright spontaneously if the first premolars are extracted. Distally angulated canines can cause incisor proclination during alignment as their crown tends to be thrown forward. It may then be anchorage-demanding to retract the labial segment into its pretreatment position, particularly if space is also required to correct crowding.

In the presence of a transverse maxillary deficiency, the upper molars may be buccally inclined and the lowers lingually inclined to compensate for the transverse skeletal discrepancy. It is important to note the inclination of the upper molars, because if they are already buccally inclined, further dental buccal inclination may not be advisable for crossbite correction. Further expansion may also be unadvisable if there is gingival recession in the molar segments.

Static and Dynamic Occlusion

The following features should be noted in the intercuspal position:

- Overjet, overbite and centrelines
- Incisor, canine and molar relationships
- Crossbites.

Angle's classification and the British Standards Institute incisor classification are described in detail in Chapter 2. The overjet is the horizontal distance between the labial surfaces of the mandibular incisors and the maxillary incisal edges. It should be measured parallel to the occlusal plane (normal = 2–4 mm) and to the most prominent point on the maxillary central incisal edges. If there is an anterior mandibular displacement, it is important to measure the overjet at initial contact before the displacement to obtain a true measure of the occlusal discrepancy. The overbite is the degree of vertical overlap of the mandibular incisors by their maxillary counterparts measured perpendicular to the occlusal plane (normal = 2–4 mm). The depth of the curve of Spee in the mandibular arch is positively correlated to the depth of the overbite.

The overbite can be classified as complete or incomplete. If complete to gingival tissues, the presence and extent of gingival trauma should be noted. In cases of anterior open bite, an assessment should be made of the symmetry of the open bite, its vertical extent in millimetres and how far it extends distally.

The coincidence and angulation of the maxillary and mandibular dental centrelines should be compared with the midfacial line. The maxillary centreline should be coincident and parallel to the midfacial line for ideal aesthetics. The lower dental centreline has less importance aesthetically, but should be corrected to establish a correct buccal segment relationship.

If a crossbite is present, it is important to check for a mandibular displacement on closure. The site of premature contact, direction and magnitude of displacement should be noted. Excessive toothwear on the tooth of premature contact may be present.

As well as the static occlusion, it is important to check for occlusal interferences during excursions of the mandible. These may predispose to later temporomandibular joint dysfunction.

Path of Mandibular Closure

A mandibular displacement is a lateral or sagittal movement of the mandible from the rest position to the position of maximum intercuspation due to a premature occlusal contact. A displacement can result in a crossbite, change in overjet, mandibular asymmetry and centreline discrepancy depending on its magnitude and direction. Orthodontic treatment should be planned to the retruded contact position.

A mandibular deviation is a sagittal movement of the mandible during closure from a habitual posture to maximum intercuspation. It is often seen in Class II division 1 malocclusion where the patient postures forwards to obtain a lip-to-lip oral seal and/or improve aesthetics. It is important that all records are taken in the intercuspal position for treatment planning.

References

1. Gonzalez-Ulloa M. Quantitative principles in cosmetic surgery of the face (profile-plasty). Plast Reconstr Surg 1962;29(2): 187–98.
2. Gonzalez-Ulloa M, Stevens E. The role of chin correction in profileplasty. Plast Reconstr Surg 1968;41:477–86.
3. Farkas LG. Anthropometry of the Head and Face, 2nd edn. Raven Press, New York, NY, 1994.
4. Ricketts RM. Esthetics, environment, and the law of lip relation. Am J Orthod 1968;54: 272–89.
5. McNamara JA Jr. A method of cephalometric evaluation. Am J Orthod 1984;86(6):449–69.

Facial aesthetics: historical and theoretical considerations

INTRODUCTION

The clinical ability to alter dentofacial form requires an understanding of facial aesthetics. This is vital for any clinician involved in treatment that will alter a patient's dentofacial appearance, whether through orthodontics, facial growth modification, corrective jaw surgery or aesthetic dentistry.

Beauty has been defined as a combination of qualities that give pleasure to the senses or to the mind. It is a philosophical concept, the aspects of which are studied under the term aesthetics, derived from the Greek word for perception (*aisthesis*). Aesthetics, therefore, is the study of beauty and, to a lesser extent, its opposite, the ugly. It involves both the understanding and evaluation of beauty, proportions and symmetry.[1]

The assessment of facial beauty is immersed in subjectivity and therefore leans towards the world of art. Facial proportions and facial symmetry, however, can be measured and therefore fit somewhere between art and science. Aesthetics itself is now essentially a science in

the formation, although obviously with a very strong philosophical and artistic background.

This chapter aims to cover the historical and theoretical aspects of facial aesthetics and their importance in contemporary dentofacial treatment.

HISTORICAL BACKGROUND

Facial Beauty

In Western literature, beauty has been described as everything from a 'social necessity' to a 'gift from God', with facial beauty being perhaps the most valued aspect of human beauty. The poet John Milton refers to the 'strange power' of beauty, describing beauty as 'Nature's brag'.

The question, 'What is beauty?' has been, and continues to be, one of the most debated and written about concepts in Western literature.[1] Beauty may be considered a mystifying quality that some faces have, or may be, 'in the eye of the beholder' as the writer Margaret Wolfe Hungerford (1878) stated. Plato (428–

Orthodontics: Principles and Practice, First Edition. Edited by Daljit S. Gill, Farhad B. Naini.
© 2011 Daljit S. Gill, Farhad B. Naini and Dental Update. Published 2011 by Blackwell Publishing Ltd.

348BC) alluded to this concept in his *Symposium*, where he described, 'Beholding beauty with the eye of the mind'. Shakespeare reiterated this view in *Love's Labour's Lost*, saying, 'Beauty is bought by judgement of the eye'. The philosopher Immanuel Kant (1790), in a treatise entitled *Critique of Judgement* stated, 'The beautiful is that which pleases universally without a concept'. Therefore, perhaps beauty as a concept can be perceived but not fully explained. This debate will no doubt continue.

What Constitutes the Human Perception of Facial Beauty?

The human perception of facial beauty may have genetic, environmental or multifactorial foundations. Evidence to support a genetic theory is that infants, from newborns until 2 years of age, when simultaneously presented with two facial photographs, have a tendency to stare longer at the face previously rated as more attractive by adults.[2] The evolutionary basis is that facial beauty is a requirement for sexual selection, leading to improved opportunity for reproduction.[3] A considerable quantitative meta-analysis undertaken by Langlois et al.[4] seems to confirm that there is also cross-cultural agreement regarding facial beauty.

Studies in the late 1800s by Sir Francis Galton, the cousin of Charles Darwin, accidentally found evidence to support what came to be known as the 'averageness hypothesis' of facial beauty, with composite facial photographs gaining higher attractiveness ratings than their individual facial photographs.[5] However, Perrett et al.[6] have shown that attractive composite faces were made more attractive by exaggerating the shape differences from the sample mean. Therefore, an average face shape is attractive but may not be optimally attractive.[7]

Facial symmetry also seems to be an important aspect of facial beauty, although mild asymmetry is essentially normal.[8] Therefore our perception of what constitutes facial beauty seems to be multifactorial.

Facial Proportions and Symmetry

The concept that 'ideal' proportions are the secret of beauty is perhaps the oldest idea regarding the nature of beauty.[9] The ancient Egyptians had a great interest in art and beauty. The famous painted limestone figure of Queen Nefertiti (*c*.1350BC) (Figure 5.1) with her harmonious facial proportions and symmetry is an example of how the Egyptians immortalised

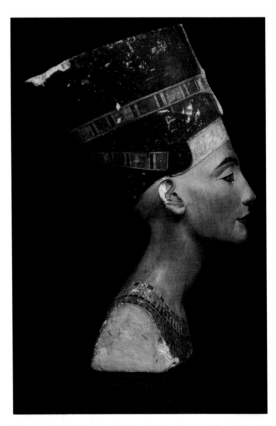

Figure 5.1 Queen Nefertiti. The famous face is well proportioned and symmetrical. (Berlin Museum). From: Naini FB. Facial Aesthetics: Concepts and Clinical Diagnosis. Oxford: Wiley-Blackwell, 2011; reprinted with permission.

the beauty of their kings and queens by depicting them, perhaps unrealistically, with 'ideal' facial proportions. In fact, the name Nefertiti literally means the 'Beautiful One'. Lesser dignitaries were not so honoured and had more realistic depictions in art and sculpture. The Egyptian proportional canons, however, used grids with meshes of equal-sized squares. This was to change with the age of Greek sculpture, which rather than featuring fixed units, described proportion between the parts of the whole human figure.

In the course of his travels the Greek mathematician Pythagoras (sixth century BC) is extremely likely to have come into contact with the mathematical treatises of the Egyptians. He postulated that beauty could be explained through mathematical laws and laws of proportion. He proposed an explanation of beauty through a significant finding, that plucking taut strings of proportionately different lengths produces harmonious notes. The difference in the proportionate lengths of the strings followed mathematical laws, and hence his explanation of laws of proportion. The term Pythagoras used to describe beauty was 'cosmos' as he felt that beauty was part of the mathematical order of the universe, hence the origin of the word 'cosmetic'. Throughout the ages, painters and sculptors have attempted to establish ideal proportions for the human form, however, possibly the most famous of all axioms about 'ideal' proportions is that of the golden proportion.[10]

Golden Proportion

This is a geometrical proportion in which a line AB is divided at a point C in such a way that AB/AC = AC/CB, i.e. the ratio of the shorter section to the longer section of the line is equal to the ratio of the longer section to the whole line. This gives AC/AB the value 0.618, termed the golden number. The point at which the line is divided is known as the golden section and is represented by the symbol Φ (phi) derived from the name of the Greek sculptor Phidias.

This proportion has classically been described as pleasing to the eye, the emphasis being upon the proportion of the parts to the whole. The prominent mathematician Euclid (c.325–265BC) described this in his treatise *The Elements*. In his edition of Euclid's Elements, the mathematician Luca Pacioli (1509) renamed the golden proportion the 'Divine Proportion' as he felt the concept could not be fully explained, and published a treatise entitled *De Divina Proportione* (*On Divine Proportion*) for which Leonardo da Vinci drew figures of symmetrical and proportionate faces and bodies.[1] Maestlin gave the first known calculation of the golden proportion as a decimal in a letter to his former pupil, the famous astronomer Johannes Kepler, in 1597.[11]

Another often quoted concept, which gives some credence to the golden proportion, is the Fibonacci sequence.[10] The distinguished mathematician Leonardo of Pisa (1170–1240), also known as Leonardo Fibonacci, devised a number sequence in which each number is the sum of the two preceding numbers, i.e. 1, 1, 2, 3, 5, 8, 13, 21, 34, 55 etc. In the nineteenth century the mathematician Edouard Lucas coined the term Fibonacci sequence, and scientists began to discover the numbers in nature, such as in the spirals of sunflower heads, the logarithmic spiral in snail shells and in animal horns. As the numbers increase in magnitude, the ratio between succeeding numbers approaches the golden proportion.

Attempts have been made to apply the concept of the golden proportion to dental aesthetics. In terms of smile aesthetics the golden proportion may be applied to the *apparent* mesiodistal width of the anterior teeth when viewed from the frontal aspect. This can be useful in designing the relative width of teeth in a beautiful smile,[12] though the evidence is certainly not conclusive.

There have also been attempts to correlate ideal facial proportions with the golden proportion.[10] However, the faces of professional models have not been found to always fit the golden proportion,[13] and a study looking at the aesthetic improvement of patients undergoing orthognathic surgery found that while most subjects were considered more aesthetic after treatment than before, the proportions were equally likely to move away from or toward the golden proportion.[14] Therefore, more evidence is required to substantiate the true significance of this concept in the clinical assessment of facial aesthetics.

Canons of Proportion

The idealisation of human proportions was a major preoccupation of Greek sculptors. One of the most famous, Polycleitus (late fifth century BC), wrote the *Canon*, a theoretical work that discussed ideal mathematical proportions for the parts of the human body. Roman copies of one of his most famous statues, the 'Doryphorus' ('Spear Bearer'), still exist. This statue is itself often referred to as the 'Canon' because it embodies Polycleitus' views on the correct proportions of the 'ideal' male form (Figure 5.2). In the second century AD the prominent Greek physician and philosopher Galen said, 'Beauty does not lie in the individual parts, but in the harmonious proportion of all the parts to all the others, as is stated in the Canon of Polycleitus.'

Phidias (*c.* 490–430 BC), a contemporary of Polycleitus, was an Athenian famous as one of the most outstanding of all sculptors. He directed the construction and design of the Parthenon, the chief temple of the Greek goddess Athena on the hill of the Acropolis at Athens. The Parthenon itself, and the statues contained within it, were said to conform to 'ideal' proportions, with Phidias *possibly* incorporating the golden proportion into the architectural design.[15] It is said of Phidias that he alone had seen the exact image of the gods, and that he revealed it to man. In ancient Greece, sculpture of the human form was used to represent the many gods. As these sculptures were constructed with ideal proportions, the belief arose that the better 'mortals' looked, the more god-like they were (Figure 5.3)!

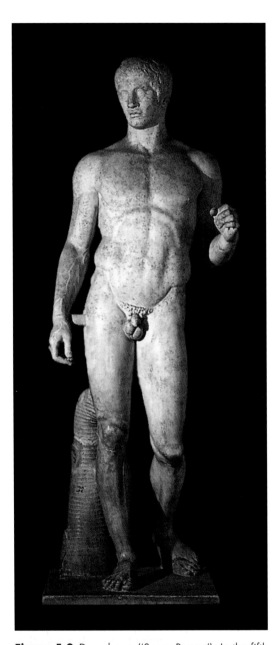

Figure 5.2 Doryphorus ('Spear Bearer'). In the fifth century BC Polycleitos wrote the *Canon* in which he laid down the guidelines for the ideal proportions of the human body. In this statue, also often referred to as the 'Canon', Polycleitos created the archetype of the Greek ideal of male beauty. (Roman copy after the Greek original, Naples Museum). From: Naini FB. Facial Aesthetics: Concepts and Clinical Diagnosis. Oxford: Wiley-Blackwell, 2011; reprinted with permission.

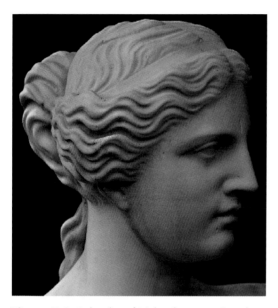

Figure 5.3 Aphrodite of Melos (known in French as 'Venus de Milo') is a representation of the classic Greek facial profile. The facial profile is orthognathic (orthos = correct; gnathos = jaw). The sweep from the forehead to the nasal tip is also almost straight. The vermilion border of the upper lip has a classic curve, which later served as the model for the Roman bow of love, termed 'Cupid's bow'. (Louvre, Paris.)

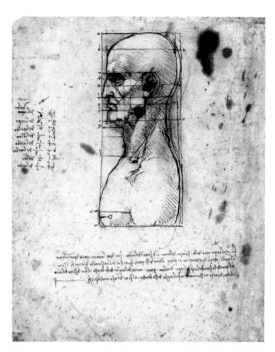

Figure 5.4 Leonardo da Vinci's *Male head in profile with proportions, c.* 1490. (Gallerie dell'Accademia, Venice.)

The Roman architect Marcus Vitruvius Pollio (first century BC) is well known for describing the facial trisection. He referred to the 'symmetrical harmony' of the 'ideal' human body and compared this to 'perfect buildings'.[16] Vitruvian concepts of proportion and symmetry were essentially Hellenistic, being based on those of the Greeks. Vitruvius' influence continued through his ten-volume work *De architectura*. Leonardo da Vinci later immortalised aspects of Vitruvian concepts regarding the proportions and symmetry of the human body.

Leonardo da Vinci (1452–1519), the Renaissance genius who excelled as a painter and sculptor, in addition to architecture, engineering, human physiology and anatomy, defined proportion as the ratio between the respective parts and the whole.[17] His notebooks reveal his quest for the ideal facial proportions. He produced studies of the proportions of the human head (Figure 5.4), a table of possible nose types, and combinations of various forms of foreheads, chins, noses and mouths. The figure of Vitruvian man (Figure 5.5), which Leonardo based on guidelines described by Vitruvius, represents 'ideal' male proportions based on man's navel as the centre of a circle enclosing man with outstretched arms. This shows the importance of proportions in the human form. The distance from the hairline to the inferior aspect of the chin (soft tissue menton) is one-tenth of a man's height. The distance from the top of the head to soft tissue menton is one-eighth of a man's height. The clinical implication is that when planning treatment changes, for example to the vertical face height of a patient, it can be misleading to base the intended result on absolute numerical

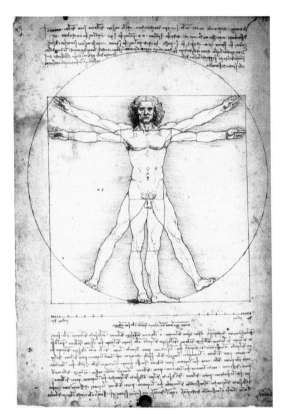

Figure 5.5 Leonardo da Vinci's *Vitruvian man, c.* 1490. This famous figure shows that the proportionate human form fits perfectly in perfect geometrical shapes, the circle and the square. The navel forms the centre. It is based on the 'ideal' male proportions described by the Roman architect Vitruvius. (Gallerie dell'Accademia, Venice.)

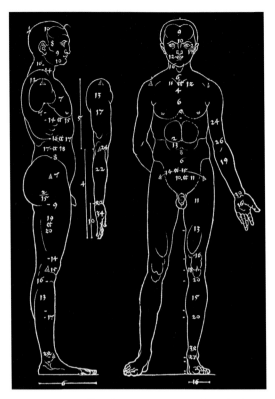

Figure 5.6 Albrecht Dürer's *Man of eight head-lengths*, representing proportions and symmetry in the human form. (Redrawn from Dürer's *Vier Bücher von Menschlicher Proportion*, 1528) (From: Naini FB. Facial Aesthetics: Concepts and Clinical Diagnosis. Wiley-Blackwell, Oxford, 2011; reprinted with permission.)

values based on population norms. People are not necessarily 'average'. It is prudent, therefore, to plan treatment bearing in mind the patient's standing height and stature, and aim to correct the individual's proportions.[18]

Albrecht Dürer (1471–1528), generally acknowledged as the greatest German Renaissance artist, maintained the importance of studying facial proportions.[19] His *Treatise on Human Proportions*, published posthumously in 1528, contained illustrations depicting perfect proportions of the aesthetically 'ideal' human face and figure (Figure 5.6). Dürer maintained

that disproportionate human faces were unattractive, whereas proportionate features were acceptable if not always beautiful.[20] Therefore clinicians can make the assessment of facial aesthetics more objective by diagnosing and helping to correct facial disproportions.

Therefore the guidelines used by clinicians today are based on those initially described in art and sculpture, albeit somewhat modified from the original.[1] What clinicians would today refer to as evidence for what constitutes 'ideal' facial measurements, based on population averages, comes from growth studies using cephalometric radiography[21] and anthropometry.[22] However, these have their own limitations.[23]

IMPORTANCE OF FACIAL AESTHETICS

Self-image and Negative Self-perception

A person's own perception of their facial appearance and any associated deformity is of great importance.[24] Of course, there is considerable individual variation in people's abilities to adapt to their facial deformity, whatever the severity. Some individuals remain comparatively unaffected, while others may have significant difficulties, which affect their quality of life.

Outsider's Perceptions

Social Disability

It has been argued that facial deformity may be a 'social disability', as its impact is not only on the individual affected, but is noticed by and reacted to by others.[25] Attractive children tend to be perceived more positively by their parents[26] and by teachers, who perceive more attractive children as being more intelligent,[27] and in professional life where less attractive adults are perceived as having fewer qualifications and less potential for employment success.[28] Although an individual's facial appearance contributes to the opinions other people form of them, obviously these opinions may well change as interpersonal relationships form. Nevertheless, an individual's first impression on others may well affect their own self-esteem and quality of life.[25]

Stereotyping

It is suggested that people tend to stereotype others based on their facial appearance.[4] For example, individuals with significant Class II malocclusions and mandibular retrognathia/retrogenia may be seen as weak and possibly idle, whereas individuals with significant Class III malocclusions and mandibular prognathism may be seen as aggressive personality types.

Teasing

Children in the school environment can be unsympathetic and hostile to those with visible differences, with teasing and bullying being everyday occurrences. The frequency of teasing directed at those with dentofacial differences is significant.[29]

Severity of Deformity

The psychological distress caused by a facial deformity is not proportional to its severity. Research seems to indicate that facial deformities of a mild to moderate nature actually cause patient's greater psychological distress than severe facial deformities.[30] This is thought to be because other people's reactions towards milder deformities are more unpredictable whereas more severe deformities tend to evoke more consistent reactions, albeit negative, allowing the patient to develop better coping strategies. The variability in people's reactions to milder facial deformities also results in considerable patient distress. It is important to note that the majority of patients seeking orthodontic treatment or orthognathic surgery fit into the mild/moderate category in terms of facial deformity, as opposed to craniofacial malformation syndromes or severe facial trauma/disease.[31]

References

1. Naini FB. Facial beauty. In: Naini FB. Facial Aesthetics: Concepts and Clinical Diagnosis. Wiley-Blackwell, Oxford, 2011.
2. Langlois JH, Roggman LA, Casey RJ, Ritter JM, Rieser-Danner LA, Jenkins VY. Infant preferences for attractive faces: rudiments of a stereotype? Dev Psychol 1987;23(3): 363–9.

3. Jones S. Almost Like a Whale: The Origin of Species Updated. Doubleday, London, 1999.
4. Langlois JH, Kalanakis LE, Rubenstein AJ, Larson AD, Hallam MJ, Smoot MT. Maxims or myths of beauty: A meta-analytic and theoretical overview. Psychol Bull 2000;126: 390–423.
5. Langlois JH, Roggman LA. Attractive faces are only average. Psychol Sci 1990;1(2):115–21.
6. Perrett DI, May KA, Yoshikawa S. Face shape and judgements of female attractiveness. Nature 1994;368:239–42.
7. Arvystas M. Orthodontic Management of Agenesis and Other Complexities: An Interdisciplinary Approach to Functional Esthetics. Martin Dunitz Ltd, New York, NY, 2003.
8. Naini FB. Facial symmetry and asymmetry. In: Naini FB. Facial Aesthetics: Concepts and Clinical Diagnosis. Wiley-Blackwell, Oxford, 2011.
9. Peck H, Peck S. A concept of facial esthetics. Angle Orthod 1970;40:284–317.
10. Ricketts RM. The biologic significance of the divine proportion and Fibonacci series. Am J Orthod 1982;81(5):351–70.
11. Herz-Fischler R. A Mathematical History of the Golden Number. Dover Publications, New York, NY, 1998.
12. Snow SR. Esthetic smile analysis for maxillary anterior tooth width: the Golden Percentage. J Esthetic Dent 1999;11:177–84.
13. Moss JP, Linney AD, Lowey MN. The use of three-dimensional techniques in facial esthetics. Semin Orthod 1995;1(2):94–104.
14. Baker BW, Woods MG. The role of the divine proportion in the esthetic improvement of patients undergoing combined orthodontic/orthognathic surgical treatment. Int J Adult Orthodon Orthognath Surg 2001;16(2):108–20.
15. Green CD. All that glitters: a review of psychological research on the aesthetics of the golden section. Perception 1995;24: 937–68.
16. Howe TN. Vitruvius: The Ten Books on Architecture. Cambridge University Press, Cambridge 1999.
17. Naini FB. Facial proportions. In: Naini FB. Facial Aesthetics: Concepts and Clinical Diagnosis. Wiley-Blackwell, Oxford, 2011.
18. Naini FB, Cobourne MT, McDonald F, Donaldson AN. The influence of craniofacial to standing height proportion on perceived attractiveness. Int J Oral Maxillofac Surg 2008;37(10):877–85.
19. Dürer A. The Art of Measurement. Alan Wofsy Fine Arts, San Francisco, CA, 1981.
20. Naini FB. Facial type. In: Naini FB. Facial Aesthetics: Concepts and Clinical Diagnosis. Wiley-Blackwell, Oxford, 2011.
21. Naini FB. Cephalometry and cephalometric analysis. In: Naini FB. Facial Aesthetics: Concepts and Clinical Diagnosis. Wiley-Blackwell, Oxford, 2011.
22. Farkas LG. Anthropometry of the Head and Face in Medicine. Elsevier, New York, NY, 1981.
23. Edler RJ. Background considerations to facial aesthetics. J Orthod 2001;28(2): 159–68.
24. Naini FB. Psychological ramifications of facial deformities. In: Naini FB. Facial Aesthetics: Concepts and Clinical Diagnosis. Wiley-Blackwell, Oxford, 2011.
25. Macgregor F. After Plastic Surgery: Adaptation and Adjustment. Praeger, New York, NY, 1979.
26. Langlois JH, Ritter JM, Casey RJ, Sawin DB. Infant attractiveness predicts maternal behaviours and attitudes. Dev Psychol 1995;31:466–72.
27. Clifford M, Walster E. The effects of physical attractiveness on teacher expectation. Sociol Educ 1973;46:248.
28. Hosoda M, Stone-Romero EF, Coats G. The effects of physical attractiveness on job-related outcomes: A meta-analysis of experimental studies. Personnel Psychol 2003;56: 431–62.

29. Shaw WC, Meek SC, Jones DS. Nicknames, teasing, harassment and the salience of dental features among schoolchildren. Br J Orthod 1980;7:75–80.
30. Macgregor F. Social and psychological implications of dentofacial disfigurement. Angle Orthod 1970;40:231–3.
31. Naini FB, Moss JP, Gill DS. The enigma of facial beauty: esthetics, proportions, deformity and controversy. Am J Orthod Dentofacial Orthop 2006;130:277–82.

Further Reading

Detailed clinical evaluation of the craniofacial complex for patients presenting with dento-facial and craniofacial deformities is beyond the scope of this book and has been described comprehensively elsewhere. For more details, see Naini FB. Facial Aesthetics: Concepts and Clinical Diagnosis. Wiley-Blackwell, Oxford, 2011.

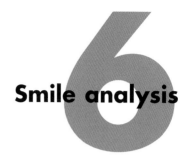

Smile analysis

INTRODUCTION

Most patients seek orthodontic treatment to improve their smile aesthetics. With modern techniques, particularly in combination with restorative dentistry, it is possible to improve the appearance of the smile assuming its individual components are understood. Knowledge of the components that contribute to an aesthetic smile are also important for informed consent reasons, as any anatomical limitations in achieving ideal aesthetics should be explained to the patient before commencing any form of treatment. Although tooth colour is a very important factor in smile aesthetics, it will not be considered within this chapter as it is considered to be more in the realms of restorative dentistry rather than orthodontics. A number of important components of the smile will be discussed including:

- The lip line
- The smile arc
- Tooth size and symmetry
- The midlines

- The buccal corridors
- Gingival aesthetics
- Contacts, connectors and embrasures.

THE LIP LINE

The lip line is the vertical relationship between the upper lip and the maxillary dentition during smiling (Figure 6.1). There are in fact two lip lines: an anterior lip line and a posterior lip line. The anterior lip line determines the amount of maxillary incisor and gingival display whilst the posterior lip line determines the amount of posterior tooth and gingival show.

Regarding the anterior lip line, ideally the full length of the upper incisors and a small amount of gingivae should be visible during smiling.[1] The lip line is high when a thick continuous band of gingival tissue is visible and low when less than 75% of the crown height of the central incisors can be seen. The lip line in females is 1–2 mm higher than in males so it is acceptable for females to show 1–2 mm of gingivae anteriorly during smiling.

Orthodontics: Principles and Practice, First Edition. Edited by Daljit S. Gill, Farhad B. Naini.
© 2011 Daljit S. Gill, Farhad B. Naini and Dental Update. Published 2011 by Blackwell Publishing Ltd.

A number of factors can influence the lip line and amount of incisor display during rest and smiling:

- *The type of smile.* There are two types of smile described within the literature. The posed smile (Figure 6.2a) is a voluntary

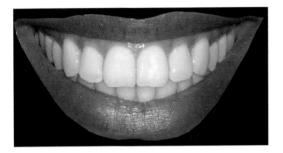

Figure 6.1 The lip line is the vertical relationship between the upper lip and the maxillary dentition during smiling. There is an anterior and posterior lip line.

smile, not linked with emotion, that is fairly reproducible. An example of a posed smile is one elicited when someone is asked to smile for a photograph. The spontaneous smile (Figure 6.2b) is an involuntary smile, linked with emotion, where there is maximal elevation of the upper lip. An example of a spontaneous smile is that elicited when somebody is told a funny joke. It is important to examine patients and take records of both the posed and spontaneous smiles, as the amount of incisor and gingival show in the latter is greater.

- *Elevation of the upper lip.* There is individual variation in upper lip elevation during smiling (mean = 7–8 mm). Excessive elevation, also termed hypermobility, results in a high lip line even if the underlying skeletal pattern is normal.
- *Vertical maxillary height.* Vertical maxillary excess can result in a high lip line. Conversely,

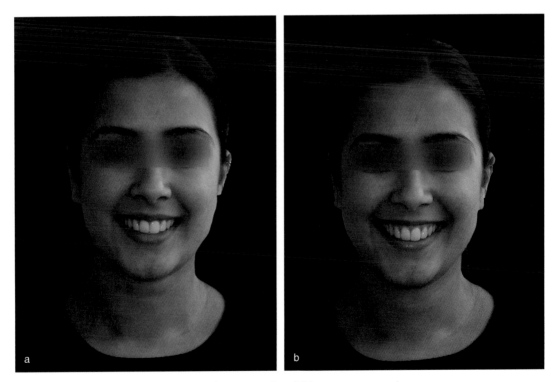

Figure 6.2 Photographs demonstrating the (a) posed and (b) spontaneous smile.

vertical maxillary deficiency, sometimes associated with maxillary retrognathia, can result in a low lip line. Orthognathic surgery can be used to address such discrepancies.

- *Vertical dental height.* A reduced vertical dental height, as seen in digit sucking, results in reduced incisor display.
- *Incisor inclination.* Proclination of the maxillary incisors results in elevation of their incisal edges and a reduction in tooth display. Conversely, retroclination increases tooth display. This is an important relationship to understand when one is altering the incisor inclination to a significant extent (e.g. presurgical orthodontics).
- *Age.* With ageing, the amount of maxillary incisor display will tend to reduce while the amount of mandibular incisor exposure increases during rest and smiling.[2] This is due to gravitational effects, as the perioral tissues tend to sag with age and the oral aperture moves inferiorly and the reduction of the maxillary incisor crown length due to toothwear.

The posterior lip line is the vertical degree of upper premolar and molar display during smiling. Population-based studies suggest that the average gingival display in the premolar region should equate to 2 mm.[3]

THE SMILE ARC

The smile arc was first described by Frush and Fisher in 1958.[4] It is the relationship between the curvature of the maxillary incisal edges and the curvature of the lower lip in the posed smile. The author feels that this definition should be slightly altered to also include the curvature of the maxillary premolar cusp tips. For ideal aesthetics, the incisal edges and premolar tips should lie parallel to the curvature of the lower lip.[5] In such cases, the smile arc is termed consonant (Figure 6.3). A number of factors are important in determining an ideal

smile arc relationship including the maxillary occlusal plane angle, the curvature of the lower lip and tooth length.

If the maxillary incisal edges do not run parallel to the lower lip or have a reverse curvature (e.g. anterior open bite), the smile arc is termed non-consonant. The smile arc flattens with age because of toothwear and because the curvature of the lower lip may reduce with ageing.[6] Poor orthodontic treatment, with incorrect positioning of the incisal edges, can also lead to flattening of the smile arc. Ideally, the maxillary central incisor and canine tips should be level while the edge of the lateral incisor should lie 1 mm apical to this position.

TOOTH SIZE AND SYMMETRY

A degree of dental symmetry is important in producing a pleasing smile. In patients with missing anterior teeth, it is important to undertake joint orthodontic-restorative planning in order to plan space redistribution to ensure correct tooth size and symmetry. A diagnostic (Kesling) set-up is an invaluable tool that aids in visualising the proposed treatment result and for informed consent.

The maxillary lateral incisor is developmentally absent in approximately 2 per cent of the population. If following a joint orthodontic-restorative consultation the decision is made to idealise the space of the missing lateral incisor for prosthodontic tooth replacement, the decision must be made as to how much space should be created for tooth replacement. The golden proportion[7] (see Chapter 5) has often been used as a guide as to how much space to create for the missing lateral incisor where the space created is 0.618 of the width of the central incisor. Evidence suggests that one aesthetic standard should not be applied to all patients as some research has found that most patients preferred a lateral incisor that was slightly bigger than suggested by the golden ratio.[8] Creating space for a larger-sized lateral incisor

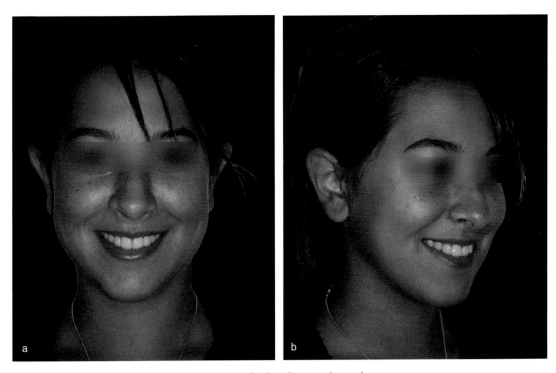

Figure 6.3a,b Photographs demonstrating an ideal smile arc relationship.

has the added benefit of helping to create adequate space between the roots of the central incisor and canine to allow future implant placement.

Central incisors that have suffered trauma, undergone toothwear or where the gingival margin has failed to migrate apically with development, can appear short and broad. For ideal aesthetics, the width of the central incisor should be approximately 80% of its length.[9] Orthodontic intrusion in combination with restorative dentistry can be used to create the ideal ratio.

THE MIDLINES

The facial midline is constructed by joining a line between soft tissue nasion and the midpoint of the upper lip. Ideally, the maxillary dental centreline should be coincident and par-

allel to this. Research suggests that parallelism is more important than coincidence. The upper midline could be displaced up to 4 mm without having a significant impact on smile aesthetics whereas if it was canted by more than 2 mm the aesthetic ranking rapidly deteriorated.[10] Aesthetically, the mandibular midline is not as important as the maxillary midline. However, it is important occlusally as good buccal interdigitation can only be achieved if the upper and lower midlines are coincident.

BUCCAL CORRIDORS

The buccal corridor is the space between the buccal surface of the premolars and molars and the angle of the mouth during smiling. Ideally, this should be minimal[11] in order to give the smile a broad appearance. The buccal corridor is dependent on a number of factors:

- Arch width and arch form. Increasing arch width will reduce the buccal corridor. For stability, the dental arches can only be expanded within acceptable limits.
- Anteroposterior maxillary position. As a wider part of the maxilla is moved forwards in relation to the inter-commissure distance with orthognathic surgery, the buccal corridor width reduces.
- The vertical dimension. There is a reported inverse relationship between the vertical dimension and the buccal corridor area.[12]
- Molar inclination. Palatally inclined premolar/molars increase the buccal corridor width.
- Inter-commissure distance during smiling. The greater this distance, the greater the buccal corridor width.

GINGIVAL AESTHETICS

Ideally, the gingival margins of the maxillary central incisors and canines should be level while those of the lateral incisors should lie 1 mm more incisal (Figure 6.4). The significance of gingival aesthetics is greatest when the lip line is high. A number of factors can produce gingival marginal discrepancies:

- Periodontal disease
- Attrition
- Ankylosis in a growing patient
- Canines substituted as laterals
- Severe crowding
- Delayed maturation of the gingival margin.

Orthodontic intrusion and extrusion can be used to correct small discrepancies.

EMBRASURES, CONNECTORS AND CONTACTS

Embrasures are the spaces between the incisal edges of adjacent teeth.[13] Ideally, embrasures should gradually increase in size from the maxillary central incisors to more distally in the arch (Figure 6.5). Toothwear can result in elimination of embrasures, which contributes to an aged smile.

Connectors are the areas between adjacent teeth where they appear to meet. Contacts are the areas where they actually meet and are smaller than connectors. Between the central incisors the connector should measure 50% of the height of the central incisor crown, between the central incisor and lateral incisor it should measure 40% of the height of the central incisor and between the lateral incisor and canine it

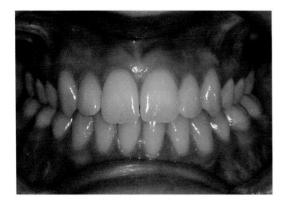

Figure 6.4 Photograph demonstrating the ideal gingival margin relationship.

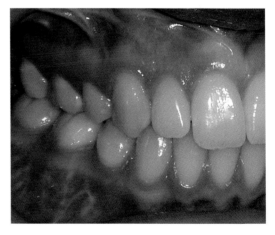

Figure 6.5 Photograph demonstrating the ideal embrasure space relationship.

should measure 30% of the height of the central incisor. This has been terms the 50–40–30 rule. A poor connector relationship can result from incorrect angulation of adjacent teeth and/or a triangular tooth shape. The latter can be corrected by interproximal enamel reduction followed by orthodontic space closure.

CONCLUSION

Some important factors contributing to the aesthetic appearance of the smile have been reviewed. Practitioners should become familiar with these components in order to undertake a comprehensive smile assessment. Numerous guidelines exist about what makes the ideal smile. It is important to appreciate that there is individual variation in what constitutes the ideal smile. It is important that treatment is individualised rather than working to prescriptive norms. In this way the individual concerns of the patient can be addressed, which will lead to greater patient satisfaction.

References

1. Van der Geld P, Oosterveld P, Van Heck G, Kuijpers-Jagtman AM. Smile attractiveness. Self-perception and influence on personality. Angle Orthod 2007;77(5):759–65.
2. Van der Geld P, Oosterveld P, Kuijpers-Jagtman AM. Age-related changes of the dental aesthetic zone at rest and during spontaneous smiling and speech. Eur J Orthod 2008;30(4):366–73.
3. Kapagiannidis D, Kontonasaki E, Bikos P, Koidis P. Teeth and gingival display in the premolar area during smiling in relation to gender and age. J Oral Rehabil 2005;32(11):830–7.
4. Frush JP, Fisher RD. The dynesthetic interpretation of the dentogenic concept. J Pros Dent 1958;8(4):558–81.
5. Parekh SM, Fields HW, Beck M, Rosenstiel S. Attractiveness of variations in the smile arc and buccal corridor space as judged by orthodontists and laymen. Angle Orthod 2006;76(4):557–63.
6. Miller CJ. The smile line as a guide to anterior aesthetics. Dent Clin North Am 1989;33(2):157–64.
7. Lombardi RE. The principles of visual perception and their clinical application to denture esthetics. J Pros Dent 1973;29:358–82.
8. Bukhary SM, Gill DS, Tredwin CJ, Moles DR. The influence of varying maxillary lateral incisor dimensions on perceived smile aesthetics. Br Dent J 2007;203(12):687–9.
9. Brisman AS. Esthetics: a comparison of dentists' and patients' concepts. JADA 1980;100(3):345–52.
10. Kokich VO Jr, Kiyak HA, Shapiro PA. Comparing the perception of dentists and lay people to altered dental esthetics. J Esthet Dent 1999;11:311–24.
11. Martin AJ, Buschang PH, Boley JC, Taylor RW, McKinney TW. The impact of buccal corridors on smile attractiveness. Eur J Orthod 2007;29(5):530–7.
12. Yang IH, Nahm DS, Baek SH. Which hard and soft tissue factors relate with the amount of buccal corridor space during smiling. Angle Orthod 2008;78(1):5–11.
13. Gill DS, Naini FB, Tredwin CJ. Smile aesthetics. Dent Update 2007;34(3):152–4, 157–8.

The psychology of facial appearance

THE IMPORTANCE OF FACIAL AESTHETICS

Facial attractiveness is recognised as being important in situations as diverse as education, relationships and employment. An individual's facial appearance is one of their most obvious characteristics and facial disfigurements are judged to be among the least desirable handicaps. Facial aesthetics clearly has universal importance but is of particular relevance in the field of dentistry.

The face has a profound social significance and any feature which causes an individual to deviate significantly from the norm can be considered a handicap. It is estimated that around 1% of the adult population has 'a scar, blemish or deformity which severely affects their ability to lead a normal life'.[1] Such deformities range from something as straightforward as a dental anomaly to a complex craniofacial deformity.

Recent years have seen advances in our views on facial aesthetics. It is now more acceptable to be concerned about facial attractiveness and it is also more acceptable for an individual to seek cosmetic procedures in an effort to improve aspects of the face which he or she dislikes. This is reflected in the increase in surgical procedures such as orthognathic treatment and also in the increased demand for orthodontics and cosmetic restorative procedures.

In today's society we tend to be subjected to many more one-off encounters than in the past. This means that people are judged constantly on the basis of their attractiveness and facial attractiveness in particular. There is considerable evidence to suggest that those who are attractive have certain advantages over less attractive people. For example, research has shown that teachers expect greater personal, academic and social success from an attractive child than from a less attractive child,[2] and, in job interviews where applicants had identical qualifications, certain personnel decisions were influenced by the attractiveness of the applicant.[3] The understanding of the importance of facial appearance in first-time encounters has developed considerably since this early research. It is now understood that, although

Orthodontics: Principles and Practice, First Edition. Edited by Daljit S. Gill, Farhad B. Naini.
© 2011 Daljit S. Gill, Farhad B. Naini and Dental Update. Published 2011 by Blackwell Publishing Ltd.

facial attractiveness is important in the first few minutes of an encounter and influences initial impressions, other qualities, such as social skills and self-esteem, also come into play. Difficulties which disfigured people have can be divided into two distinct areas: social and cultural (i.e. the view from outside) and the impact on individual perceptions of self-concept and emotional well-being (i.e. the view from the inside).[4,5] For this reason some researchers have recommended psychological interventions, including social interaction skills training, for facially disfigured people in an attempt to counteract the stigma of facial disfigurement.[6]

The severity of a facial disfigurement is not a good predictor of the extent of psychological distress. Macgregor[7] and Lansdown et al.[8] noted that individuals who have obvious facial deformity tend to be treated with compassion, whereas those with lesser deformities (for example, a marked overjet) are more likely to be subjected to teasing and ridicule. These individuals may then feel anxious in social situations because they are not sure how others will respond to them. This, in turn, can have profound effects on their ability to socialise and develop positive self-esteem. It is possibly due to this that the demand for cosmetic dentistry and orthodontics has increased in recent years. Improved dentofacial appearance is usually the motivating factor for these forms of treatment, ahead of the desire for improved dental health or function.[9]

DENTOFACIAL DEFORMITY AND ITS MANAGEMENT

Dentofacial Deformity and Orthodontic Treatment

Individuals are frequently stereotyped based on dental features, especially during childhood and adolescence, and dental and facial features are significant targets for nicknames, harassment and teasing among children.[10,11] Shaw[12] studied the influence of certain dentofacial features on a child's social attractiveness and the hypothesis that children with normal dental appearance would be judged better looking, more intelligent and more desirable as a friend was upheld. Findings such as these, along with society's emphasis on aesthetics, are undoubtedly a driving force for the ever-increasing demand for orthodontic treatment.

The effect that malocclusion has on body image and self-esteem remains the subject of some controversy. It is often assumed that individuals with malocclusions will possess low self-esteem and that intervention will improve this, although it appears that the relationship between perceptions of attractiveness and self-esteem is complex and nowhere near as clear-cut as it may initially appear.[13] Albino et al.[14] found that parent-, peer- and self-evaluations of dental-facial attractiveness significantly improved following orthodontic treatment but there was no evidence that treatment improved self and parental evaluations of social competency and self-esteem.

Studies have shown that dental practitioners tend to be more critical of dentofacial aesthetics than are the general public.[15,16] It is therefore important that treatment is not forced on those patients who do not perceive a problem, as they are unlikely to cooperate. It is also important not to allow parents to dictate treatment for a child; the child's cooperation is required if treatment is to be successful and unfortunately an enthusiastic parent does not always have an enthusiastic and motivated child!

Dentofacial Deformity and Restorative Treatment

Patients who request restorative treatment to improve their appearance have motivating factors similar to those pursuing orthodontic treatment, namely improvement in aesthetics. However, the dentist's perceptions of ideal aesthetics are not necessarily the same as those of the patient. Neumann et al.[17] asked patients to complete questionnaires about personal aesthetic satisfaction and oral self-image. Their results showed discrepancies between clinical findings and the patients' self-perception and satisfaction, which reinforces the necessity for clinician and patient to plan together for aesthetic treatment. This area is further complicated by the fact that there are no 'aesthetic norms' and clinicians therefore have to be guided partly by their professional judgement and partly by what the patient wishes to achieve. The patient's wishes need to be taken into account but the clinician should ascertain that these are achievable. If not, the patient should be told at the outset if post-treatment dissatisfaction is to be avoided.

Facial Deformity and Orthognathic Treatment

More severe dentofacial problems or craniofacial malformations frequently require orthognathic intervention (a combination of orthodontics and surgery). The source of motivation is one of the most important factors in patients undergoing orthognathic treatment and, again, one of the primary motivating factors is an improvement in aesthetics.[18,19] Patients who present with long-standing inner feelings about deficiencies in their appearance (internal motivation) are more likely to have satisfactory treatment outcomes than those patients who seek treatment to please someone else (e.g. a parent or spouse) or because they believe that surgery will make their external environment easier (external motivation). The latter group usually requires a change in their personal environment before treatment is likely to be successful. Other patient characteristics may provide some indication of how the patient is likely to react to treatment. For example, those patients who present with unrealistic expectations of treatment (e.g. expecting a

better job, new relationships) are more likely to express dissatisfaction postoperatively, as are those patients who have only very recently become concerned about a certain aspect of their facial features. Any features which give the clinician cause for concern[20,21] should be taken seriously and referral to a liaison psychiatrist or clinical psychologist should be considered before any active treatment is undertaken.

It is, however, encouraging to note that orthognathic treatment has been shown to result in positive psychosocial outcomes, such as improved self-esteem, self-confidence, body image and social functioning, as well as reduced anxiety and self-consciousness, although the extent of these benefits remains difficult to quantify.[22]

Patients with more severe facial deformities (including patients with clefts of the lip and/or palate and craniofacial syndromes, e.g. Crouzon syndrome) present with a whole range of additional problems and these individuals may therefore be at greater risk of experiencing psychosocial problems.[23] Sarwer and colleagues[24] showed that adults with craniofacial anomalies reported significantly lower levels of self-esteem and quality of life compared with non-facially disfigured adults, and more than one-third of the patients in their study had experienced discrimination in employment or social settings. Improved mental well-being is cited as a major benefit for facial reconstruction in patients with craniofacial malformations and those who support early surgery during childhood do so on the grounds that normalisation of appearance before the child develops a sense of deformity has major benefits.[25]

Acquired Facial Deformity

Facial deformities may occur as a result of various injuries, including surgery for head and neck cancer and traumatic injuries due to assault or road traffic accidents. Patients who experience disfiguring surgery for head and neck cancer are particularly vulnerable to depression, especially in the immediate postoperative phase. Many functions are centred around the head and neck area: eating, drinking, speaking and non-verbal communication. It is therefore not surprising that adjusting to the dramatic change in facial form and function is extremely difficult.[26] Studies have shown the ability of these patients to adapt to their facial deformity in a wide range of situations including work and social activities. However, loss of facial function and form has massive implications for both the patient and their family,[27] and counselling should be available to all concerned.

It has been realised relatively recently that facial injuries acquired through trauma (e.g. assault or road traffic accidents) may also have psychological effects. Mayou et al.[28] found that 8% of road traffic accident victims had post-traumatic stress disorder up to 1 year later. Therefore, in certain cases, care from both maxillofacial surgeons and psychiatrists or psychologists may be necessary.

If surgical management is required to correct an acquired facial deformity, counselling and careful management are necessary. Individuals with acquired deformities tend to be more critical and express greater dissatisfaction postoperatively than those with developmental deformities. Patients with developmental problems have never had an image of normality (although to some extent they acquire this from the media) whereas those with acquired problems tend to expect to look exactly as they did before the injury; an expectation that is frequently unrealistic.[20]

ABNORMAL RESPONSES TO FACIAL/DENTOFACIAL DEFORMITY

Of equal importance are those patients who present with abnormal or inappropriate concerns regarding their dental or facial appearance. One group, in particular, is that of individuals with body dysmorphic disorder (BDD). These individuals present with an imagined, or relatively minor, defect and a level of concern that is exaggerated out of all proportion. A large percentage of those with BDD present with concerns affecting the head/face area, which stresses the need to be vigilant in patient assessment.[29] They may present to a wide range of clinicians including general dental practitioners, orthodontists,[30] maxillofacial surgeons and plastic surgeons. Patients with BDD develop preoccupations which are distressing and time consuming. For example, they may spend hours thinking about the defect, studying it in the mirror or attempting to camouflage it. This preoccupation can reach such proportions that the a patient can become housebound or even attempt suicide.

Patients with BDD may be reluctant to discuss their problems at initial consultation, embarrassed by what they perceive to be a dreadful defect. Alternatively, they may be intrusive and present with photographs and diagrams in an attempt to illustrate the defect. They may also send letters and make numerous phone calls for the same reason. A feature which is frequently noted in patients with BDD is that they have often seen a number of other clinicians, an issue which the individual may conceal if treatment has been refused several times already.

The importance of careful assessment of these individuals cannot be overemphasised. It is important to recognise such patients at an early stage if inappropriate and potentially damaging treatment is to be avoided and it is important that clinicians are not pressured into treating patients against their better judgement; treatment should be provided only where there is clinical justification. There are reports of patients with minimal deformities who have benefited from surgery when treated in conjunction with psychiatric preparation,[31] however, the majority of clinicians support the view that surgical (or dental) intervention is not usually helpful in the long term. Management of patients with BDD is extremely difficult; referral to the patient's general medical practitioner or to a liaison psychiatrist/clinical psychologist is a vital first step and pharmacological treatment[32] or cognitive behavioural therapy[33] are likely to have better outcomes than dental or surgical treatment.

CONCLUSION

The importance of facial attractiveness in modern society cannot be overlooked. It may be that patients who request treatment are not merely seeking aesthetic improvements but are, subconsciously, reacting to society's view that facial attractiveness is important. Dental practitioners have a vital role to play in the management of patients who have concerns about their dental or facial appearance. However, it is also important not to unnecessarily reinforce the myth that facial attractiveness is all important and that, if one's teeth are perfect, life will be better. Patients should be encouraged to realise that other features of their personality are also important.

Careful initial assessment is essential if problems such as body dysmorphic disorder are to be detected and managed appropriately. Although this is time consuming, it may prevent problems at a later date.

References

1. Office of Population Censuses and Surveys. The prevalence of disability among adults. HMSO, London, 1988.
2. Clifford MM, Walster E. The effects of physical attractiveness on teacher expectations. Sociol Educ 1973;46:248–58.
3. Dipboye RL, Fromkin HL, Wiback K. Relative importance of applicant sex, attractiveness and scholastic standing in evaluation of job applicant resumés. J Appl Psychol 1975;60:39–43.
4. Cash TF. The psychology of physical appearance: aesthetics, attributes and images. In: Cash T, Pruzinsky T (eds) Body Images. Guilford Press, New York, NY, 1990:51–79.
5. Thompson A, Kent G. Adjusting to disfigurement: Processes involved in dealing with being visibly different. Clin Psychol Rev 2001;21:663–82.
6. Kleve L, Rumsey N, Wyn-Williams M, White P. The effectiveness of cognitive behavioural interventions provided at outlook: a disfigurement support unit. J Eval Clin Pract 2002;8:387–95.
7. Macgregor FC. Social and psychological implications of dentofacial disfigurement. Angle Orthod 1970;40:231–3.
8. Lansdown R, Lloyd J, Hunter J. Facial deformity in childhood: severity and psychological adjustment. Child Care Health Dev 1991;17:165–71.
9. Kerosuo H, Hausen H, Laine T, Shaw W. The influence of incisal malocclusion on the social attractiveness of young adults in Finland. Eur J Orthod 1995;17:505–12.
10. Shaw WC, Meek S, Jones D. Nicknames, teasing, harassment and the salience of dental features among school children. Br J Orthod 1980;7:75–80.
11. Hunt O, Burden D, Hepper P, Stevenson M, Johnston C. Self-reports of psychosocial functioning among children and young adults with cleft lip and palate. Cleft Palate-Craniofac J 2006;43:598–605.
12. Shaw WC. The influence of children's dentofacial appearance on their social attractiveness as judged by peers and lay adults. Am J Orthod 1981;79:399–415.
13. Kenealy PM, Kingdon A, Richmond S, Shaw WC. The Cardiff dental study: a 20-year critical evaluation of the psychological health gain from orthodontic treatment. Br J Health Psychol 2007;12:17–49.
14. Albino JEN, Lawrence SD, Tedesco LA. Psychological and social effects of orthodontic treatment. J Behav Med 1994;17: 81–98.

15. Kerr WJS, O'Donnell JM. Panel perception of facial attractiveness. Br J Orthod 1990;17: 299–304.

16. Cochrane SM, Cunningham SJ, Hunt NP. Perceptions of facial appearance by orthodontists and the general public. J Clin Orthod 1997;31:164–8.

17. Neumann LM, Christensen C, Cavanagh C. Dental esthetic satisfaction in adults. J Am Dent Assoc 1989;118:565–70.

18. Stirling J, Latchford G, Morris DO, Kindelan J, Spencer RJ, Bekker HL. Elective orthognathic treatment decision making: a survey of patient reasons and experiences. J Orthod 2007;34:113–27.

19. Kiyak HA, Hohl T, Sherrick P, West RA, McNeill RW, Bucher F. Sex differences in motives for and outcomes of orthognathic surgery. J Oral Surg 1981;39:757–64.

20. Edgerton MT, Knorr NJ. Motivational patterns of patients seeking cosmetic (aesthetic) surgery. Plast Reconstr Surg 1971;48: 551–7.

21. Peterson LJ, Topazian RG. Psychological considerations in corrective maxillary and midfacial surgery. J Oral Surg 1976;34: 157–64.

22. Hunt OT, Johnston CD, Hepper PG, Burden DJ. The psychosocial impact of orthognathic surgery: A systematic review. Am J Orthod Dentofacial Orthop 2001;120: 490–7.

23. Thomas PT, Turner SR, Rumsey N, Dowell T, Sandy JR. Satisfaction with facial appearance among subjects affected by a cleft. Cleft Palate-Craniofac J 1997;34:226–31.

24. Sarwer DB, Bartlett SP, Whitaker LA, Paige KT, Pertschuk MJ, Warren TA. Adult psychological functioning of individuals born with craniofacial anomalies. Plast Reconstr Surg 1999;103:412–18.

25. Lefebvre A, Munro I. The role of psychiatry in a craniofacial team. Plast Reconstr Surg 1978;61:546–69.

26. David DJ, Barritt JA. Psychosocial implications of surgery for head and neck cancer. Clin Plast Surg 1982;9:327–36.

27. Vickery LE, Latchford G, Hewison J, Bellew M, Feber T. The impact of head and neck cancer and facial disfigurement on the quality of life of patients and their partners. Head and Neck 2003;25:289–296

28. Mayou R, Bryant B, Duthie R. Psychiatric consequences of road traffic accidents. BMJ 1993;307:647–51.

29. Veale D, Boocock A, Gournay K, et al. Body dysmorphic disorder: A survey of fifty cases. Br J Psychiatry 1996;169:196–201.

30. Hepburn S, Cunningham SJ. Body dysmorphic disorder in adult orthodontic patients. Am J Orthod Dentofacial Orthop 2006;130: 569–74.

31. Thomas CS. Dysmorphophobia: A question of definition. Br J Psychiatry 1984;144: 513–16.

32. Phillips KA, McElroy SL, Keck PE, Pope HG, Hudson JI. Body Dysmorphic Disorder: 30 cases of imagined ugliness. Am J Psychiatry 1993;150:302–8.

33. Rosen JC, Reiter J, Orosan P. Cognitive-behavioral body image therapy for body dysmorphic disorder. J Consult Clin Psychol 1995;63:263–9.

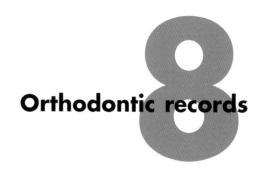

Orthodontic records

INTRODUCTION

It is incumbent on all of us as practitioners of clinical orthodontics to keep the highest possible standard of clinical records. These will assist us to provide as efficient and effective treatment as possible for our patients, as well as pre-empting any medicolegal or clinical governance issues that may arise during treatment. Typical clinical records should include study models, radiographs and clinical photographs, all of which can now be obtained digitally, and in specific situations cone-beam computed tomography (CT) scans. The advent of digital records has been a major leap forwards for orthodontics and the advantages of digital records are manifold.

DIGITAL PHOTOGRAPHS

- *Immediate viewing of the images.* This is an irresistible feature to every clinician, as they can instantly see whether the area of interest has been recorded and whether the image is of sufficient quality. In a teaching situation, immediate feedback is invaluable to the photographer and if required, a better quality image can be obtained without delay.
- *Major financial savings.* From an economic point of view moving to digital photography is an absolute must as, after the initial purchase price of the equipment, there is almost no cost to recording each image.
- *Storage and filing problems are history.* Storage of patient images can be carried out efficiently using one of many different storage systems on the market. An enormous volume of clinical images can be stored on one hard disc, giving the clinicians instant access to all their patient images, throughout treatment, at the touch of a button.
- *File sharing.* Duplication of images is extremely simple and these can be transferred to presentational software or patient letters as well as allowing easy production

Orthodontics: Principles and Practice, First Edition. Edited by Daljit S. Gill, Farhad B. Naini.
© 2011 Daljit S. Gill, Farhad B. Naini and Dental Update. Published 2011 by Blackwell Publishing Ltd.

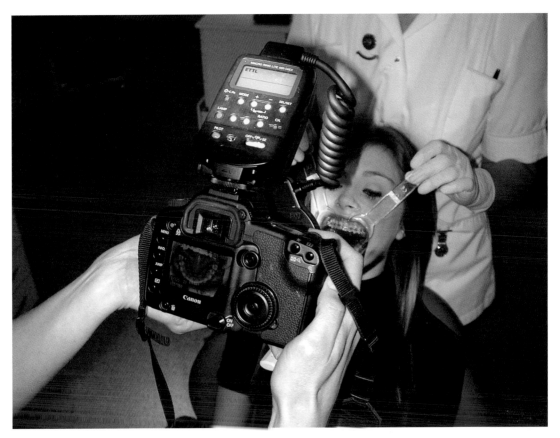

Figure 8.1 LCD screen in 'live view' mode to allow shot to be composed easily.

of hard copies, which is of use to both the patient and their general dental practitioner. These images can be used as teaching material or as motivational tools for the individual patients both before, during and after treatment.

Production of High-quality Digital Photographs

A high-quality, robust camera body and versatile lenses are essential, to allow both intraoral and extraoral photographs to be taken, at a convenient distance from the patient, without changing lenses. A typical recommendation of

a high-quality camera body would be the Canon 60D. This should be used in combination with a Canon 100 mm macro lens and Canon Ring Flash for the best results. The 60D has a 10 m pixel CMOS sensor and the largest LCD monitor (3.0 inches) on any SLR camera currently available. A new feature on the Canon 60D is that it has a LCD 'live view' which means that the LCD screen, on the back of the camera, can be used for setting up the shot rather than the photographer having to look through the view finder (Figure 8.1). This will offer significant advantages for composing the shot correctly, and when used in combination with the zoom feature on the screen the photographer can review images, checking focus and depth

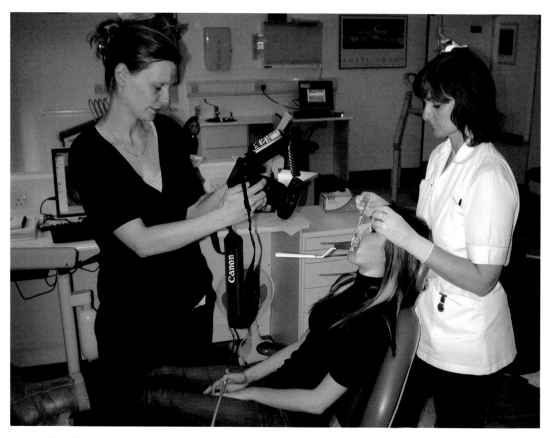

Figure 8.2 Digital zoom feature allows focusing to be confirmed before patient leaves.

of field immediately after the picture is taken (Figure 8.2). The only disadvantage of this high-quality set up is the weight of the system, which necessitates some training and practice by the clinicians to ensure the best results are consistently achieved.

Other Essential Equipment

The types of retractor used for clinical photography make an enormous difference to the quality of the results obtained.[1] It is essential to use two pairs of retractors when taking a series of clinical photographs for each patient (Figure 8.3). The correct end of the larger retractor must be selected to achieve vertical or horizontal retraction of the soft tissues, as appropriate, and the small end of the smaller retractors are used to retract soft tissues when taking occlusal photographs (Figure 8.4).

To allow high-quality occlusal photographs to be taken careful selection of occlusal mirrors is also essential. The recommended occlusal mirrors are the ones produced by 'Filtrop AG'.[2,3] The large 'panhandles' allow complete control of the occlusal view by the clinician taking the photographs (Figure 8.5). It is essential that the photographer takes control of the mirror handles for occlusal photographs and of the retractor on the side being photographed when taking buccal intraoral views (Figure 8.6). The

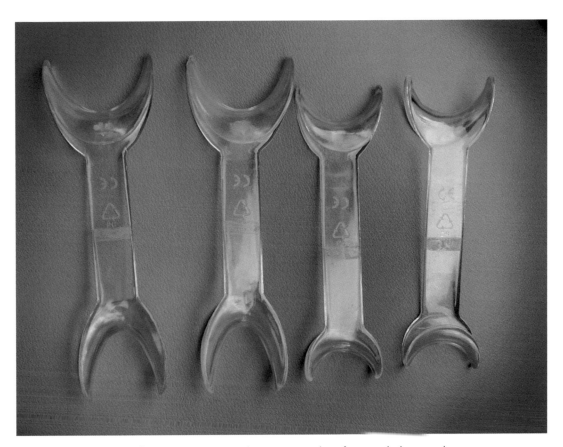

Figure 8.3 Four types of retractor are essential to ensure quality of intraoral photographs.

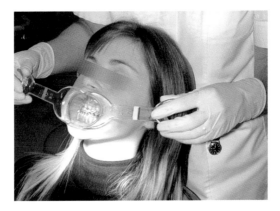

Figure 8.4 Retraction of soft tissues for taking frontal intraoral photograph.

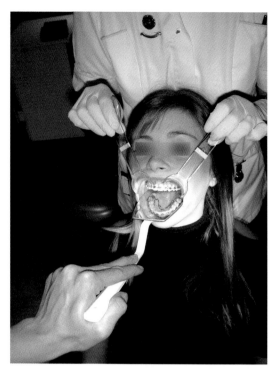

Figure 8.5 Mirror with large 'panhandle' to allow complete control with no fingers on the photograph.

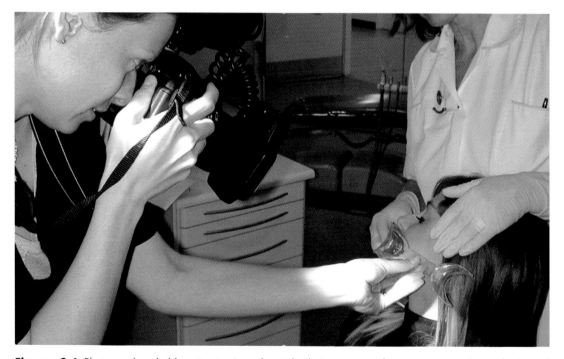

Figure 8.6 Photographer holds retractor on the side being captured to ensure maximum horizontal retraction.

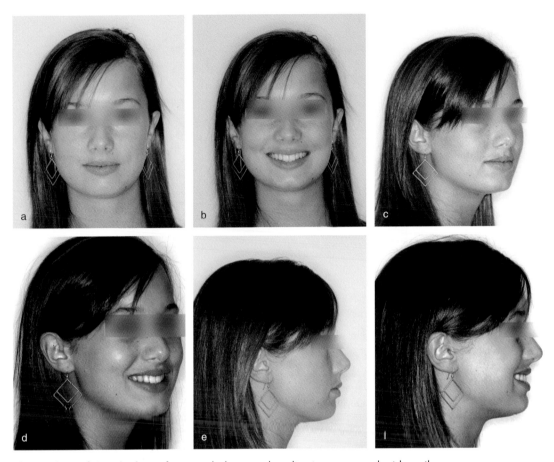

Figure 8.7a–f Standard set of extraoral photographs – lips in repose and wide smile.

lens choice recommended for both intraoral and extraoral photography is a Canon EF 100 mm F2.8 macro USM lens, which is perfectly suited for dental application. The aperture range can be reduced to F32, which gives maximum depth of field for the front intraoral shot and increased to F5.6 to allow the required amount of light to enter through the lens for the extraoral photographs. The Canon ring flash will allow 'through the lens' metering which maximises the quality of the result in different lighting situations.

Extraoral Photographs

A full set of extraoral photographs should include front, three-quarter and profile views, each with lips in repose and on full smiling (Figure 8.7). These are recommended at the start and the end of active orthodontic treatment as well at any other treatment milestone, such as the end of functional appliance therapy or immediately preceding and following orthognathic surgery. An attempt should always be made to get the lips completely at

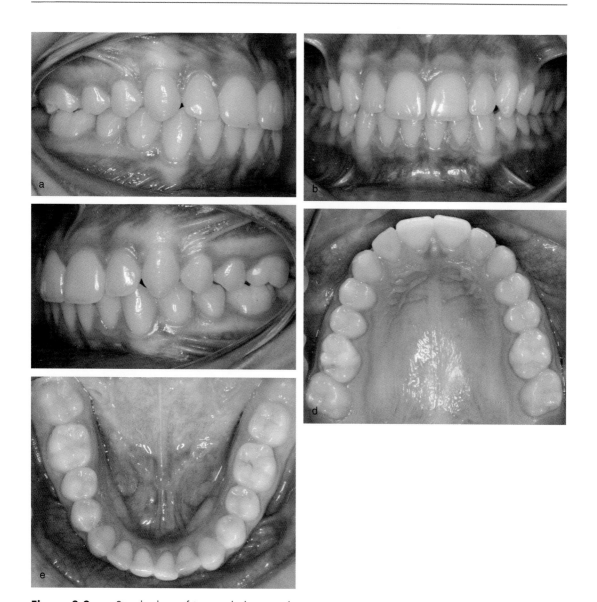

Figure 8.8a–e Standard set of intraoral photographs.

rest and also in a wide smile, showing the maximum amount of dentition, as this is the view that will be most affected by orthodontic treatment. When taking all the extraoral photographs, the photographer must focus on the lower eyelid on the eye closest to the photographer to ensure that the rest of the area of interest is in sharp focus.

Intraoral Photographs

A full set of intraoral photographs, which include left and right buccal shots, a front intraoral view as well as upper occlusal and lower occlusal views should be taken at the start and the end of treatment as well as any treatment milestones (Figure 8.8). For those working in a

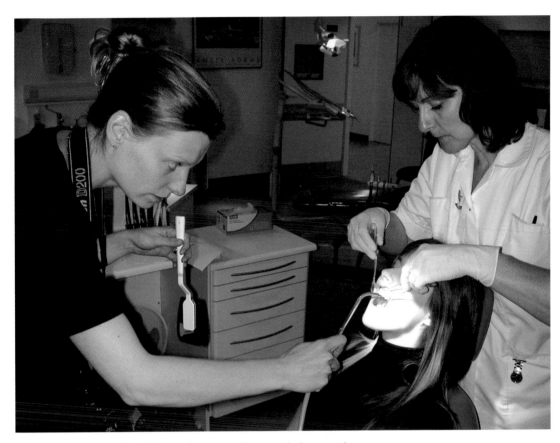

Figure 8.9 Suction should be used prior to all intraoral photographs.

teaching environment it is advisable for all clinicians to take photographs with each arch wire change, so that the trainee and the supervisor can follow stage by stage progress of treatment in some detail.

One final tip for obtaining the highest possible quality photographs is to use the saliva ejector on each and every case before capturing the photograph (Figure 8.9).

There is absolutely no substitute for high-quality clinical photographs. The reasons for satisfactory progress of every case can be instantly identified. Also if treatment is not progressing well then it should be immediately apparent from the photographs why this is the case. Clinical photographs rapidly become an

essential tool and will allow the clinicians and the supervisors to derive the maximum possible benefit from the experience of treating each individual case. They also serve to remind the patient and the parent of the enormous progress that is being made during treatment.

CLINICAL MEASUREMENTS

It is essential that clinicians take a series of measurements at regular intervals so that they have an objective measure of the progress of treatment. A typical clinical measurement sheet is shown in Table 8.1. It is incumbent on all clinicians, particularly when in training, to

Table 8.1 Typical measurement sheet to be filled in by clinician every visit

STRAIGHT WIRE RECORD SHEET

NAME:		Patient Ref. No:									
Date											
Overjet (tooth number) (mm)											
Overbite (mm)											
Centreline (mm)		-/-	-/-	-/-	-/-	-/-	-/-	-/-	-/-	-/-	-/-
Reverse overjet (mm)											
Intercanine width (mm)											
Canine relationship	Left										
	Right										
Intermolar width (mm)	Upper										
	Lower										
Molar relationship	Upper										
	Lower										
Spaces (mm)	-/-	-/-	-/-	-/-	-/-	-/-	-/-	-/-	-/-	-/-	-/-
Archwire	← →										
Elastics	-/-	-/-	-/-	-/-	-/-	-/-	-/-	-/-	-/-	-/-	-/-
Extraoral traction requested/worn											
Photos											
Oral hygiene (1–10), 1 = Poor, 10 = Fantastic											
Comments											

routinely measure, overjet, overbite, centrelines, canine and molar relationships on a visit-by-visit basis. If there is lack of improvement in any of these parameters then the reason for this should be ascertained as soon as possible. Only by combining high-quality photographs with meticulous recording of the clinical measurements, on a visit-by-visit basis, will the reasons for lack of progress with any particular case become obvious.

STUDY MODELS

High-quality study models are also an essential record to allow us to measure the improvement of orthodontic cases. Traditionally study models are constructed in plaster. The Peer Assessment Rating (PAR) system, which is the objective grading used to assess improvement in occlusion as a result of treatment (see also Chapter 11), is dependent on measurement of a number of features of the malocclusion from the study models. Recently, digital study models have been made available to the orthodontic profession by many different orthodontic companies. One of the first systems on the market to produce three-dimensional electronic models was 'Orthocad' and this development may revolutionise the use of study models. It is a very simple task to take a couple of alginate impressions, cast some models, box them and then post them to a supplier who can arrange digitisation of these models and then return the digital information via the internet (Figure 8.10).

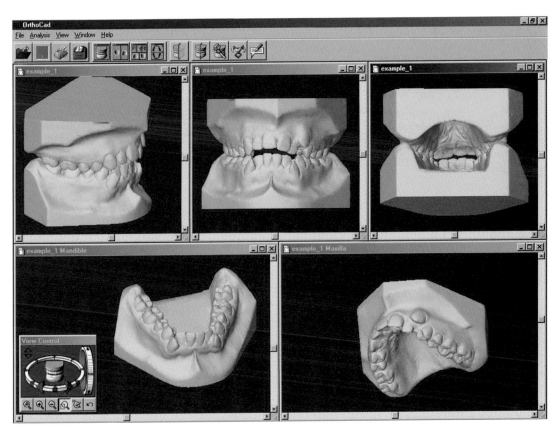

Figure 8.10 Digital three-dimensional models will soon replace conventional plaster models.

Digital study models can be used in place of traditional study models for case assessment,[4] formal space analysis and Kesling set-ups.[5] It has been demonstrated in a number of papers that the measurements taken from these electronic models are as accurate as those taken from traditional plaster study models. Should conventional models be required at any stage in the future then these can be easily reconstructed from the digital data using a three-dimensional printer. The vast amounts of landfill space that will be required for millions of plaster models stored all over the world will hopefully be a thing of the past, as all this information is simply recorded electronically in streams of ones and zeros.

SUMMARY

Digital technology is here to stay, and it has certainly revolutionised our approach to radiographs, clinical photographs and study models. The way we record, analyse, store and transfer patient records has changed beyond recognition in the past decade. Storage of these clinical records is no longer a problem, and particularly in this age of 'big brother' and obsession with data protection, the increased security demanded for all clinically sensitive information is easily possible, now that the records can be made in digital form.

References

1. McKeown HF, Sandler PJ, Murray AM. How to avoid errors in clinical photography. J Orthod 2005;32:43–54.
2. Sandler PJ, Murray AM. Clinical photography in an orthodontic practice environment – Part 1. Orthodontic Update 2010;3:75–80.
3. Sandler PJ, Murray AM. Clinical photography in an orthodontic practice environment – Part 2. Orthodontic Update 2010;3:107–9.
4. Sandler PJ, Murray AM, Bearn D. Digital records in orthodontics. Dent Update 2002;29:18–24.
5. Sandler PJ, Sira S, Murray AM. A photographic 'Kesling' setup. J Orthod 2005;32: 85–8.

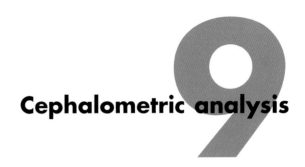

Cephalometric analysis

INTRODUCTION

A lateral cephalogram is a standardised lateral skull view with known magnification (Figure 9.1) which is taken to aid orthodontic diagnosis and treatment planning. A posteroanterior (PA) cephalogram is a standardised anterior view taken when a skeletal asymmetry is present. The origins of cephalometry stem from the work of anthropology (study of living subjects) and craniometry (dry skulls) where measurements were taken to assess craniofacial form. The first lateral head film was taken by Pacini in 1922 but it was the independent invention of the cephalostat by Broadbent (USA) and Hofrath (Germany) in 1931 that allowed accurate radiographic measurements to be taken from lateral skull views.

THE CEPHALOSAT

The cephalostat is a machine that holds the head in a set position in relation to the X-ray tube and the film/digital receptor (Figure 9.2).

For a lateral cephalogram ear rods are placed in the external auditory meati and the patient's midsagittal plane is vertical and parallel to the film. Broadbent originally used the Frankfort plane (keeping it parallel to the floor) to orientate the head in the cephalostat and this is still widely used in radiographic departments. Solow and Tallgren[1] (1971) suggested use of 'natural head position' (NHP) as being a more physiological method and from a practical point of view this is most easily simulated by asking the patient to look into their own eyes in a mirror on the opposite side of the room when taking the cephalogram. The teeth are kept in centric occlusion with lips at rest.

Knowledge of the exact distances between tube, patient and film enables the magnification of the image to be known (usually 7–8%). The reproducibility of the head position enables sequential images to be superimposed on each other. This makes the cephalogram of great importance to the orthodontist because it allows growth and treatment effects to be accurately assessed.

Orthodontics: Principles and Practice, First Edition. Edited by Daljit S. Gill, Farhad B. Naini.
© 2011 Daljit S. Gill, Farhad B. Naini and Dental Update. Published 2011 by Blackwell Publishing Ltd.

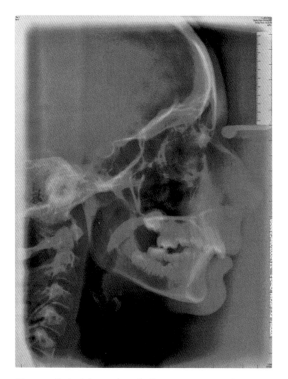

Figure 9.1 A lateral cephalogram. Image taken with patient in the 'natural head position'. There is a skeletal II pattern due to mandibular retrognathia and a distoangularly impacted lower second premolar. A rule allows image magnification to be calculated.

USES OF CEPHALOMETRY

The original purpose of cephalometry was to study growth patterns in the craniofacial complex. An excellent example of this use is in the Bolton Growth Study, carried out in Cleveland, USA, which comprises the world's most extensive source of longitudinal human growth data (http://dental.case.edu/bolton-brush).

Current uses include:

- *Morphological analysis* – sagittal and vertical relationship of dentition, facial skeleton and soft tissue profile. This aids diagnosis particularly where there is a skeletal discrepancy or where anteroposterior movement of the incisors is planned. However, it may not be required in some Class I malocclusions and the benefits need to be weighed against the potential damaging effects of ionising radiation.[2]
- *Growth analysis* – superimposition of cephalograms taken over a period of time. This may help in deciding the timing of treatment in a small number of patients, especially those with skeletal III malocclusions.

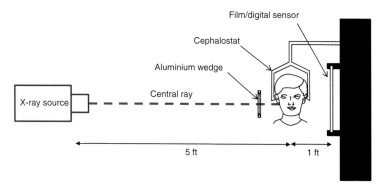

Figure 9.2 The relationship of the X-ray tube, patient's head and image receptor when taking a lateral cephalogram

However, the radiation dose to the patient must be justifiable.[2]

- *Treatment analysis* – a lateral cephalogram can be taken during treatment to assess progress by comparing it to the pretreatment view, e.g. after functional appliance therapy or towards the end of fixed appliance treatment.
- *Assessment of unerupted teeth.* For example, to show the relationship of impacted maxillary canines to the incisor roots.
- *Research.* For example, post retention records to assess stability of orthognathic procedures.
- *Other* – assessment of growth stage (cervical spine maturation); assessment of patients with OSA (airway analysis); identification of pathology. For example pathology of the pituitary gland, cervical spine.

CEPHALOMETRIC ANALYSIS

Skeletal and dental relationships are measured by reference to a landmark or plane drawn on the lateral cephalogram. These can be either 'hand traced' or more commonly now digitised using specialised cephalometric software (e.g. QuickCeph (Mac), Dolphin Imaging (Windows)). Common cephalometric landmarks, planes and angles are shown in Tables 9.1–9.3 and Figures 9.3 and 9.4.

The aim of cephalometric analysis is to compare a patient's measurements taken from a cephalogram against 'standard values'. These values are a useful guide in both diagnosis and treatment planning. The first published comprehensive analysis was by Downs[4] (1948) and since then many different analyses have been formulated often based on wildly different sample sizes (Table 9.4).

The analysis is usually given in tabular form with data expressed either as a linear measurement (in mm or a proportion (%)) or as an angle (degrees). The advantage of angular measurements is that they are not influenced by image magnification or patient size. Standard deviation for each measurement allows the clinician to easily see where their patient differs most

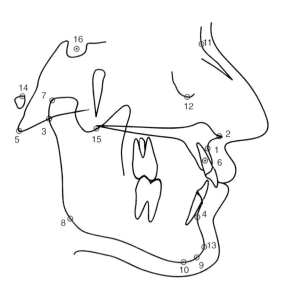

Figure 9.3 Cephalometric landmarks (see Table 9.1 for key).

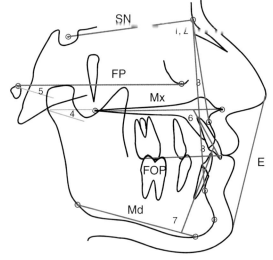

Figure 9.4 Common cephalometric planes and angles (see Tables 9.2 and 9.3 for key; APo line not shown to aid clarity).

Table 9.1 Cephalometric landmarks

Number in Figure 9.3	Landmark	Definition
1	A-point	Deepest concavity on anterior profile of maxilla
2	Anterior nasal spine	Tip of anterior process of maxilla
3	Articulare	Intersection of the posterior border of the neck of the mandibular condyle and the lower margin of the posterior cranial base
4	B-point	Deepest concavity on anterior surface of mandibular symphysis
5	Basion	Posterior limit of midline cranial base
6	Upper incisor centroid	Midpoint of the most prominent upper incisor root
7	Condylion	Most superior posterior point on the condylar head
8	Gonion	The most posterior inferior point on the angle of the mandible
9	Gnathion	The most anterior inferior point on the mandibular symphysis
10	Menton	Lowest point on mandibular symphysis
11	Nasion	Most anterior point on frontonasal suture
12	Orbitale	Most inferior point on orbital margin
13	Pogonion	Most anterior point on bony chin
14	Porion	Upper and outermost point on bony external auditory meatus
15	Posterior nasal spine	Tip of posterior nasal spine of maxilla
16	Sella	Midpoint of sella turcica

Adapted from Houston et al.[3]

Table 9.2 Cephalometric planes

Abbreviation	Plane/line	Definition
FP	Frankfort plane	A line joining porion and orbitale
Md	Mandibular plane	A line joining gonion and menton
Mx	Maxillary plane	A line joining the anterior and posterior nasal spines
FOP	Functional occlusal plane	A line drawn between the cusp tips of the permanent molars and the premolars or deciduous molars
E	Ricketts' E-line	A soft tissue line tangential to chin and nasal tip
SN	SN line	A line joining sella and nasion representing the anterior cranial base
	APo line	A line joining A-point and pogonion

Table 9.3 Cephalometric angles

Number in Figure 9.4	Angle	What it represents
1	SNA	AP position of maxilla relative to cranial base
2	SNB	AP position of mandible relative to cranial base
3	ANB	AP position of mandible relative to maxilla
4	MMPA	Angle between the maxillary and mandibular planes
5	FMPA	Angle between the Frankfort and mandibular planes
6	UI /Mx	Inclination of upper incisors to maxillary plane
7	LI/Md	Inclination of lower incisors to mandibular plane
8	UI/LI	Interincisal angle
9	SN/Mx	Angle between the SN line and maxillary plane

Table 9.4 Cephalometric analyses

Author	Year
Downs	1948
Wylie	1947, 1952
Riedel	1952
Steiner	1953
Tweed	1954
Sassouni	1955
Bjork	1961
Eastman	1970
Jarabak	1972
Harvold	1974
Wits	1975
Ricketts	1979
Pancherz	1982
McNamara	1983
Holdaway (soft tissue)	1983
Bass (aesthetic)	1991

Table 9.5 Eastman standard values

Measurement	Mean Value	Standard Deviation
SNA	81°	3°
SNB	78°	3°
ANB	3°	2°
MMPA	27°	4°
UI/Mx	109°	6°
LI/Md	93°	6°
UI/LI	135	10°
LI/APo	+1 mm	2 mm
LAFH %	55%	2%
SN/Mx	8°	3°

significantly from the norm. In the UK, the most widely used analysis is that based on a study of children and adults at the Eastman Dental Hospital by Ballard.[5] The values were later rounded to the nearest whole number by Mills and became the Eastman standard values[6] (Table 9.5).

An alternative presentation of normative data is to express it graphically in the form of a template. This is superimposed on the patient's cephalogram to see where the patient varies from the norm. An example is the Proportionate Template,[7] which is useful in determining the degree of anteroposterior (AP) and vertical skeletal dysplasia present in adult patients. This can then be used as a guide for planning for orthognathic (jaw) surgery (Figure 9.5).

It is of note that all these cephalometric analyses quote values based on samples derived from white Caucasian populations. For validity a patients cephalometric values should be com-

SMALL

Jacobson
PROPORTIONATE
TEMPLATE

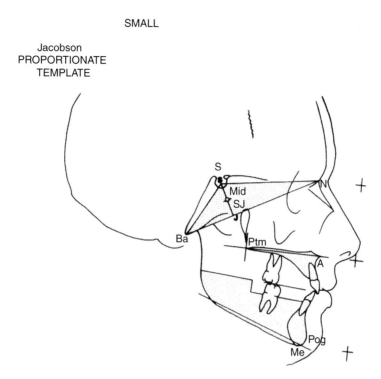

Figure 9.5 The Proportionate Template. S, sella; Ba, basion; N, nasion; Ptm, pterygomaxillare; A, A-point; J, J-point; Me, menton; Mid SJ, point midway between sella and J-point; Pog, pogonion.

pared with the norms for their ethnic group and there are now published data for Chinese,[8] Black American,[9] and other ethnic groups[10].

ASSESSMENT OF ANTEROPOSTERIOR SKELETAL PATTERN

Using the ANB angle

- ANB <2° Class III
- 2° ≤ANB ≤4° Class I
- ANB >4° Class II

An allowance is made for the ANB angle (the 'Eastman correction') if SNA is abnormally high or low. This compensates for an abnormal position of nasion in the vertical plane:

- Add 0.5° to ANB for every 1° SNA is <81°
- Subtract 0.5° from ANB for every 1° SNA is >81°.

For this correction to be valid the angle between the SN line and the maxillary plane (SN/Mx) must lie in the range of 5–11°.

The Wits appraisal[11]

This assesses the skeletal pattern without reference to the anterior cranial base. Perpendicular lines are drawn from A point on the maxilla and B point on the mandible to intersect the functional occlusal plane (FOP) at points AO and BO (Figure 9.6). The distance between AO and BO indicates the skeletal pattern. For a skeletal I pattern the difference is 0 mm (SD 1.7) in females while AO is 1 mm (SD 1.9) behind BO

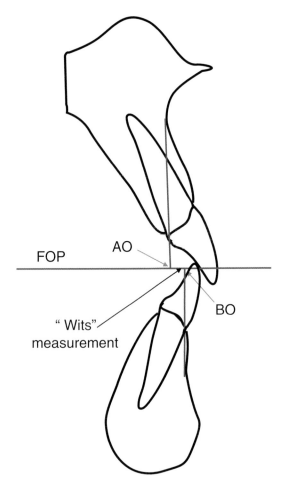

Figure 9.6 The Wits appraisal. FOP, functional occlusal plane.

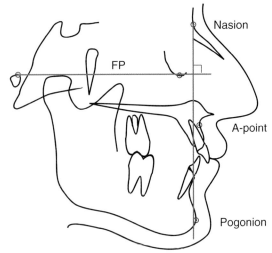

Figure 9.7 The nasion perpendicular reference line. FP, Frankfort plane.

pogonion to the line indicates the mandibular position; the normal value is 0–2 mm posterior to the line.

ASSESSMENT OF VERTICAL SKELETAL PATTERN

The Maxillary-mandibular Planes Angle

- MMPA <23° Low angle
- 23° ≤MMPA ≤31° Normal angle
- MMPA >31° High angle

This gives an indication of the degree of vertical dysplasia present. It indicates the ratio of anterior to posterior lower facial heights (Figure 9.8). Hence an increased MMPA could be due to an increased lower anterior face height, a reduced posterior lower face height or a combination of the two. A high MMPA is often associated with a posterior pattern of mandibular growth rotation and a low angle with an anterior growth rotation. Clinically the vertical facial pattern is assessed by estimating the patient's FMPA, which has the same range of values as the MMPA.

in males. For a skeletal II pattern AO is ahead of BO and for skeletal III BO is ahead of AO. Unusual orientation of the FOP can affect the reliability of this method.

The nasion perpendicular reference line

This is part of the McNamara analysis.[12] A line is dropped from nasion perpendicular to the Frankfort plane (Figure 9.7). The relationship of A point to this line gives an indication of the AP position of the maxilla; the normal value is 1 mm forward of the line. The relationship of

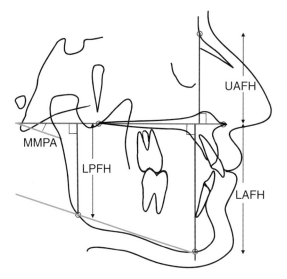

Figure 9.8 The measurement of facial heights and the MMPA. UAFH, upper anterior face height; LAFH, lower anterior face height; LPFH, lower posterior face height.

Facial Proportions

This is the ratio of the lower facial height to the total anterior facial height expressed as a percentage. Perpendicular lines are drawn from the maxillary plane to nasion and menton to measure upper and lower anterior face heights, respectively (Figure 9.8).

- Increased vertical proportions >57%
- 53% ≤average vertical proportions ≤57%
- Reduced vertical proportions <53%

ASSESSMENT OF INCISOR POSITION

Incisor Inclination

The average inclination of the upper incisors to the maxillary plane is 109° (SD 6°). Angles above this suggests proclination and below retroclination. However, the clinical appearance will also depend on the orientation of the maxillary plane, crown/root angle and head

posture. Tebbett[13] has suggested that optimum aesthetics are achieved by making the labial surface of the upper incisor parallel to the true vertical, when the patient is in NHP.

The average inclination of the lower incisors to the mandibular plane (LI/Md) is 93° (SD 6°). However, the MMPA should also be taken into consideration as this influences the incisor position – as the MMPA increases the lip musculature tends to retrocline the lower incisors; conversely if the MMPA is reduced the incisors become relatively more proclined. This relationship is expressed by the equation:

$$MMPA + LI/Md = 120°.$$

Relationship of lower incisors to APo line

Williams[14] advocated using a reference line drawn between A-point and pogonion as a treatment goal for lower incisor position. He found that in well-balanced faces with good occlusions the lower incisor edges lay on or just in front of this line. However, this is an aesthetic objective and not a predictor of stability.

Lower incisor edge to upper incisor centroid distance[15]

The horizontal distance between the lower incisor edge and the midpoint of the root of the upper central incisor is important when considering the incisor relationship and in particular the depth of the overbite. For overbite stability at the end of treatment the lower incisor edge should be 0–2mm ahead of upper incisor centroid.

SOFT TISSUE ANALYSIS

The zero meridian

A line dropped from soft tissue nasion perpendicular to the Frankfort plane. The soft tissue chin should lie within 2mm of this line.

Ricketts' E-line[16]

A line joining soft tissue chin and tip of nose (Figure 9.3). This is used to assess whether lips are well positioned, retrusive or protrusive. Ideally the lips should lie close to but behind the line (−2 mm, SD 2 mm).

The Nasolabial Angle

The angle between the columella and the upper lip. The normal range is 90–110°. This gives an indication of lip support by the upper incisors and should be taken into consideration when contemplating reduction of an overjet. The angle can be described as either normal, acute or obtuse.

EVALUATION OF GROWTH AND TREATMENT CHANGES

An evaluation of growth and/or treatment change can be determined by superimposing two sequential lateral cephalograms on stable reference structures

Superimposition on the Anterior Cranial Base

The SN line registered at sella gives a reasonably accurate picture of overall facial growth and also demonstrates any change in the incisor relationship brought about by orthodontic treatment.[17] A more valid method is to use the outline of the anterior cranial base itself (de Coster's line) and other adjacent structures which are stable after fusion of the sphenoethmoidal synchondrosis at age 6–7 years.[18] However, this is not as easy or reproducible as using the SN line.

Maxillary superimposition

There are no true stable structures in the maxilla as all undergo periosteal remodelling. A common method is to superimpose on the contour of the palate at the base of the alveolar process.[3] This will demonstrate growth and dental changes occurring during the course of treatment with reasonable accuracy. In addition superimposition on the anterior surface of the zygomatic process of the maxilla (the 'key ridge' as identified by Bjork and Skieller, 1979)[19] can be used to aid AP registration. This is the one site in the maxilla which appears to undergo little change with growth as demonstrated by implant growth studies.

Mandibular Superimposition

The mandible can be superimposed on Bjork's stable structures,[20] which consist of: the anterior contour of the bony chin; inner contour of the cortical plates at the symphysis; the mandibular canal; and a molar tooth germ (from mineralisation until start of root formation). This is used to demonstrate the amount and location of mandibular growth occurring between serial radiographs and also to show the dental changes as a result of treatment mechanics.

References

1. Solow B, Tallgren A. Natural head positioning in standing subjects. Acta Odontol Scand 1971;29:591–607.
2. Isaacson KG, Thom AR, Horner K, Whaites E. Orthodontic Radiographs: Guidelines, 3rd edn. British Orthodontic Society, London, 2008.
3. Houston WJB, Stephens CD, Tulley WJ. A Textbook of Orthodontics, 2nd edn. London: Wright, 1992.
4. Downs WB. Variations in facial relationships: Their significance in treatment and prognosis. Am J Orthod 1948;34:812–40.
5. Ballard CF. Morphology and treatment of Class II division 2 occlusions. Trans Eur Orthod Soc 1956;32:44–54.

6. Mills JRE. Principles and Practice of Orthodontics. Churchill Livingstone, Edinburgh, 1982.

7. Jacobsen A. The proportionate template as a diagnostic aid. Am J Orthod 1979;75: 156–72.

8. Chan GKH. A cephalometric appraisal of the Chinese (Cantonese). Am J Orthod 1972;61:279–85.

9. Fonseca RJ, Klein WD. A cephalometric evaluation of American Negro women. Am J Orthod 1978;73:152–60.

10. Hamdan AM, Rock WP. Cephalometric norms in an Arabic population. J Orthod 2001;28:297–300.

11. Jacobsen A. The 'Wits' appraisal of jaw disharmony. Am J Orthod 1975;67:125–38.

12. McNamara JA Jr. A method of cephalometric evaluation. Am J Orthod 1984;86: 449–69.

13. Tebbett PM. The labial face of the maxillary central incisor as an aesthetic and repro-ducible assessment of its inclination. MSc University, London, 1990.

14. Williams R. The diagnostic line. Am J Orthod 1969;55:458–76.

15. Houston WJB. The incisor edge-centroid relationship and overbite depth. Eur J Orthod 1989;11:139–43.

16. Ricketts RM. Planning treatment on the basis of facial pattern and an estimate of its growth. Angle Orthod 1957;27:14–37.

17. Athanasiou A. Orthodontic Cephalometry. London, Mosby-Wolfe, 1995.

18. Melsen B. The cranial base. Acta Odont Scand 1974;32(suppl 62):126.

19. Bjork A, Skieller V. Growth of the maxilla in 3 dimensions as revealed radiographi-cally by the implant method. Br J Orthod 1979;4:53–64.

20. Bjork A. Prediction of mandibular growth rotation. Am J Orthod 1969;55:585–99.

Space planning for the dentition (space analysis)

INTRODUCTION

One way of viewing the clinical practice of orthodontics is to see it as the redistribution of space with, in addition, provision for the impact of growth in children and adolescents. In a majority of patients, where the skeletal elements are not particularly adverse, ideal positioning of the teeth is a reasonable expectation. However, an understanding of the available space is critical to orthodontic planning if the objectives are to be achieved. Various analyses have been described that measure one or more aspects of a malocclusion that impact on space[1,2] but these offer only part of the information required to analyse space or are tied to specific techniques.[3] By contrast, a space planning system used in the permanent dentition has been developed at the Royal London Hospital[4,5] over many years, which allows for all the factors which can contribute to space distribution (Box 10.1).

Apart form achieving the six keys of ideal occlusion,[6] the dentition should be placed in an ideal position in the face in all three planes. However, the requirements of aesthetics may conflict with the requirements for stability, and therefore the space planning exercise for any individual is inextricably linked with the treatment objectives. Thus, space planning needs to be used in a flexible manner to allow for various treatment options to be explored. For example, while it may be necessary in some patients to achieve aesthetic objectives by tooth movements that are potentially unstable, space planning can identify the need to obtain patient consent for long-term retention.

ROYAL LONDON SPACE PLANNING

The space analysis system consists of two parts, the first identifying space requirements and, the second, the creation and utilisation of space. Both parts involve measurements of reference models and cephalograms, and incorporation of the space implications of treatment objectives and planning decisions.

Orthodontics: Principles and Practice, First Edition. Edited by Daljit S. Gill, Farhad B. Naini.
© 2011 Daljit S. Gill, Farhad B. Naini and Dental Update. Published 2011 by Blackwell Publishing Ltd.

Box 10.1 Benefits of comprehensive space planning

- A disciplined approach to treatment planning
- Defining whether the objectives are attainable
- Anticipating shortage of anchorage or excess of space
- Identifying whether extractions are necessary
- Planning the mechanics of anchorage
- Planning the mechanics of arch relationship correction
- Improving pretreatment patient information
- Obtaining valid informed consent

Table 10.1 Space requirements

	Lower	Upper
Crowding and spacing	___ mm	___ mm
Levelling occlusal curve	___ mm	___ mm
Arch width change	___ mm	___ mm
Incisor A/P change	___ mm	___ mm
Inclination change	___ mm	___ mm
Total	___ mm	___ mm

+ = space available or gained
− = space required or lost
A/P, anteroposterior.

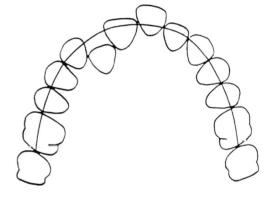

Figure 10.1 The arch form selected for the assessment of crowding reflects the majority of teeth, not necessarily the most prominent central incisor.

Space Requirements

A shortage or consumption of space is recorded as a negative and a surplus or creation of space as a positive. There are fives factors to be considered in space requirement, the first three determined from the models and the other two based on the cephalogram. It is preferable to analyse each arch separately with the lower considered first as it is the template around which the upper arch is fitted. The only occlusal factor not assessed in the space requirements is the correction of the molar relationship, which is considered in the second part of the analysis (Table 10.1).

Crowding and Spacing

Crowding can only be quantified in relation to an arch form, but this is not always obvious as the irregularity of the teeth can mean that more than one arch form could be used as a measuring reference. The simplest is to use an arch form passing through the majority of the buccal cusps and incisal tips (Figure 10.1). Individual teeth that do not lie on the arch form are easily identified. It is important to note that this arch form is used purely to quantify crowding and need not coincide with the intended post-treatment arch form as separate assessments

will be made for arch width and labiolingual position of incisors.

Teeth anterior to the first molars that do not lie on the selected arch form are measured mesiodistally using a clear ruler and crowding is calculated by subtracting the space available. The process is repeated for the upper arch. This method of assessing crowding has been shown to be accurate and repeatable.[7] It is important to ensure that the incisors which contribute to the arch form are the same as those which are traced on the cephalogram and used to measure the overjet. In contrast, spacing is straightforward to measure as the alignment of the teeth in most cases is good and the process is simply one of adding up the spaces available for a (+) score of space.

Levelling of Occlusal Curve

Generally, in the growing child, a small curve will exist between the lower first molars and the incisors (Figure 10.2). Provided the depth of curve is no more than a couple of millimetres, there is no need to make an allowance for space. A steeper curve, however, will have implications for the available space as there will be vertical contact point displacements. A level arch will produce the maximal space requirement with all the contact areas lined up. A curve of 3 or 4 mm, as measured against a flat plane from the distal cusps of the first molars to the incisal edges generally requires 1 mm of additional space to flatten the arch. Curves of 5 mm or more are likely to require 2 mm of space for the whole arch. The levelling of the second molars is not considered as this occurs as a process of distal movement[8] and does not impact on space in the anterior or mid-arch segments.

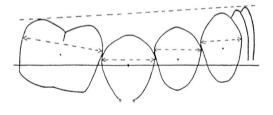

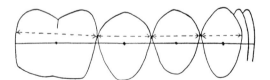

Figure 10.2 Increased occlusal curves are due to slipped contacts in the vertical plane. Levelling the occlusal plane involves restoring the contact point relationships.

Arch Width Change

Posterior crossbites can be corrected by the contraction of one arch, expansion of the other, or a combination of both. It is necessary to identify any premature occlusal contacts and mandibular displacements, and to assess the shape and symmetry of the arches and whether any individual teeth are displaced. In terms of transverse arch relationship, the arch width between the tips of the mesiobuccal cusps of upper first molars should be 2 mm greater than the width between the buccal grooves of the lower molars. This can be determined by the use of dividers or by direct measurements with a ruler on the models. There is no evidence that more than 5 mm of expansion of the upper first molars can be achieved with a stable result. If the differential between the upper and lower intermolar widths is greater than 5 mm, a degree of lower arch contraction across the molars will be required if stable correction is to be achieved.

It has been shown in a number of studies that expansion also leads to a change of arch form with less widening across the premolars than across the first molars. The overall effect of 1 mm expansion across the upper intermolar width is the creation of 0.6 mm space.[9–11] A 5 mm expansion of the upper intermolar width will result in approximately 3 mm additional space in the arch ($5 \times 0.6 = 3.0$ mm). Similarly, contraction of the lower intermolar width will reduce the available space using the same formula. A space requirement to contract an arch will necessitate either enamel reduction, extraction or incisor protrusion.

Incisor Anteroposterior Position

This requires cephalometric assessment. The treatment objective at the outset will determine whether the existing lower incisor position is acceptable. If a forward movement of the lower incisors is desired, for example in a Class II division 2 malocclusion, space will be created

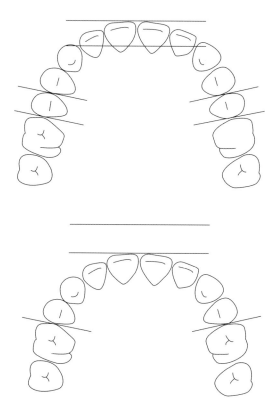

Figure 10.3 The retraction of incisors by a distance requires the same amount of space in each buccal segment. In the lower diagram, the inter-molar distance is equivalent to the distance between second premolars in the upper diagram.

by this movement. If all four lower incisors are advanced by 1 mm, additional space will be created distal of the incisors by an equivalent amount on each side, totalling 2 mm space. Conversely, retraction of either the upper or lower incisors is a space requirement; a 1 mm retraction of all four incisors will require 2 mm space (see also Figure 10.3). It is essential that the incisors which are measured cephalometrically are the same incisors which are used for measurement of the overjet and for the assessment of the crowding or spacing when deciding on the arch form.

The overjet will be altered by any proposed movement of the lower incisors forwards or backwards. The target overjet for an individual will depend on several variables including size of teeth, anticipated depth of overbite and ethnicity (target inclinations) with a range of 1.5–4 mm, most commonly 3 mm. For each millimetre of overjet reduction, 2 mm space will be required for upper incisor retraction or will be created by lower incisor advancement. Larger overjets requiring upper retraction of 6 mm or more require slightly less space, as retraction will also result in a change of arch form (mainly upper canine expansion). It has been shown that an additional 1 mm of space on either side will be created in these cases.[9] In the 6 mm retraction example, the space required is 10 mm not 12 mm.

Incisor Inclination

The space occupied by the teeth is determined by the contact areas. It has been shown that changes in the inclination of upper incisor teeth will result in altered labiolingual positions of the contact areas in relation to the incisal edges. The effect of this is most commonly seen in Class II division 2 patients. In these patients, it is generally necessary to change the inclination of the teeth, moving the contact areas to more palatal positions. If the upper incisors are torqued, and the overjet remains unchanged as shown in Figure 10.4, there is an overall space requirement. Where the change in inclination is 10° for all four incisors, 2 mm is required.[12] This would only be 1 mm if only two incisors required torquing.

In contrast, where the teeth are significantly proclined, the overjet is corrected by tipping the teeth until a normal inclination is achieved. This occurs with less palatal movement of the contact areas than of the incisal tips. Paradoxically, this equates to a space gain. If all four upper incisors are tipped backwards by 10°, the gain is +2 mm. Changes of inclination have to be considered independently of incisor retraction: this can be demonstrated more simply with an example. Suppose proclined

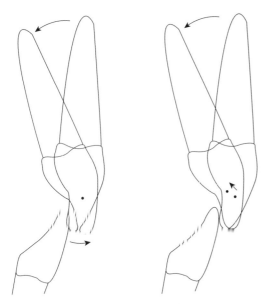

Figure 10.4 Superimposition of upper incisors before and after palatal root torque. Registration on the contact point (left) shows an increase in overjet whereas registration on the point of occlusal contact with the lower incisor (right) shows a palatal and gingival movement of the contact point. In either case, additional space is required in the arch to accommodate the effects of palatal root torque.

incisors need retracting by 5 mm to reduce an overjet and that it is intended to upright them by 10°; the analysis records this as two separate events – retraction of the incisal edges is recorded as −10 mm (2 × 5 mm) and the change in inclination is recorded as +2 mm.

This part of the analysis is undertaken for the upper arch only; the smaller space implications of inclination changes in the lower arch are not assessed.

Integration of Space Requirement Components

A composite score is calculated for each arch from the various components. Among the factors considered, only crowding and spacing and incisor anteroposterior change can have significant space implications, whereas curve of Spee, arch width and incisor inclination affect space by no more than 2 or 3 mm in either arch.

The difference in the total space required for the upper and lower arches requires clarification. The assessment, thus far, has taken into consideration all the variables on which alignment and occlusion depend, with the exception of the molar relationship, and it is this which is reflected in the difference between the space required for upper and lower arches. Class I molars are associated with a space requirement which is equal in both upper and lower arches, unless there is a disproportion in the size or number of teeth between the arches (e.g. small or absent maxillary lateral incisors). Assuming 7 mm premolars, a bilateral full unit Class II occlusion will have a 14 mm greater upper space requirement (more negative) than lower; a 7 mm discrepancy will indicate half unit Class II molars etc. The reconciliation of upper and lower space difference with the molar relationship is very useful as it frequently highlights either an error in analysis or a Bolton discrepancy[13] in tooth size.

Additional Space Creation and Utilisation

The second part of the space planning process is concerned with any additional space to be created or utilised during treatment. This is recorded in the lower part of the space planning form (Table 10.2).

Tooth Reduction and Enlargement

Individual teeth of incorrect size in relation to the others (e.g. small lateral incisors) may appear not to present problems for alignment, but good occlusion can only be achieved when the amount of tooth material in both arches is

Table 10.2 Space creation/utilisation

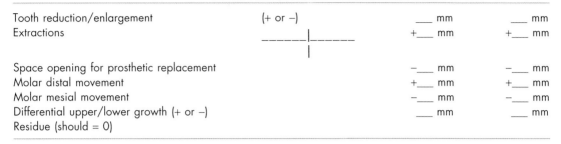

Tooth reduction/enlargement	(+ or –)	___ mm	___ mm
Extractions		+___ mm	+___ mm
Space opening for prosthetic replacement		–___ mm	–___ mm
Molar distal movement		+___ mm	+___ mm
Molar mesial movement		–___ mm	–___ mm
Differential upper/lower growth (+ or –)		___ mm	___ mm
Residue (should = 0)			

in proportion. There is therefore a space requirement for the creation of space alongside small teeth for eventual enlargement.

Conversely, space is gained from reducing the mesiodistal width of an unusually broad tooth or from approximal enamel reduction. In an intact arch, there are 11 contact areas mesial of the first molars. A 0.5 mm reduction in each of these contact areas requiring a 0.25 mm of enamel reduction per tooth surface results in a potential 5.5 mm space. It is unlikely that more than this space can be created by tooth reduction without damage to the patient's dentition, but this is potentially valuable space, particularly in mature teeth with favourable morphologies (narrow, parallel-sided incisors are not suitable for enamel reduction).

Absent Teeth

The initial assessment of crowding and spacing does not take absent teeth into consideration. Thus, the decision to open space for the prosthetic replacement of absent teeth is an extension of the principle of building up small teeth. For example, the space to be taken up by a prosthetic upper lateral incisor is recorded as –6 to –7 mm.

Extractions

The whole mesiodistal width of the permanent teeth to be extracted is recorded, as the mesial

movement of posterior teeth is recorded separately. Typically, the loss of two premolars will create 14 mm of space. The loss of distal units, second or third molars, is not recorded.

Molar Distal Movement

Distal movements of the molars results in arch lengthening. A millimetre of distal movement of the molar on either side will produce an overall increase in arch length of 2 mm. This is particularly likely to be applicable in the upper arch, where headgear or temporary anchorage devices are used to produce distal movement.

Molar Mesial Movement

The space gained by extraction is not entirely available for relief of anterior crowding or incisor retraction as some of this space will be occupied by forward movement of the posterior teeth.

Where no anchorage reinforcement is used, the net space available is determined by several factors as listed in Box 10.2. For example, correcting the angulation and inclination of teeth in the labial segments may be associated with only small amounts of space, but these factors may be very significant in terms of anchorage with greater mesial movement of the molars during treatment unless additional measures are taken to control anchorage.

These wide ranging variables make it difficult to recommend a percentage space available following loss of first or second premolars and it is therefore wise to think in terms of a range of space availability from extractions and to apply clinical judgement on the anchorage demands of each case.

However, typically, around 60% of mandibular first premolar space is available for the benefit of the labial segment without anchorage reinforcement. This reduces to around 40% for second premolar extractions. The net space available is less in the upper arch than for the equivalent lower extraction as the tendency is for greater upper molar mesial movement. Thus, if the lower first premolars are extracted, it would be expected that the molars would move forwards by perhaps 3 mm; if the lower second or upper first premolars are extracted, molar mesial movement could be in the region of 4 mm and this could be 5 mm when upper second premolars are removed as shown in Figure 10.5.

In the upper arch, it is critical this is considered as there is a tendency for the upper poste-

---

Box 10.2 Factors that affect the availability of space following premolar extractions

- Whether first or second premolars are extracted
- Whether the upper or lower arch is considered
- Whether second molars are bonded
- Whether the patient is a child or an adult
- Whether the crowding is located anteriorly or in the buccal segments
- Degree of incisor crowding and therefore the amount of canine retraction
- Angulation and inclination changes needed mesial of the extraction spaces
- Angulation of teeth distal to the extraction spaces

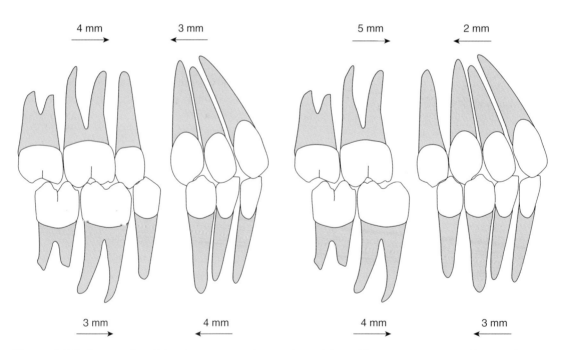

Figure 10.5 Amount of mesial molar movement that can be anticipated in an average case without anchorage reinforcement or intermaxillary elastics following the loss of 7 mm wide first premolars (left) or second premolars (right).

rior teeth to move forwards more than in the mandible. If forward movement of the molars is not desirable, anchorage should be correctly planned by adding extraoral anchorage or temporary anchorage devices to ensure that all of the available space from extractions can be utilised for alignment or retraction of incisors and canines.

This aspect of space planning is undertaken at the same time as decisions are made on mechanotherapy. For example, should Class II correction in a given case involve intermaxillary elastics or functional appliances, allowance should be made for additional lower molar mesial movement (say 2 mm per side, equivalent to −4 mm space for the arch).

Effects of Growth on Space

In the growing patient, provision needs to be made for the likely effects of growth. Although the amount of growth is unpredictable, we can take advantage of the known average growth changes, and also the likely effects of treatment on growth. Growth studies have shown that additional forward movement of the mandible of 1–2 mm is to be expected between the ages of 9 and 16 years.[14] To be more precise, what really matters in Class II cases is growth in relation to the occlusal plane; the steepness of the occlusal plane means that even vertical growth helps improve occlusion.

The effect of favourable mandibular growth in Class II cases is to reduce the overjet. However, in space planning terms, there is a paradox as this mandibular growth has no bearing on lower arch space requirements but is equivalent to reducing upper arch space requirements. Thus, growth of 1–2 mm per side is scored as a +2 to +4 mm upper arch gain in space. This is in addition to the changes anticipated from treatment.

This additional growth of the mandible can be a problem in Class III cases in which the lower arch will advance by a millimetre or

more in relation to the upper arch. This will increase the requirements for retraction of the lower incisors to maintain a positive overjet. The deterioration in Class III cases has no impact on the upper arch but can significantly increase the space requirement in the lower arch. 1–2 mm growth will need additional lower incisor compensation and score as −2 to −4 mm.

The prediction of space gain or requirement as a result of growth is the least reliable part of the analysis as it is based on estimation. However, provision should be made for these growth effects in patients with skeletal discrepancies where there may be significant implications for the fulfilment of treatment goals.

Residual Space on Completion of the Analysis

Once all the aspects of treatment planning and the space implication of the mechanics are assessed, the residual space requirement for each arch should be zero. If this cannot be achieved, it signifies that the treatment objectives are not attainable or that different treatment mechanics and space utilisation are necessary.

CONCLUSIONS

A space planning technique has been developed that is not linked to any particular treatment philosophy or appliance technique and is summarised in Appendices 10.1 and 10.2. It takes into account all the significant features contributing to space and the correction of malocclusions. A disciplined approach to orthodontic treatment planning will result in more efficient treatment, better results, and a satisfactory record of the decision-making process, allowing informed consent at the outset.

References

1. Tanaka MM, Johnston LE. The prediction of the size of unerupted canines and premolars in a contemporary orthodontic population. J Am Dent Assoc 1974;88:798–801.
2. Braun S, Hnat WP, Johnson BE. The curve of Spee revisited. Am J Orthod Dentofacial Orthop 1996;110:206–10.
3. Merrifield LL. Dimensions of the denture: Back to basics. Am J Orthod Dentofacial Orthop 1994;106:535–42.
4. Kirschen RH, O'Higgins EA, Lee RT. The Royal London Space Planning: an integration of space analysis and treatment planning Part I: Assessing the space required to meet treatment objectives. Am J Orthod Dentofacial Orthop 2000;118:448–55.
5. Kirschen RH, O'Higgins EA, Lee RT. The Royal London Space Planning: an integration of space analysis and treatment planning. Part II: The effect of other treatment procedures on space. Am J Orthod Dentofacial Orthop 2000;118:456–61.
6. Andrews LF. The six keys to normal occlusion. Am J Orthod 1972;62:296–309.
7. Johal AS, Battagel JM. Dental crowding – A comparison of three methods of assessment. Eur J Orthod 1997;19:543–51.
8. Woods M. A reassessment of space requirements for lower arch levelling. J Clin Orthod 1986;20:770–8.
9. O'Higgins EA, Lee RT. How much space is created from expansion or premolar extraction? J Orthod 2000;27:11–13.
10. Adkins MD, Nanda RS, Currier GF. Arch perimeter changes on rapid palatal expansion. Am J Orthod Dentofacial Orthop 1990;97:194–9.
11. Akkaya S, Lorenzon S, Üçem TT. Comparison of dental arch and arch perimeter changes between bonded rapid and slow maxillary expansion procedures. Eur J Orthod 1998;20:255–61.
12. O'Higgins EA, Kirschen RH, Lee RT. The influence of maxillary incisor inclination on arch length. Br J Orthod 1999;26:97–102.
13. Bolton WA. Disharmony in tooth size and its relation to the analysis and treatment of malocclusion. Am J Orthod 1958;28:113–30.
14. Pollard LE, Mamandras AH. Male postpubertal facial growth in Class II malocclusion. Am J Orthod Dentofacial Orthop 1995;108:62–8.

Appendix 10.1 Orthodontic space planning

Patient's name: .... **Date:** ....

Treatment objectives

1. ....
2. ....
3. ....
4. ....
5. ....

Space requirements

	LOWER	UPPER
Crowding and spacing:	___ mm	___ mm
Levelling occlusal curve:	___ mm	___ mm
Arch width change:	___ mm	___ mm
Incisor A/P change:	___ mm	___ mm

Appendix 10.1 *(Continued)*

Inclination change:	___ mm	___ mm
TOTAL	___ mm	___ mm

Space creation/utilisation in addition to any planned
above

Tooth reduction/enlargement:	(+ or −)	___ mm	___ mm
Extractions:	_____|_____	+___ mm	+___ mm
	|		
Space opening for prosthetic replacement:		−___ mm	−___ mm
Molar distal movement:		+___ mm	+___ mm
Molar mesial movement:		−___ mm	−___ mm
Differential upper/lower growth: (+ or −)		___ mm	___ mm
RESIDUE (should = 0)		___ mm	___ mm

+ = *Space available or gained.*
− = *Space required or lost.*

Appendix 10.2 Guidance notes

Space requirements

Crowding and spacing	Measure in relation to the line of arch which reflects the majority of teeth.
Level occlusal curve	Assess depth of *lower* curve from premolar cusps to flat plane on distal cusps of *first* molars and incisors. Only one value is given for the arch, and only if the premolars have not been assessed separately as crowded. Allow 1 mm space for 3 mm depth of curve, 1.5 mm for 4 mm depth, and 2 mm space for a 5 mm curve (usually no allowance is necessary). In the *upper* arch, 1 mm space is recorded in Class II division 2 cases with a significant occlusal curve
Arch width change	Allow 0.5 mm space for each mm posterior arch width change. More space creation can be recorded in cases of rapid palatal expansion (max 0.7 mm/mm expansion)
Incisor A/P change	Allow 2 mm space for each mm change. Assess lower arch first and then correct the upper incisors to an overjet of 3 mm. When the upper first premolars are extracted and the incisors are being retracted by 5 mm or more, 1 mm less space is required due to change in arch form
Angulation change	Applies only to maxillary incisors. Although 0.5 mm space is appropriate for correction of each parallel-sided vertical tooth, no allowance is entered as angulation corrections tend to be included in the crowding assessment
Inclination change	Applies only to maxillary incisors. Allow 1 mm space for every 5° change affecting all four incisors, and 0.5 mm space if only two teeth affected

Space creation/ utilisation

Tooth reduction	Record the total mesiodistal enamel reduction for each arch. This may be to reshape an individual tooth or to relieve small amounts of crowding

(Continued)

Appendix 10.2 *(Continued)*

Tooth enlargement	Record the space to be used by building up teeth pretreatment, or to be created if the build up is to be undertaken post treatment
Extractions	Record the mesiodistal width of the permanent teeth to be extracted (excluding second and third molars). The extraction of primary teeth is not recorded except if the permanent successors are absent
Space opening	Record any space to be created or kept in the arches for prostheses
Molar distal change	Estimate the amount of distal movement required from molars during treatment. This frequently has to be adjusted in order to achieve a zero residue at the end of the space analysis. It is then necessary to assess whether the anticipated molar movements are realistic
Molar mesial change	Estimate the anticipated forward migration of molars, either due to active appliance treatment or due to anchorage loss
Differential growth	Estimate A/P growth differences between the maxilla and mandible during treatment (not necessary for most patients). A positive upper space assessment applies to forward growing Class II cases, but a negative lower assessment applies for the creation of additional space in Class III cases where a deterioration in arch relationship is anticipated during and after treatment
Residue	This should be zero in both arches. It may be necessary to adjust the treatment objectives to achieve this, but these must remain attainable and not simply manipulated to achieve the zero residue

Notes:
1. The occlusal curve score is never more than 2 mm and usually 0 or 1.
2. The arch width and inclination scores are never more than 3 mm and usually 0, 1 or 2.
3. The difference between the upper and lower space requirements reflects the molar relationship unless there is an upper/lower Bolton discrepancy.

The index of orthodontic treatment need

Indices to assess orthodontic treatment need and outcome are not a recent development. Some have been around for over 35 years.[1] Others look at specific regions of the occlusion such as the lower incisors[2] while others limit themselves to the assessment of certain groups of patients.[3]

Since the introduction of the new National Health Service (NHS) primary care dental contract in April 2006, the index of orthodontic treatment need (IOTN) has been used to assess whether or not a patient can receive NHS orthodontic treatment. As such, all general dental practitioners are required to have a working knowledge of this index and anyone providing orthodontic treatment within the NHS must have detailed knowledge to know who they can accept for treatment and who they cannot.

A comprehensive review of all types of orthodontic index is beyond the scope of this chapter and the content will be limited to IOTN, which is currently widely used in the UK. The aim is to give the reader some background in how the index was developed and to enable application of the index in clinical practice.

DEVELOPMENT OF THE IOTN

In 1986 the UK government published a report into unnecessary dental treatment.[4] Within this report, orthodontics received a lot of criticism stating that much of it was unnecessary and carried out for appearance only. As a result of this the orthodontic profession thought the development of a treatment priority index would be useful. After reviewing the literature, it was felt that an index with two components, one evaluating appearance and one evaluating dental health would be the best way forward, and details were first published in 1989.[5] A modification of the index used by the Swedish Dental Health Board was used to record the need for orthodontic treatment on dental health and functional grounds. This index was modified by defining five grades, with precise dividing lines between each grade. A visual analogue scale was used to assess independently the aesthetic treatment need of the patients. This scale was constructed using dental photographs of 12 year olds collected during a large multidisciplinary survey. From this, the dental health

Orthodontics: Principles and Practice, First Edition. Edited by Daljit S. Gill, Farhad B. Naini.
© 2011 Daljit S. Gill, Farhad B. Naini and Dental Update. Published 2011 by Blackwell Publishing Ltd.

component (DHC) and the aesthetic component (AC) of IOTN were developed.

CLINICAL APPLICATION OF IOTN

Application of the AC is very simple. The patient is asked to close the front teeth together and the examiner compares the appearance of the patient's teeth with the visual 1–10 scale (Figure 11.1). Factors such as poor oral hygiene and fractured or discoloured teeth should be ignored. Morphological similarity should not be sought. The examiner should think what number on the AC does this patient's teeth look 'as bad as' or 'as good as' rather than what they look like. The AC is also useful for patient counselling. Patients and parents may be invited to

suggest how they think their own teeth would score on the scale. It is, however, important to note that it is the dental professional's score that should be recorded as the AC score and *not* the patient's/parent's opinion.

Application of the DHC involves following a hierarchical scale using the acronym 'MOCDO' as a prompt. Further details can be found in the booklet 'An introduction to occlusal indices'.[6] MOCDO stands for:

- *M* – Missing teeth (5,4)
- *O* – Overjet (5,4,3,2)
- *C* – Crossbites (4,3,2)
- *D* – Displacement of contact points or crowding (4,3,2,1)
- *O* – Overbite (4,3,2).

The aim is to ensure the examiner surveys the dentition in a systematic manner and scores the

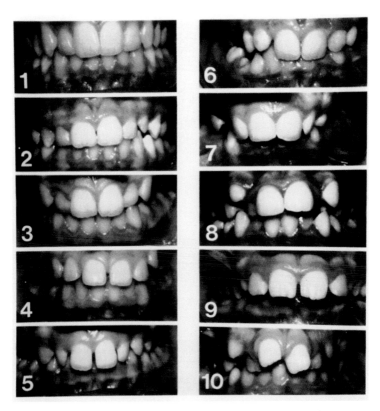

Figure 11.1 The visual analogue scale used to score the aesthetic component of the IOTN.

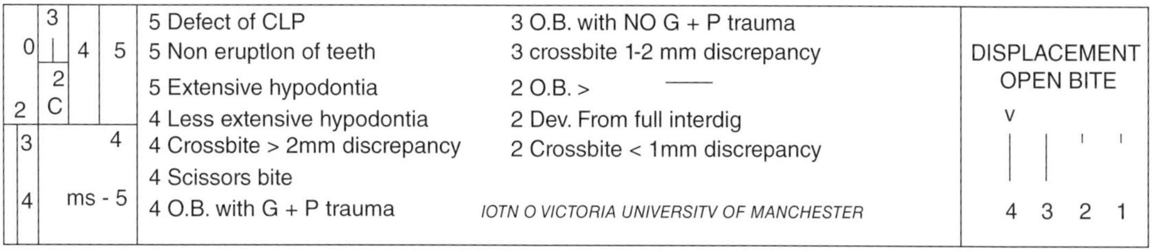

				5 Defect of CLP	3 O.B. with NO G + P trauma	
0	3	4	5	5 Non eruptlon of teeth	3 crossbite 1-2 mm discrepancy	DISPLACEMENT OPEN BITE
	2			5 Extensive hypodontia	2 O.B. > ———	
2	C			4 Less extensive hypodontia	2 Dev. From full interdig	v
3			4	4 Crossbite > 2mm discrepancy	2 Crossbite < 1mm discrepancy	
				4 Scissors bite		
4	ms - 5			4 O.B. with G + P trauma	*IOTN O VICTORIA UNIVERSITV OF MANCHESTER*	4 3 2 1

Figure 11.2 The IOTN ruler.

correct grade. The numbers in parenthesis after each occlusal feature represents the DHC grade which can be given in that section. The aim is to award the highest number highest up the scale. For example, if a patient scores grade 4 in the missing teeth *and* overjet section, the IOTN grade relating to the missing teeth section is the one awarded. The majority of the information required to score IOTN can be found on the IOTN ruler (Figure 11.2). A comprehensive list of all IOTN grades is shown in Appendix 11.1.

M – Missing Teeth

Absent and impacted teeth are scored in this section. The grades are as follows

- 5i – Any ectopic tooth *or* a tooth which has less than 4 mm of space to erupt and is still totally unerupted.
- 5h – Congenital absence of *more* than one tooth in any quadrant, which will require some form of orthodontic treatment as a result of these teeth being congenitally absent.
- 4h – Congenital absence of only one tooth in any quadrant, which will require some form of orthodontic treatment as a result of this tooth being congenitally absent.

Figure 11.3 shows a case with congenital absence of the upper right lateral incisor. It does not matter if the orthodontic treatment plan is to open or close this space, as some form of orthodontic treatment is required, this is an example of a 4h grade. If, however, in this case,

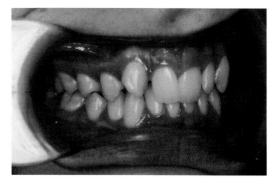

Figure 11.3 Patient with a congenitally absent upper right lateral incisor with an IOTN grade of 4h.

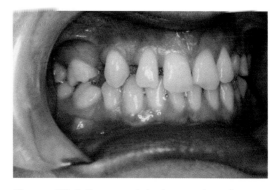

Figure 11.4 Patient with both premolars absent in the upper right quadrant with an IOTN grade of 5h.

the lower right second premolar was present and impacted, the correct score would be 5i as it has less than 4 mm of space to erupt and 5i is higher up the hierarchical scale than 4h.

Figure 11.4 shows a case with congenital absence of both premolars in the upper right quadrant. Again, regardless of whether the plan is to space close, leave space for a single

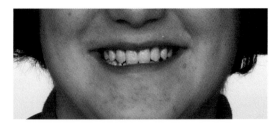

Figure 11.5 An untreated patient with congenital absence of both upper lateral incisors who is not a 4h IOTN grade as no orthodontic treatment is required.

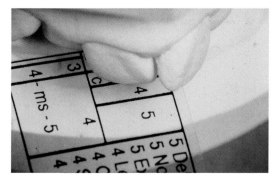

Figure 11.6 The IOTN ruler being used to measure overjet. If the tooth falls on the line, the lower grade is recorded. In this case it is 4a.

tooth pontic or a double tooth pontic, some orthodontic treatment need exist.

Figure 11.5 shows an untreated case with congenital absence of both upper lateral incisors. As the aesthetics are good and no space opening or closing is required, this should *not* be scored as an example of a grade 4h.

The grade 5i can also be awarded in the mixed dentition if the space between the distal aspect of the lateral incisor and the mesial aspect of the first permanent molar is less than or equal to 17 mm in the mandible and 18 mm in the maxilla.

O – Overjet

The patient should be asked to close their teeth together and the most prominent aspect of the most prominent incisor is measured from the lower incisors, exactly in the same way one would measure overjet clinically except the IOTN ruler is used and the lines on the top left hand section of the ruler are used (Figure 11.2). Figure 11.6 shows the IOTN ruler being used. If, as is shown in Figure 11.6, the most prominent point of the teeth lands on the line, the lower grade should be scored. In Figure 11.6, this would therefore be a grade 4a. With overjet between 3.5 mm and 6.0 mm, the competence of the lips must be noted. If the lips are incompetent, 3a is the grade. If they are competent, the grade 2a should be scored. An overjet below 3.5 mm does not score in this section.

Reverse overjet is scored using the lines on the bottom left hand corner of the IOTN ruler. All incisors must be in reverse overjet to score in this section. Both the magnitude of the reverse overjet and whether or not the patient has any masticatory or speech problems must be noted to score the correct grade. A reverse overjet of greater than −3.5 mm would score 4b unless the patient reported masticatory or speech problems, which is what the letters m and s refer to on the ruler. If they do report such problems, the grade would be 5m. Again, for a reverse overjet between −1.0 mm and −3.5 mm, the grade would be 3b without the masticatory or speech difficulties. If these are reported, the grade would be 4m. A reverse overjet less than −1.0 mm would score a grade of 2b.

C – Crossbite

The patient is asked to close their teeth together until the teeth first contact and then into their final occlusion. Any displacement, forwards, laterally or posteriorly, is noted and the magnitude of this displacement is noted. The DHC grade is then awarded as follows:

- None or <1 mm: 2c
- ≥1 mm but <2 mm: 3c
- ≥2 mm: 4c.

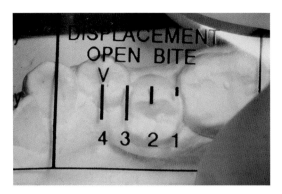

Figure 11.7 The IOTN ruler being used to measure contact point displacements in the buccal segments. In this case the grade is 3d.

D – Displacements of Contact Points or Crowding

The examiner looks for the worst area of crowding in the mouth from the last standing molar on both sides. The magnitude of this displacement is then scored in the occlusal plane using the lines on the right hand end of the ruler illustrated in Figure 11.2. Figure 11.7 shows the IOTN ruler being used to score contact point displacements between two lower premolars. It can be seen that the contact point displacement is longer than the '2' line but less than the '3' line. This would score a grade 3d. If the worst contact point displacement was longer than the 1 line but less than or equal to the '2' line, the grade would be 2d. On the ruler, the lines '3' and '4' are the same length but the '4' line has a 'greater than' symbol above it (Figure 11.2). Contact points longer than lines '3' and '4' would therefore score 4d.

O – Overbite

In practice, very few patients are ever scored in the overbite section because if they do have a deep bite, they often have another occlusal feature which has already been picked up in the M, O, C or D sections above. It is, however, a simple section to score. If the overbite is complete with any evidence of gingival trauma, the grade is 4f. If the overbite is complete to the mucosa with no gingival trauma, the grade is 3f. If the overbite is complete, deeper than 3.5 mm but with no gingival contact, the grade is 2f. There is a line in the middle of the IOTN ruler (Figure 11.2) next to the symbol '2 O.B. >' which is 3.5 mm long to assist measurement of such overbites.

Open bites are also scored in this section using the same lines used in the 'D' section above using the same criteria. For example, if the worst open bite was longer than the 2 line and less than the 3 line, the grade would be 3. The possible grades awarded in this section are grade 2e, 3e, 4e (see Appendix 11.1).

NOT MANAGED TO AWARD AN IOTN GRADE?

Patients with well-aligned, untreated arches or with high-quality treatment results often do not score in any of the above sections. Before awarding an IOTN grade 1, the examiner should look critically at the buccal occlusion from both the lingual and buccal sides. Any deviation *whatsoever* from an absolutely perfect anatomical occlusion should be recorded at a grade 2g. In practice therefore, it is highly unlikely that one would ever see a patient with a grade 1 DHC score. Details of the more uncommon grades can be found in Appendix 11.1.

References

1. Summers CJ. The occlusal index: a system for identifying and scoring occlusal disorders. Am J Orthod 1971;59:552–67.
2. Little RM. The irregularity index: a quantitative score of mandibular anterior alignment. Am J Orthod 1975;68:554–63.
3. Mars M, Plint DA, Houston WJ, Bergland O, Semb G. The Goslon Yardstick: a new system

of assessing dental arch relationships in children with unilateral clefts of the lip and palate. Cleft Palate J 1987;24:314–22.

4. Schanschieff SG, Shovelton DS, Toulmin JK. Report of the Committee of Enquiry into Unnecessary Dental Treatment. London, HMSO, 1986.

5. Brook PH, Shaw WC. The development of an index of orthodontic treatment priority. Eur J Orthod 1989;11:309–20.

6. Richmond S, O'Brien K, Buchanan I, Burden D. An Introduction to Occlusal Indices. Victoria University of Manchester, Manchester, 1992.

Appendix 11.1 IOTN Categories: the Dental Health Component

Grade1	**No treatment required**	
	1	Extremely minor malocclusions, including contact point displacements less than 1 mm
Grade 2	**Little**	
	2a	Increased overjet >3.5 mm but ≤6 mm (with competent lips)
	2b	Reverse overjet greater than 0 mm but ≤1 mm
	2c	Anterior or posterior crossbite with ≤1 mm discrepancy between retruded contact position and intercuspal position
	2d	Contact point displacement of teeth >1 mm but should be as symbol in 3e 2 mm
	2e	Anterior or posterior open bite >1 mm but ≤2 mm
	2f	Increased overbite ≥3.5 mm (without gingival contact)
	2g	Prenormal or postnormal occlusions with no other anomalies. Includes up to half a unit discrepancy
Grade 3	**Borderline need**	
	3a	Increased overjet >3.5 mm but ≤6 mm (incompetent lips)
	3b	Reverse overjet greater than 1 mm but ≤3.5 mm
	3c	Anterior or posterior crossbites with >1 mm but ≤2 mm discrepancy between the retruded contact position and intercuspal position
	3d	Contact point displacement of teeth >2 mm but ≤4 mm
	3e	Lateral or anterior open bite >2 mm but ≤4 mm
	3f	Deep overbite complete onto gingival or palatal tissues but no trauma
Grade 4	**Treatment required**	
	4a	Increased overjet >6 mm but ≤9 mm
	4b	Reverse overjet >3.5 mm with no masticatory or speech difficulties
	4c	Anterior or posterior crossbites with >2 mm discrepancy between the retruded contact position and intercuspal position
	4d	Severe contact point displacements of teeth >4
	4e	Extreme lateral or anterior open bites >4 mm
	4f	Increased and complete overbite with gingival or palatal trauma

Appendix 11.1 *(Continued)*

	4h	Less extensive hypodontia requiring prerestorative orthodontics or orthodontic space closure to obviate the need for a prosthesis
	4l	Posterior lingual crossbite with no functional occlusal contact in one or more buccal segments
	4m	Reverse overjet >1 mm but <3.5 mm with recorded masticatory and speech difficulties
	4t	Partially erupted teeth, tipped and impacted against adjacent teeth
	4x	Presence of supernumerary teeth
Grade 5	**Treatment required**	
	5a	Increased overjet >9 mm
	5h	Extensive hypodontia with restorative implications (more than one tooth missing in any quadrant requiring pre-restorative orthodontics)
	5i	Impeded eruption of teeth (apart from third molars) due to crowding, displacement, the presence of supernumerary teeth, retained deciduous teeth, and any pathological cause
	5m	Reverse overjet >3.5 mm with reported masticatory and speech difficulties
	5p	Defects of cleft lip and palate and other craniofacial abnormalities
	5s	Submerged deciduous teeth

Uncommon IOTN Grades

Using the 'MOCDO' system, most IOTN grades will be identified. There are, however, a few grades which should be mentioned to ensure the examiner does not miss when awarding the IOTN grade.

5p – Defect of cleft lip and palate. In practice, virtually all cleft patients would however score 5i, 5h or 4h. The 5p grade is included to ensure all cleft patients are identified as high need for treatment.

5s – Submerged deciduous teeth. To award this grade, only two of the cusps of the deciduous tooth should be above the mucosa or the adjacent teeth should be severely tipped. In practice, such a situation would usually have been intercepted at an earlier stage so again this is an uncommon grade.

4l – Lingual crossbite with no occlusal contact. This is a full scissors bite, sometimes seen in severe Class II malocclusions. No tooth in a buccal segment should have any occlusal contact, so again it is rarely seen.

4x – Presence of supernumerary teeth.

4t – Partially erupted tooth tipped/ impacted against another. This is used when a tooth is clinically impacted but partially erupted, which means the 5i grade cannot be applied.

Principles of orthodontic treatment planning

Of all the skills that an orthodontist must develop, competent treatment planning is undoubtedly both the most difficult and the slowest to acquire. It not only requires that an individual develops a spatial awareness of how the teeth, jaws and face are to be reconfigured in three dimensions, but the effects of time, the fourth dimension, on both dentofacial growth and the planned treatment mechanics must be fully appreciated and understood as well. It is therefore imperative that the clinician is completely thorough in the examination of the patient and meticulous with record collection.

For example, to commence treatment without first defining precisely where the patient is starting from is fraught with risk. Chapter 4 has already described the importance of identifying whether a mandibular displacement from centric relation to centric occlusion exists, either as a result of a premature occlusal contact from an edge-to-edge incisor occlusion (Figure 12.1), a palatal upper lateral incisor (Figure 12.2), or a bilateral cusp-to-cusp crossbite (Figure 12.3). Missing such a possibility would otherwise lead to some serious miscalculations about how much space would be

required to correct the malocclusion, as well as whether posterior anchorage would need to be reinforced or not.

Therefore, the key to success is to follow a methodical approach in the following areas:

- Patient concerns
- Patient motivation
- Medical history
- General dental health
- Growth estimation
- Problem list
- Treatment aims
- Treatment options
- Informed consent.

PATIENT CONCERNS

The most important question to have answered satisfactorily when planning a course of treatment is what the patient is truly concerned about. This then ensures that their concern will be completely addressed in whatever treatment options are offered later. However, when examining young patients this can prove to be

Orthodontics: Principles and Practice, First Edition. Edited by Daljit S. Gill, Farhad B. Naini.
© 2011 Daljit S. Gill, Farhad B. Naini and Dental Update. Published 2011 by Blackwell Publishing Ltd.

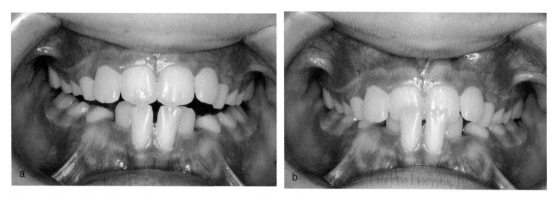

Figure 12.1 (a) Edge-to-edge incisors in centric relation. (b) Reverse overjet in centric occlusion.

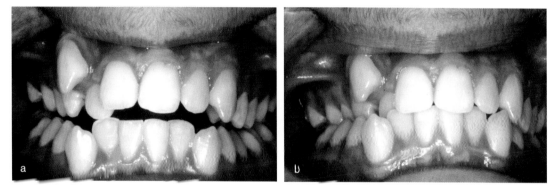

Figure 12.2 (a) Edge-to-edge occlusion on the palatal lateral incisor in centric relation. (b) Lateral incisor anterior crossbite in centric occlusion.

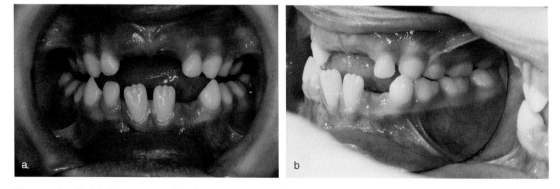

Figure 12.3 (a) Cusp-to-cusp deciduous canine occlusion in centric relation. (b) Left unilateral crossbite in centric occlusion.

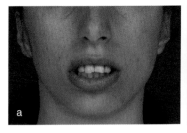 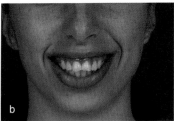 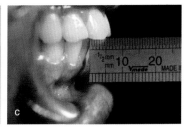

Figure 12.4 (a) Excessive incisor show at rest. (b) Gummy smile during animation. (c) 5 mm overjet.

difficult as they will often use contemporary colloquialisms, such as having 'goofy' teeth to describe a problem with incisor protrusion, or more ambiguously as having 'wonky' teeth to describe either their dental crowding, rotational irregularity or even spacing.

Older patients may use more descriptive terminology, but with a different perception of the meaning of the word from the one the clinician has. For example, they may describe their incisor protrusion as having an 'overbite'. Conversely, they may use a term which accurately reflects their concern but which the clinician misinterprets. Figure 12.4 illustrates such a case, where the patient primarily complained of upper incisor prominence, which the clinician misconstrued to mean as the mild 5 mm incisor protrusion. Instead, her concern was related to the excessive vertical incisor show beneath her upper lip, and had her treatment plan not included some measures to correct her vertical maxillary excess she would have finished treatment still dissatisfied.

Lastly, when examining minors, after their concerns have been identified it is as important to ascertain whether their accompanying parent has the same, additional or different areas of concern, since these should also be taken into account when planning the young child's treatment.

PATIENT MOTIVATION

The next most important key in treatment planning is to ascertain the level of patient motiva-

tion for change because invariably it will correlate with the level of their potential treatment compliance. One way to achieve this is to ask the patient to score out of 10 how distressed they feel about each of their concerns, where a score of 10 is maximal and a score of 0 is none. Alternatively, a more sophisticated way of ascertaining this could be to apply the Aesthetic Component of the Index of Orthodontic Treatment Need, as described in Chapter 11. In either case, a lower score of self-concern will probably relate to an individual who is either unlikely to comply with, or unwilling to consent to a complex, prolonged course of treatment.

However, occasionally, a patient may persistently focus on either a real or imaginary cause of concern to which their level of dissatisfaction appears to exceed what would be considered to be either socially or clinically justifiable. In such circumstances, the rare possibility that the patient may have a body dysmorphic disorder (BDD) should be considered, and the expertise of a clinical psychologist should be sought.[1]

MEDICAL HISTORY

The vast majority of young patients who present for treatment are fit and healthy. However, certain medical conditions can affect the provision and outcome of treatment, and as such should be borne in mind. For example, patients with a type IV delayed hypersensitivity reaction to either nickel or rubber chemicals will require special orthodontic management, and even more so for patients with type I immediate natural rubber latex allergies.[2,3]

Under the 2008 National Institute for Health and Clinical Excellence, UK, guidelines, patients at risk of developing infective endocarditis no longer require pre-procedure antibiotic prophylaxis, but the stringent importance of maintaining an excellent level of oral hygiene around the teeth being orthodontically corrected is paramount, in order to minimise the occurrence of any bacteraemia.[4]

In terms of physical access for treatment, patients with spinal abnormalities such as scoliosis may find it difficult to lie supine in a dental chair to receive prolonged episodes of fixed appliance adjustments,[5] while patients with cerebral palsy may not have adequate coordination or manual dexterity[6] (e.g. be unable to comply with wearing a headgear, attaching intraoral elastics, or to maintain a satisfactory level of oral hygiene around a fixed appliance). Equally, patients with epilepsy should not be supplied with acrylic removable orthodontic appliances for fear that they might fracture during a grand mal seizure, with the subsequent risk that the fragments could either cause an upper aero-digestive injury or be completely swallowed or inhaled.[7]

Many older patients with a history of polypharmacy are now beginning to present for orthodontic treatment and they may require special consideration. For example, postmenopausal women with osteoporosis may be taking bisphosphonates which will affect the orthodontic movement of teeth through the suppression of osteoclastic activity in normal bone physiology.[8]

GENERAL DENTAL HEALTH

It is essential that a good standard of oral health exists before the provision of any advanced dental treatment. The risk of undertaking complex orthodontic treatment in an individual

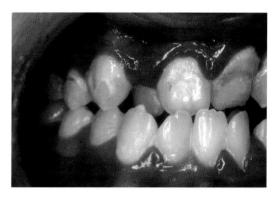

Figure 12.5 Enamel decalcifications (abandoned fixed appliance treatment).

who has poor oral hygiene is that there is a greater risk of inducing either enamel decalcifications or caries around the fixed appliance brackets (Figure 12.5). Indeed, insufficient pre-treatment improvement in the calibre of oral hygiene after appropriate education in a capable individual can often provide a reliable indicator of the overall importance they place on their teeth. Clearly, an individual with a low value of dental worth is unlikely to commit to completing a course of complex treatment.

GROWTH ESTIMATION

Treatment success using many orthodontic approaches such as myofunctional and orthopaedic appliances is dependent on facial growth, and therefore this needs to be assessed when planning treatment. Indeed, timing the start of routine orthodontic treatment to coincide with the maximal pubertal growth spurt is advantageous, and this can be achieved either by plotting standing height measurements on to a gender-specific growth chart (Figure 12.6), or by examining the patient's lateral cephalogram for a change in the morphology of the second and third cervical vertebrae, specifically for the caudal surfaces to progress from being flat to becoming concave[9] (Figure 12.7).

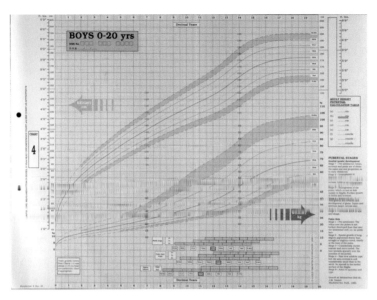

Figure 12.6 Growth Foundation standing height chart for males. © Child Growth Foundation, reproduced with permission.

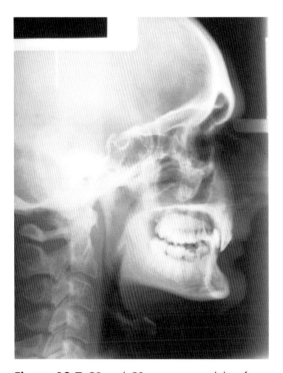

Figure 12.7 C2 and C3 concave caudal surfaces on a lateral cephalogram.

PROBLEM LIST

Constructing a list of problems that need attention helps the clinician consider how best to resolve the patient's malocclusion. As with the sequence followed in the initial examination of the patient, this should list in turn any problematic features of relevance regarding:

* The soft tissues of the face and mouth
* The skeleton of the jaws, in any of the three dimensional planes (coronal, sagittal and transverse)
* The status of the teeth, as well as their alignment, occlusion and position.

Soft tissues

The presence of an obtuse naso-labial angle, and a pronounced labio-mental fold in a patient with incisor protrusion could contraindicate upper incisor retraction, for fear that this might result in an aesthetically displeasing concave lower facial third profile (Figure 12.8).

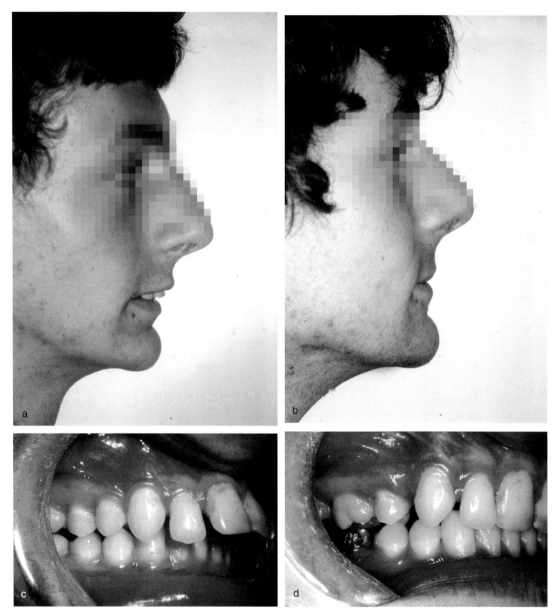

Figure 12.8 (a) Pretreatment profile view of obtuse naso-labial angle, and pronounced labio-mental fold in a patient with Angle's Class II malocclusion. (b) Post-treatment concave lower face profile. (c) Pretreatment incisor protrusion. (d) Incisor retroclination following treatment with an upper removable appliance.

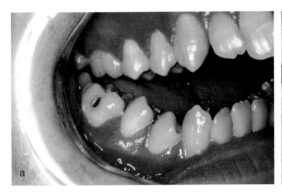
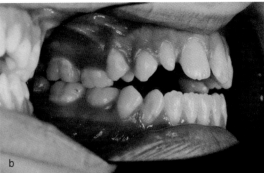

Figure 12.9 (a) Severe anterior open bite of skeletal origin. (b) Modest anterior open bite of local origin.

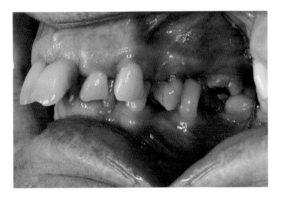

Figure 12.10 Overeruption of unopposed maxillary and mandibular premolars.

Skeleton

Equally, an anterior open bite of skeletal origin would require a different treatment approach to one that arose from a localised dentoalveolar distortion through a digit sucking habit (Figure 12.9).

Teeth

Similarly, a previously extracted tooth might result in a dysfunctional occlusion as a consequence of the overeruption of the antagonist tooth (Figure 12.10).

TREATMENT AIMS

The aims of orthodontic treatment are usually crystallised from those features in the problem list which have been identified as requiring correction, and they should:

- Address the patient's concerns
- Establish and maintain an ideal, functionally stable occlusion and an improved dentofacial appearance
- Prioritise and determine the sequence of any planned stages of correction.

For example, implementing treatment to first arrest the trauma associated with an increased overbite in an Angle's Class II division 2 malocclusion (Figure 12.11), to organising the surgical exposure of impacted upper canines in an Angle's Class II division 1 case, before a functional appliance with acrylic covering the palate is made to correct the increased overjet (Figure 12.12).

TREATMENT OPTIONS

Once the treatment aims have been established, the next stage is to prepare a number of treatment options that will deal with perhaps only some, most or all of the objectives. This usually results in a selection of potential treatments of ascending complexity that can then be presented for consideration. The principle being that clinical practice has moved away from a benign paternalistic approach where the clinician decides what treatment should best be provided, to a patient-centred approach which allows the patient to choose instead (Figure 12.13).

To facilitate the creation of each treatment option, the following need to be considered, of which two are discussed here with the remainder being covered in more detail elsewhere in the book:

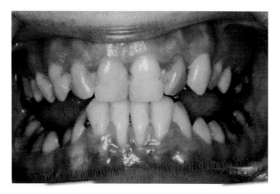

Figure 12.11 Lower incisor labiogingival trauma related to the deep overbite.

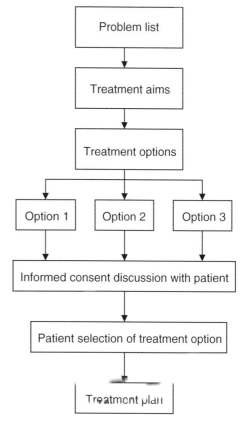

Figure 12.13 Algorithm for devising a treatment plan.

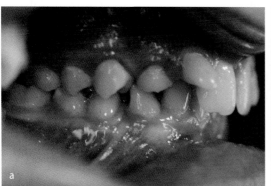

Figure 12.12 (a) Incisor protrusion and retained deciduous canines. (b) Surgically exposed impacted upper canines.

- Treatment timing
- Space analysis
- Severity of the malocclusion
- Anchorage
- Retention.

Treatment timing

While randomised controlled trials have proved that early treatment in the mixed dentition stage confers no advantage to the final orthodontic outcome, nevertheless, in selected circumstances it still may be beneficial, even though it imposes on the patient a more prolonged course of overall treatment.[11] For example, the early correction of a Class II incisor relationship can reduce both the incidence of subsequent dental trauma (Figure 12.14), and/or psychosocial ridicule the child may otherwise remain exposed to[11] (Figure 12.15).

Severity of the malocclusion

For the correction of Angle's Class I malocclusions on a skeletal Class I base, treatment planning is undertaken for the lower arch first, where in general, the anteroposterior position of the lower labial segment and the transverse intercanine and intermolar widths are preserved. This is because the lower arch is considered to develop in a zone of neutral pressure, where the muscle forces of the lips and cheeks labio-buccally are counterbalanced by those generated from the tongue lingually. The concept is that consciously moving the lower teeth out of this zone will subject them to subsequent relapse.[12] Although research has shown that maintaining these lower arch dimensions as sacrosanct does not always confer postretention stability, in the absence of any other reliable predictors, it is still considered clinically prudent so to do.[13,14]

Once a decision has been made as to whether the lower arch can be corrected with an orthodontic

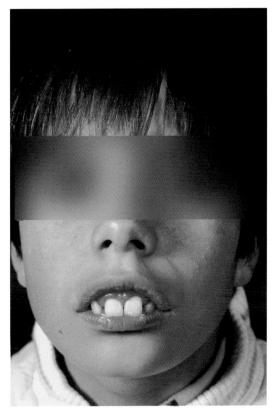

Figure 12.15 Grossly incompetent lips and protruding upper incisors.

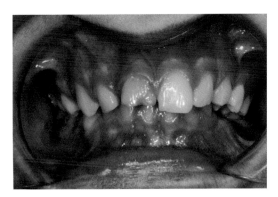

Figure 12.14 Traumatised protrusive upper central incisor.

any dental extractions, then the upper arch mechanics to achieve a Class I canine and incisor relationship can be planned accordingly. In contrast, for the correction of Angle's Class II or Class III malocclusions which arise as a consequence of an underlying skeletal base discrepancy, three treatment approaches may be considered:

• Growth modification
• Orthodontic camouflage
• Combined orthodontic and orthognathic surgery

These are covered later in sections 3 and 4 of the book.

INFORMED CONSENT

For patients to have autonomy in whatever treatment they consent to undergo, they must be provided with sufficient information that will allow them to make an informed choice. In this regard, during an informed consent discussion a clinician must therefore explain;

• What each treatment option will involve
• What each will or will not deliver
• Outline the risks and benefits associated with each of the choices
• The potential consequences of not undergoing treatment.

After all of the above explanations have been given, for the clinician to be certain the patient has the capacity to give valid consent, the patient's ability to understand and retain the information must be evident together with their ability to use and weigh it in the decision-making process.[15] Once these conditions have been satisfied, and the patient has made their selection, the option they have chosen then becomes the definitive treatment plan to be followed (Figure 12.13).

References

1. Hepburn S, Cunningham S. Body dysmorphic disorder in adult orthodontic patients. *Am J Orthod Dentofacial Orthop* 2006;130: 569–74.
2. Hain MA, Longman LP, Field EA, Harrison JE. Natural rubber latex allergy: implications for the orthodontist. *J Orthod* 2007;34:6–11.
3. Noble J, Ahing SI, Karaiskos NE, Wiltshire WA. Nickel allergy and orthodontics, a review and report of two cases. *Br Dent J* 2008;204:297–300.
4. National Institute for Health and Clinical Excellence. Prophylaxis Against Infective Endocarditis: Antimicrobial Prophylaxis Against Infective Endocarditis in Adults and Children Undergoing Interventional Procedures. NICE Clinical Guideline 64, London, 2008.
5. Dougall A, Fiske J. Access to special care dentistry – part 1. Access. *Br Dent J* 2008;204:605–16.
6. Lewis D, Fiske J, Dougall A. Access to special care dentistry, part 8. Special care dentistry services: seamless care for people in their middle years – part 2. *Br Dent J* 2008;205:359–71.
7. Dougall A, Fiske J. Access to special care dentistry – part 5. Safety. *Br Dent J* 2008;205: 177–90.
8. Rinchuse DJ, Rinchuse DJ, Sosovicka MF, Robinson JM, Pendleton R. Orthodontic treatment of patients using bisphosphonates: a report of 2 cases. *Am J Orthod Dentofacial Orthop* 2007;131:321–6.
9. Baccetti T, Franchi L, McNamara JA. An improved version of the cervical vertebral maturation (CVM) method for the assessment of mandibular growth. *Angle Orthod* 2002;72:316–23.
10. O'Brien K. Is early treatment for Class II malocclusion effective? Results from a randomised controlled trial. *Am J Orthod Dentofacial Orthop* 2006;(4 Suppl):S64–5.

11. O'Brien K, Wright J, Conboy F, Chadwick S, Connolly I, Cook P. Effectiveness of early orthodontic treatment with the twin-block appliance: a multicenter, randomized, controlled trial. Part 2: Psychosocial effects. *Am J Orthod Dentofacial Orthop* 2003;124: 488–94.

12. Mills JRE. The stability of the lower labial segment. *Dent Pract* 1967;18:293–306.

13. Little RM. Stability and relapse of dental arch alignment. *Br J Orthod* 1990;17: 235–41.

14. Houston WJ, Edler R. Long-term stability of the lower labial segment relative to the A-Pog line. *Eur J Orthod* 1990;12:302–10.

15. Department of Health. Reference Guide to Consent for Examination or Treatment. Department of Health, London, 2001.

Orthodontically related root resorption

INTRODUCTION

Orthodontic treatment can be associated with a number of iatrogenic changes including decalcification, periodontal problems and root resorption. Orthodontically induced inflammatory root resorption (OIIRR) is a common unavoidable adverse effect of treatment which is the focus of this chapter. It is a pathological process that results in a loss of substance from mineralised cementum and dentine[1,2] (Figure 13.1) due to the removal of hyalinised tissue during orthodontic tooth movement.[3,4] Fortunately, a reparative process in the periodontium commences when the applied orthodontic force is discontinued or reduced below a certain level.[5,6] This healing process can occur as early as the first week of retention following orthodontic treatment and increases over time.[7-9] There are biological and mechanical factors that influence the severity of OIIRR. Mechanical causative factors can be controlled by the clinician to minimise the adverse effect of OIIRR and allow initiation of repair.

INCIDENCE, DISTRIBUTION AND SEVERITY OF OIIRR

OIIRR occurs in almost all orthodontically treated individuals. However, significant root resorption following orthodontic treatment is a rare event. Lupi et al.[10] radiographically investigated a sample of 88 ethnically diverse adults and showed that 15% of the teeth had resorption prior to orthodontic treatment. After 12 months of orthodontic treatment, the incidence of OIIRR increased to 73%. Two percent showed moderate to severe root resorption before treatment and 24.5% showed the same degree of severity after orthodontic treatment. More recently, Smale et al.[11] showed that 24% of the teeth had root shortening, but only 3.6% had shortening of more than 2 mm.

Generally, the distribution of root resorption is dictated by the pressure zone created by different types of tooth movement. Therefore, for tipping movement, it is usually found in the marginal and apical parts of the tooth.[12] OIIRR

Orthodontics: Principles and Practice, First Edition. Edited by Daljit S. Gill, Farhad B. Naini.
© 2011 Daljit S. Gill, Farhad B. Naini and Dental Update. Published 2011 by Blackwell Publishing Ltd.

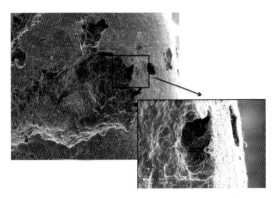

Figure 13.1 Scanning Electron Microscopy of a root resorption crater.

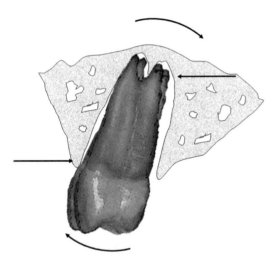

Figure 13.2 Majority of orthodontic movements are not translatory but tipping in nature, therefore, root resorption occurs at the apical part of the tooth root.

tends to occur preferentially in the apical region because (Figure 13.2):

- Orthodontic tooth movement is not entirely translatory and the fulcrum is usually occlusal to the apical half of the root[13]
- The orientation of the periodontal fibres in the apical end is different which increases the stress in the region[14]
- More friable acellular cementum covers the apical third of the root, which can be easily

injured in the case of trauma and concomitant vascular stasis.[13–15]

There are three levels of OIIRR severity:[16]

1. Cemental or surface resorption with remodelling
2. Dentinal resorption with repair
3. Circumferential apical root resorption.

Significant resorption of the root apex results in root shortening with no evidence of regeneration. However, with time, the sharp edges formed by resorption craters may be levelled. Surface reparation only occurs in the cemental layer.

RADIOGRAPHIC DIAGNOSIS OF OIIRR

Radiographs have been widely used to clinically diagnose OIIRR. The dental panoramic tomograph (DPT) provides an overall view of the dentition with a lower radiation dose than a full-mouth series of intraoral radiographs.[17] However, due to the narrowness of the focal trough, the apices and palatal structures can be out of focus in the incisor region. Therefore, additional radiographs such as periapical radiographs or occlusographs may be needed to supplement the DPT. Sameshima and Asgarifar[18] compared periapical radiographs with DPTs and found the amount of root resorption was exaggerated by 20% or more on a DPT. The paralleling technique for periapical radiography is preferable as it provides a geometrically accurate image, and, together with the use of a film holder and aiming device, radiographs can be standardised at two different time points. The two-dimensional nature of radiography limits its accuracy because buccal and lingual root defects are not detectable.[19] With the advance of technology, cone-beam computed tomography will be more readily used in future root resorption studies. It will provide a more accurate three-dimensional image with a lower dosage of radiation, which can be used for qualitative and quantitative assessment.

PATHOGENESIS OF OIIRR

Orthodontic tooth movement is associated with local over-compression of the periodontal ligament (PDL), which results in hyalinisation. Resorption of the cementum occurs simultaneously with the removal of hyalinised tissue.[5,20–22] Resorption starts at the periphery of the hyalinised periodontal membrane and is followed by resorption of surrounding root and bone surfaces[4,23] and invasion of blood vessels.[24] The resorption process propagates until no hyalinised tissue is present and/or the force level diminishes. The resorption crater expands the root surfaces involved and thereby indirectly decreases the pressure exerted through force application. Decompression alters the process to reverse and cementum reparative process begins. It has also been documented that OIIRR initiated 10–20 days after force onset[12,21,25] continued even during extended retention periods of up to 1 year.[7,8,26] The resorbing areas on a root surface may show signs of concurrent active resorption and repair.[7,12]

The cellular process of OIIRR involves three sequences of events in the periphery and main hyalinised zones.[4,24] First, tartrate resistant acid phosphatase (TRAP)-negative mono-nucleated fibroblast-like cells initiate root resorption from the periphery of the main hyalinised zone by the nearest viable cells in the presence of adequate vascularity. Second, TRAP-positive multinucleated cells participate in the removal of main hyalinised tissue and resorption of the adjacent root structure. This phase commences only after a considerable amount of hyalinised tissue between alveolar bone and the root surface has been eliminated and continues even after the initial root resorption has terminated. The cells involved during this resorptive phase are derived from adjacent marrow spaces.

Lastly, active root resorption continues to occur in areas of hyalinised tissue even after orthodontic force has ceased to be applied. Reparative processes start from the periphery of the resorption craters and extend to the central part.

PHYSICAL PROPERTIES OF OIIRR CEMENTUM

Cementum at the cervical and middle thirds of the root has greater hardness and elastic modulus than that of the apical third[27,28] (Figure 13.3). This is because of the variable mineral content of cellular and acellular cementum.[29] Chutimanutskul et al.[29] showed the hardness and elastic modulus of cementum were affected by the application of orthodontic forces whereby the mean hardness and elastic modulus of cementum was greater in the light force group than the heavy force group. The mean hardness and elastic modulus of cementum also gradually decreased from the cervical to apical regions.[27,28]

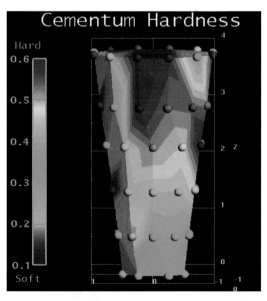

Figure 13.3 Cementum hardness distribution along the tooth root.

Rex et al.[30] studied the mineral composition (calcium [Ca], phosphorus [P] and fluoride [F]) of human premolar cementum following the application of orthodontic forces. The results showed limited change in the mineral composition of cementum after the application of light force. There was a trend towards an increase in the Ca and P concentration of cementum at various areas of PDL compression. The application of heavy force caused a significant decrease in the Ca concentration of cementum at certain areas of PDL tension. Orthodontic force did not appear to influence the F concentrations in cementum.

FACTORS INFLUENCING THE DEGREE OF OIIRR

OIIRR can be influenced by a wide range of shared biological and or mechanical factors. Biological factors are directly related to the individual and can be genetic or environmental. Mechanical factors are attributed to the nature of the orthodontic appliance and could be controlled by both the clinician and the patient.

Biological Factors

Root resorption can occur in individuals without orthodontic treatment and is related to one's tissue response and metabolic activity. The metabolic signals (e.g. hormones, body type and metabolic rate) influence the relationship between osteoblastic and osteoclastic activity which modifies cell metabolism, an individual's reaction pattern to disease, trauma and ageing.[5] Root resorption can vary among individuals and within the same person at different times.

Genetic Factors

Genetic influence on the susceptibility to root resorption remains controversial. Previously, a sib-pair model was used to investigate the genetic influence on root resorption and reported 70% heritability for resorption of maxillary incisor roots and the mesial and distal roots of the mandibular first molars. This accounted for approximately half of the total phenotypic variation.[31] This meant that siblings experienced similar levels of OIIRR. A further study also revealed a familial association of OIIRR.[32]

One of the difficulties in assessing the genetic contribution to OIIRR is the ability to separate genetic factors from environmental factors such as orthodontic treatment.[33] Ngan et al.[33] investigated the genetic contribution to OIIRR by retrospectively assessing the pre- and post-treatment records of 16 monozygotic and 10 dizygotic twins. Each twin pair had the same malocclusion and the same type of appliance treatment with the same clinician. Panoramic radiograph tooth root measurements were used to obtain quantitative and qualitative estimates of concordance for OIIRR. The concordance estimate for root resorption in monozygotic twins was 44.9% for qualitative measurements and 49.2% for quantitative measurements. The concordance estimate for root resorption in dizygotic twins was 24.7% for qualitative measurements and 28.3% for quantitative measurements. The authors thus confirmed the presence of a genetic component to OIIRR. However, they advised that a larger sample was required before a model of heritability could be used to determine the components contributing to the variance.[33]

Ethnicity can also influence the susceptibility to OIIRR. Sameshima and Sinclair[34] have found that Caucasians and Hispanics are more prone to OIIRR than people from the Far East.

Environmental Factors

- *Asthma and allergy.* An increased incidence of OIIRR, especially blunting of maxillary molars, has been found in patients with chronic asthma.[35,36] This could be attributed to the close proximity of the roots to the inflamed maxillary sinus and/or the presence of inflammatory mediators in these patients. Allergy may increase the risk of OIIRR.[36,37] Nishioka et al.[38] investigated the association between excessive root resorption and immune system factors in a sample of Japanese orthodontic patients. The result showed that the incidence of allergy, asthma and root morphology abnormality was significantly higher in the root resorption group. Corticosteroids are commonly used to treat allergy, asthma, dermatitis and eczema. They have been shown to interfere with orthodontic tooth movement rate and tissue reaction in animal studies.[39-42] Research of the effects of corticosteroids on orthodontic induced root resorption remains controversial. This could be due to different dosages of corticosteroids used and also different animal models studied. Verna et al.[43] investigated the effect of acute and chronic corticosteroid treatment on OIIRR. The results showed more root resorption at the mesial coronal level in the acute treatment group than in the chronic treatment and control groups. The less resorption found in the chronic group may have been due to faster remodelling of bone, less hyalinisation and less remodelling of root tissue.

- *Endocrine and hormone imbalance.* Imbalance of the endocrine system due to hypothyroidism, hypopituitarism, hyperpituitarism, hyperparathyroidism,[44] Paget's disease[45] and hypophospataemia[46] is hypothesised to be related to OIIRR.[44,47,48] Goldie and King[49] reported an association with a decrease in OIIRR and secondary hyperparathyroidism. An excess of thyroid hormones, which increases bone turnover, have been found to reduce root resorption during orthodontic tooth displacement in a rat model.[50] In contrast, hypothyroidism has been associated with increased root resorption in the absence of orthodontic load.[51] Calcitonin can inhibit odontoclast activity.[52] The action of calcito-

nin on osteoclasts occurs at later stages of osteoclast development and it inhibits the fusion of pre-osteoclasts to form mature multinucleated cells.

- *Nutrition.* Root resorption has been demonstrated in animals deprived of dietary calcium and vitamin D.[44,48] Engstrom et al.[44] found the experimental rat group that was fed with a diet deficient in calcium and vitamin D had hypocalcaemia, increased alkaline phosphatase activity and increased circulating parathyroid hormone when compared with the control group, which was fed with a normal diet. Orthodontic tooth movement produced greater and more rapid bone resorption and more severe OIIRR in the experimental group. The study also showed an increased number of osteoclasts in the PDL of the test group, which was suggested to be due to the increased parathyroid hormone levels.

- *Drugs.* Inhibition of cyclo-oxygenase and the subsequent production of prostaglandins by non-steroidal anti-inflammatory drugs (NSAIDs) can be useful in decreasing bone and root resorption. Villa et al.[53] investigated the effect of nabumetone, a type of NSAID, on root resorption during intrusive orthodontic tooth movement and discovered less root resorption when patients received nabumetone, and the drug did not impede tooth movement. This was supported by Kameyama et al.,[54] in whose study the rats were prescribed aspirin and which led to a suppression of root resorption caused by mechanical injury. Bisphosphonates are potent inhibitors of bone resorption that are widely used to treat osteoporosis. Bisphosphonates directly or indirectly induce apoptosis in osteoclasts, which plays a role in the inhibition of bone resorption.[55] The effects on orthodontic tooth movement includes slower tooth movement and less root resorption due to decreased number of osteoclasts.[56] Clodronate has also been shown to inhibit the production or release of pro-inflammatory molecules in macrophages and or osteoblastic cells.[57–61]

Age

The ageing process results in changes to the hard and soft tissues of the dentoalveolus. The PDL becomes less vascular, aplastic and narrow with age. The bone becomes more dense, avascular and aplastic and the thickness of cementum increases." Mirabella and Artun[62] evaluated a large sample of adult patients for investigating the prevalence and severity of OIIRR in maxillary anterior teeth. Forty percent of the adults had one or more teeth with ≥2.5mm resorption. This indicated that the sample of adults had a higher mean value of severely resorbed teeth per patient than the comparable group of adolescents which was 16.5%.[63] On the other hand, Harris and Baker[64] reported that 61% of adult patients had some degree of root resorption after orthodontic treatment, which was not significantly different from the 58% of adolescent patients experiencing root resorption in that same study.

Partially formed roots have been found to develop normally during orthodontic treatment and it has been suggested that teeth with open apices may be more resistant to OIIRR.[63,65–67] Linge and Linge[63] found less resorption in patients treated before the age of 11. They suggested that resorption could be avoided if tooth movement was completed before the roots were fully developed, before the age of 11.5 years, but treatment at this age may not be suitable for many patients.

Habits

A number of habits have been reported to result in an increased risk of OIIRR. Finger sucking beyond the age of 7 years has been suggested to be a risk factor.[63] Nail biting,[68] forward tongue pressure and tongue thrust[63,69] have also been proposed to be linked to OIIRR. Long-term orthopaedic tongue thrusting forces that result in anterior open bite may promote root resorption,[70] particularly when vertical elastics are used in an attempt to close open bites associated with tongue problems.

History of Trauma

Orthodontic tooth movement of a severely traumatised tooth may result in increased resorption.[63,67,71–73] Linge and Linge[67] found that teeth which had previously experienced trauma had an average loss of root structure after orthodontic movement of 1.07mm compared with a loss of 0.64mm in untraumatised teeth. However, Kjaer[74] proposed that teeth with slight or moderate injuries may not have any greater tendency towards OIIRR than uninjured teeth. Malmgren[72] suggested a waiting period of 1 year after a traumatic incident before the initiation of orthodontic tooth movement.

Cortical and Alveolar Bone

It has been suggested that OIIRR is amplified in dense alveolar bone compared with less dense alveolar bone, especially if there is an increased number of resorptive cells associated with the increased number of marrow spaces.[6,22] Reitan[22] proposed that a strong continuous force on low density alveolar bone caused an equivalent amount of OIIRR to that of a mild continuous force on high density alveolar bone.

Kaley and Phillips[75] identified the risk of root resorption was 20 times greater when upper incisors were in close proximity to cortical plate. On the contrary, Otis et al.[76] found that the amount of alveolar bone present around the root, the thickness of cortical bone, the density of trabecular network and fractal measurements on the bony trabeculae had no significant correlation with the amount of root resorption.

Verna et al.[77] investigated the impact of bone turnover rate on the amount of tooth movement and the incidence of OIIRR in rats. High bone turnover increased the amount of tooth movement compared with the normal or low bone turnover state. The untreated side in the low bone turnover group showed more root resorption suggesting that in clinical situations where turnover of alveolar bone was delayed, root surfaces could already be affected by root resorption at baseline condition.

Type of Malocclusion

A number of studies have found a relationship between OIIRR and malocclusion.[31,34,63,70] Severe malocclusion requires greater tooth movement, for example, greater overjet requires greater retraction and deeper overbite needs greater intrusion,[31,78] with hence greater amounts of root resorption.

Kaley and Phillips[75] reported that Class III patients showed severe root resorption with the root apex approximating the palatal cortical plate. They suggested that tipping forward of maxillary incisors to compensate for the Class III jaw relationship forces the roots against the palatal cortical plate during orthodontic treatment.

Harris and Butler[70] demonstrated that open bite patients experienced significantly greater degrees of root resorption. It was believed that the orthopaedic forces of tongue thrusting generated the same physiological responses as mechanotherapy intended to torque or intrude a tooth. This study also suggested that:

- The greater the overjet, the greater the in-treatment root loss
- The greater the skeletal discrepancy, the greater the resorption
- The more the maxillary plane was tipped up anteriorly, the greater the resorption
- The steeper was Down's occlusal plane, the greater was the observed degrees of incisor root shortening.

Hypofunctional Periodontium

A hypofunctional periodontium results in a narrowed periodontal space and derangement of functional fibres, which eliminates the normal cushioning effect of the PDL,[79] thus resulting in a high concentration of force. This leads to stimulation of inflammation by the promotion of inflammatory mediators secreted from local cells to induce destruction of tooth and bone.[80] Sringkarnboriboon et al.[81] found that the amount of root resorption was significantly greater in teeth with a hypofunctional periodontium than in those with a normal periodontium, which suggested that orthodontic movement of non-occluding teeth should be performed with caution.

Specific Tooth Vulnerability to Root Resorption

The teeth most frequently affected by OIIRR according to severity are the maxillary lateral incisors, maxillary central incisors, mandibular incisors, the distal root of mandibular first molars, mandibular second premolars and maxillary second premolars.[34,82–84] Maxillary lateral incisors are more susceptible to root resorption if they have abnormal root shape.[34] Paetyangkul et al.[85] showed in a micro-CT study that the maxillary premolars were more susceptible to orthodontic root resorption than mandibular premolars when these teeth were subjected to buccally directed force for 12 weeks.

Dental Invagination

Dental invagination is the most prevalent dental anomaly in orthodontic patients.[86] Maxillary lateral incisors are most often affected followed by maxillary central incisors. It has been claimed that dental invagination was one of the predisposing factors for OIIRR.[74,86] However, there is no general agreement concerning the role of dental invagination as a risk factor for orthodontic root resorption.[87] Mavragani et al.[88] investigated the association between dental invagination and root shortening during orthodontic treatment and found invaginated teeth often displayed deviated root form, which was considered a risk factor for OIIRR. However, invaginated teeth had delayed development and immature roots which seemed to protect against root resorption.[89] The authors concluded that the mild form of dental invagination confined within the crown and not extended beyond the level of the cementoenamel junction was not a risk factor for OIIRR.

Abnormal Root Morphology

The tendency of OIIRR was found to be greater in teeth with aberrant shaped roots.[34,74,90-92] Sameshima and Sinclair,[34] in a comparative study using radiographs taken before and after orthodontic treatment, reported that tooth with abnormal root morphology, for example, pipette-shaped, pointed, dilacerated and slender roots, frequently showed OIIRR when compared with teeth with a normal root shape.

Oyama et al.[93] investigated in a variety of root shapes the stress distribution at the root apex during orthodontic force application, using finite element method. They discovered that during orthodontic force application, short, bent and pipette root shapes resulted in a greater loading of the root than normal root shapes, which suggested root deviations tended to promote root resorption.

Root Resorption Prior to Orthodontic Treatment

Patients with pre-existing evidence of root resorption have been found to be at greater risk of developing further severe OIIRR with treatment.[70,94]

Previous Endodontic Treatment

Conflicting reports remain in the literature regarding the susceptibility of non-vital endodontically treated teeth to OIIRR. One group has found a greater incidence of OIIRR in endodontically treated teeth.[95] The increase in root resorption in the study appeared to be biased as the non-vital teeth were treated endodontically as a result of trauma.[95] Spurrier et al.[96] found vital incisors resorbed to a significantly greater degree than endodontically treated incisors. Many other authors believe that endodontically treated teeth are more resistant to root resorption due to an increase in dentine hardness and density.[6,92,96,97]

The disagreement among these studies may be due to the presence or absence of active inflammation related to residual infection during the orthodontic movement. Orthodontic tooth movement itself creates an inflammatory response that may increase an already existing resorptive process. A successful endodontically treated tooth with healthy periodontal support, in the absence of inflammation, should not be more susceptible to resorption than a normal tooth.

Mechanical Factors

Orthodontic tooth movement and biomechanics have been found to account for approximately a tenth to a third of the total variation in OIIRR.[15,98] One study showed up to 90% of variation has been attributed to the extent of tooth movement.[99]

Duration of Treatment

Most studies agree that the severity of OIIRR is directly related to the duration of orthodontic treatment.[78,82,91,100-105] Paetyangkul et al.[106] compared the quantitation amount of root resorption with micro-CT (Figure 13.4) following 4, 8 and 12 weeks of orthodontic forces and discovered substantially more resorption with longer duration of force (Figure 13.5).

Smale et al.[11] radiographically assessed the amount of apical root resorption on average 6 months post initiation of fixed orthodontic appliance therapy. The results showed that root resorption began in the early levelling stages of orthodontic treatment. About 4.1% of patients studied had an average resorption of ≥1.5 mm of the maxillary incisors and about 15.5% had one or more maxillary incisors with resorption of ≥2.0 mm from 3 to 9 months after initiation of fixed appliance therapy.

In a randomised clinical trial, Brin et al.[83] compared the amount of OIIRR in Class II malocclusions treated with one phase versus two phases of treatment. The results showed that 11% of central incisors and 14% of lateral incisors demonstrated moderate to severe, i.e. 2 mm, external apical root resorption (EARR). The proportion of incisors with moderate to severe EARR was slightly greater in the one phase treatment group.

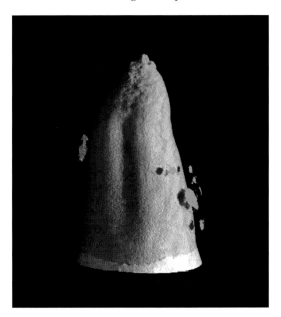

Figure 13.4 Micro-CT image of tooth root subjected to 12 weeks of orthodontic force. The green zones are the resorption craters extracted from the tooth image.

Distance of Tooth Movement

As previously discussed, teeth that are moved large distances have extended exposure to the resorptive process. Therefore, the severity of OIIRR may be regarded to be positively related to the distance of tooth movement.[104,107–110]

Magnitude of Applied Force

Many animal studies[111–113] and human studies[25,114–117] have agreed that the force magnitude is directly proportional to the severity of OIIRR. Heavy force induces excessive

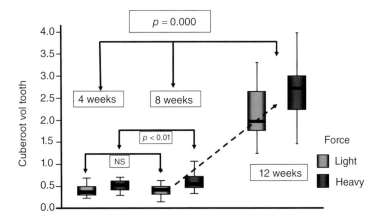

Figure 13.5 Box-plot comparing the amount of root resorption between 4, 8 and 12 weeks of force application.

hyalinisation and interferes with the repair process of resorption craters.[5,12,22,25,112,118] Studies on human upper first premolars involved 25 g and 225 g of buccal force in a scanning electronic microscopy (SEM) study and 25 g and 225 g intrusive force in a micro-CT study found an increased amount of OIIRR with an increased force level[119,120] (Figures 13.6, 13.7).

Different Appliances and Treatment Techniques

Numerous studies have compared the extent of root resorption following treatment with differ-ent types of orthodontic appliances. Parker and Harris[99] compared the EARR among cases treated with the Tweed standard edgewise technique, Begg light-wire technique and Roth-prescription straight-wire technique and found no difference between them. In contrast, McNab et al.[121] found more EARR in patients treated with Begg appliances than edgewise appliance. The excessive lingualisation of the maxillary incisor root by the torquing forces applied at the end of stage III of Begg technique may explain the higher incidence of EARR in this group.

Blake et al.[122] compared radiographically the amount of apical root resorption after orthodontic treatment with edgewise and self-ligating Speed appliances. The Speed system provides a continuous rotatory and torque action through its spring-clip mechanism in contrast with the edgewise appliance, which may provide an interrupted force. There was no statistically significant difference in root resorption between the two appliance systems. On the contrary, a recent radiographic study found that the Speed appliance caused more root resorption when compared with the Tip-Edge and MBT straight-wire techniques.[123]

Barbagallo et al.[124] compared the extent of root resorption between conventional orthodontic appliance and clear plastic aligners and

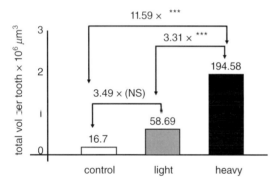

Figure 13.6 Bar chart comparing the amount of root resorption between heavy and light buccally directed orthodontic force.

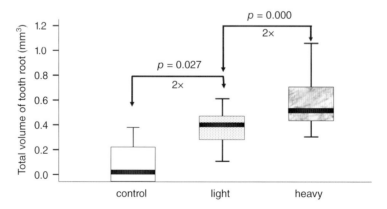

Figure 13.7 Box-plot comparing the amount of root resorption between heavy and light intrusive orthodontic force.

discovered that teeth that are subjected to light orthodontic force of 25g displayed similar amount of root resorption as those induced by the clear plastic aligners.

Direction of Force

The type and direction of tooth movement have a considerable role in OIIRR. It is expected that intrusion and torque have a higher force per unit area and thus cause more tissue necrosis and OIIRR.[6] Some authors have suggested there is less root resorption associated with bodily movement compared with tipping due to the different stress distribution.[6,125] Han et al.[126] compared the amount of root resorption in the same individual after application of continuous intrusive and extrusive forces using SEM. The study showed intrusion of teeth caused about four times more root resorption than extrusion. Weekes and Wong[127] observed root resorption at the interproximal region of the cervical third part of the root after extrusion indicating orthodontic extrusion was not without risk.

Neitzert et al.[128] comparatively evaluated the amount of root resorption following the application of buccal root torque (15°), distal root tip (15°) and axial rotation (using 225g) for 4 weeks and concluded that 225g of rotating force causes more root resorption than 15° buccal root torquing force, 15° tipping force causes greater amounts of root resorption than 15° torquing force, and 225g of rotating force causes similar amounts of root resorption as 15° tipping force (Figure 13.8).

Intermittent Versus Continuous Force Application

There are conflicting reports as to whether continuous or discontinuous force produces a difference in the amount of OIIRR. A pause in tooth movement allows the resorbed cementum to heal, which may produce less root

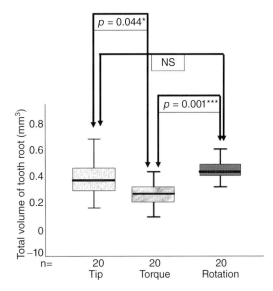

Figure 13.8 Box-plot comparing the amount of root resorption between tipping, torquing and rotational orthodontic force.

resorption.[125,129-133] There were a number of studies with varying durations and frequencies of interruption in the applied forces, which have led to varied results.

Reitan[6,134,135] advocated the use of intermittent forces to prevent the development of root resorption by allowing reparative processes to occur during periods with little or no force. Levander et al.[130] radiographically evaluated the effect of a treatment pause of 2–3 months, on teeth in which EARR was discovered after an initial treatment period of 6 months with fixed appliances. The amount of root resorption was significantly less in patients treated with a pause than in those treated without interruption. The intermission of the forces facilitated reorganisation of damaged periodontal tissue and reduced root shortening. Maltha and Dijkman[131] compared the amount of root resorption after continuous (24 hours per day) and discontinuous (16 hours per day) force application and reported more resorption in dogs when using continuous than intermittent forces. Ballard et al.[136] have also quantified the volume of root resorption crater following intermittent orthodontic forces to be significantly lower than continuous orthodontic forces.

Extraction Versus Non-extraction Treatment Protocols

There are studies which have discussed the amount of OIIRR associated with extraction treatments.[103,104,121] The approach of categorising an extraction or non-extraction plan as being associated with OIIRR is overly simplistic. Attention should be drawn to the distance the teeth are moved. Extractions for severe crowding do not have as much impact on movement of the maxillary incisors as the displacement following extractions for overjet reduction.

ORTHODONTIC RELAPSE AND OIIRR

Following active appliance removal, there is a conversion of the former pressure side of the active treatment period into the tension side during the relapse period.[137] Langford[8] showed that relapse forces were capable of causing significant root resorption for up to three months after RME.

REPAIR OF OIIRR

Repair of root resorption craters begins when the applied orthodontic force is discontinued or reduced below a certain level.[5,6] According to Schwarz,[138] when the orthodontic force reduces below the optimal force of 20–26 g/cm², root resorption stops. Many studies have demonstrated that the resorptive defects are repaired by deposition of new cementum and re-establishment of new PDL.[7,8,22,139–141]

Henry and Weinmann[14] defined two types of repair: anatomical repair was characterised by

the restoration of the root surface to its original contour; and a functional repair occurred when the exposed dentin has been covered by a thin layer of repair cementum, resulting in a deficient root outline. In both types, the PDL was restored to its original width.

The amount of root resorption repair increases with time.[7–9,142] Owman-Moll and Kurol[143] demonstrated more reparative cementum in the resorption cavities after 6 and 7 weeks of retention when compared with 2 and 3 weeks of retention. The reparative process increased during the first 4 weeks of retention and after 5–6 weeks, the process slowed down and reached a steady phase.[9] The reparative process seemed to continue for a long period of time.

Owman-Moll et al.[9] documented the amount of root resorption cavities repaired at different retention periods following 6 weeks of light buccally directed orthodontic force of 50 cN. After the first week of retention, 28% of the resorption craters showed some degree of repair. The repair rose to 75% after 8 weeks of retention. Partial repair was recorded more often (17–31%) than functional or anatomical repair during the first four weeks of retention. After 5–8 weeks of passive retention, functional repair dominated the repair process (33–40%). Resorptive areas with anatomical repair were registered six times more often after 8 weeks of retention (12%) than they were after the first week of retention (2%). In a later study, Owman-Moll and Kurol[143] found 38%, 44% and 82% of resorption craters repaired after 2, 3 and 6–7 seven weeks of retention, respectively.

A recent micro-CT study has shown that root resorption continues for another 4 weeks after orthodontic force has ceased.[144] The reparative processes seems to be different for different levels of force application. In the study, reparative process reached a steady rate after 4 weeks of passive retention following the application of 4 weeks of light force whereas the majority of the reparative process occurred after 4 weeks of passive retention following the application of 4 weeks of heavy orthodontic force.

CLINICAL CONSEQUENCES OF OIIRR

A long-term radiographic evaluation of root resorption after active orthodontic therapy revealed progressive remodelling of the root surface.[97] The jagged resorbed edges were smoothed and sharply pointed root ends were round with time. However, the original root contours and lengths were never re-established. Severely resorbed teeth can still function in a reasonable manner with the worst outcome of hypermobility being a rare event.[97] Vlaskalic et al.[105] reviewed six articles published between the years 1914 and 1997 that discussed cases of OIIRR which caused a problem to the patient and the clinician. There were no reports found with tooth loss from severe apical root resorption after orthodontic treatment unless there was some other form of trauma to the tooth.

A reduction in root length due to apical resorption has been described as less detrimental than an equivalent loss of periodontal attachment at the alveolar crest especially in cases with ≤3 mm of early root resorption.[10] Kalkwarf et al.[145] showed a nearly linear relationship between root length and percentage of periodontal attachment. Results indicated that 4 mm of root resorption translates into 20% of total attachment loss and 3 mm apical root loss equals only 1 mm crestal bone loss. After the initial 2 mm apical root loss, calculations revealed every additional 2 mm root loss equalled to only 1 mm of crestal bone loss. Therefore, patients who are susceptible to marginal periodontal breakdown may have a higher risk of losing severely resorbed teeth prematurely. This emphasises the importance of periodontal disease control in patients with severely resorbed teeth. In addition, teeth with abnormally short roots and loss of periodontal attachment may not be suitable as future bridge abutments.

PREVENTION AND MANAGEMENT OF OIIRR

Clinically, a number of approaches have been suggested in the literature to minimise OIIRR. These include decreased treatment duration,[12,91] the use of light intermittent forces,[5,12,22,25] avoidance of sustained jiggling intermaxillary elastics,[63] limited tooth movement for OIIRR-prone teeth, e.g. intrusion and torque,[99] habit control[68] and a thorough assessment of familial tendency and medical history.[34,69,103,146]

It was strongly suggested that periapical radiographs should be taken at least every year to determine the presence of root resorption.[147] The original treatment goals must be reassessed depending on the extent of root resorption detected. The results may have to be compromised depending on the amount of root resorption, or at least the force levels should be modified or a two to three month pause in treatment with passive arch wires should be implemented.[130] Additional radiographs should be taken every 3 months in at-risk patients to monitor the progress of root resorption.[90,147] It may be advisable to take final radiographs prior to the removal of fixed appliances.[19] In the case of teeth with severe OIIRR, follow-up radiographs have been recommended until additional root loss is no longer detected.[148]

Numerous animal studies have been conducted to investigate the possibility of reducing the risk of OIIRR by applying drugs that modulate the activity of osteoblasts, osteoclasts and odontoclasts. Arginine-glycine-aspartic acid-containing peptides inhibit the resorptive activity of isolated clast cells by targeting the integrin receptor expressed by odontoclasts and have shown to be effective in reducing root resorption during tooth movement.[149] Low-dose systemic administration of doxycycline in rats may have an inhibitory effect on OIIRR via reduction of odontoclasts, osteoclasts, mononuclear cells and TRAP-positive cells on the root.[150] Low doses of thyroid hormone have also been shown to play a protective role on the root surface against OIIRR.[151] In addition, steroid-treated rats have displayed significantly less root resorption on the compression side and fewer TRAP-positive cells within the PDL space on the same side.[42] However, many of these drugs also altered the activity of osteoblasts and osteoclasts in alveolar bone, which may interfere with the rate of tooth movement.

Recent research has focused on identifying biological markers in the gingival crevicular fluid in the light of relating these markers and the risk of OIIRR.[152,153] If successful, this technique could be easily implemented in identifying patients at risk of OIIRR prior to orthodontic treatment and treatment planning could be modified accordingly.

References

1. Cohen S, Burns RC. Pathways of the Pulp, 7th edn. Mosby, St. Louis, 1998.

2. Brudvik P, Rygh P. Non-clast cells start orthodontic root resorption in the periphery of hyalinized zones. Eur J Orthod 1993;15(6):467–80.

3. Brudvik P, Rygh P. Root resorption after local injection of prostaglandin E2 during experimental tooth movement. Eur J Orthod 1991;13(4):255–63.

4. Brudvik P, Rygh P. Root resorption beneath the main hyalinized zone. Eur J Orthod 1994;16(4):249–63.

5. Rygh P. Orthodontic root resorption studied by electron microscopy. Angle Orthod 1977;47(1):1–16.

6. Reitan K. Biomechanical principles and reactions. In: Graber TM, Swain BF (eds) Orthodontics. Current Principles and Techniques. Mosby, St. Louis, 1985: 101–92.

7. Barber AF, Sims MR. Rapid maxillary expansion and external root resorption in man: a scanning electron microscope study. Am J Orthod 1981;79(6):630–52.

8. Langford SR, Sims MR. Root surface resorption, repair, and periodontal attachment following rapid maxillary expansion in man. Am J Orthod 1982;81(2):108–15.

9. Owman Moll P, Kurol J, Lundgren D. Repair of orthodontically induced root resorption in adolescents. Angle Orthod 1995;65(6):403–8.

10. Lupi JE, Handelman CS, Sadowsky C. Prevalence and severity of apical root resorption and alveolar bone loss in orthodontically treated adults. Am J Orthod Dentofacial Orthop 1996;109(1):28–37.

11. Smale I, Artun J, Behbehani F, Doppel D, van't Hof M, Kuijpers-Jagtman AM. Apical root resorption 6 months after initiation of fixed orthodontic appliance therapy. Am J Orthod Dentofacial Orthop 2005;128(1): 57–67.

12. Stenvik A, Mjor IA. Pulp and dentine reactions to experimental tooth intrusion. A histologic study of the initial changes. Am J Orthod 1970;57(4):370–85.

13. Harris EF, Boggan BW, Wheeler DA. Apical root resorption in patients treated with comprehensive orthodontics. J Tenn Dent Assoc 2001;81(1):30–3.

14. Henry JL, Weinmann JP. The pattern of resorption and repair of human cementum. J Am Dent Assoc 1951;42(3):270–90.

15. Baumrind S, Korn EL, Boyd RL. Apical root resorption in orthodontically treated adults. Am J Orthod Dentofacial Orthop 1996;110(3):311–20.

16. Brezniak N, Wasserstein A. Orthodontically induced inflammatory root resorption. Part I: The basic science aspects. Angle Orthod 2002;72(2):175–9.

17. Leach HA, Ireland AJ, Whaites EJ. Radiographic diagnosis of root resorption in relation to orthodontics. Br Dent J 2001;190(1):16–22.

18. Sameshima GT, Asgarifar KO. Assessment of root resorption and root shape: periapi-

cal vs panoramic films. Angle Orthod 2001;71(3):185–9.

19. Brezniak N, Wasserstein A. Orthodontically induced inflammatory root resorption. Part II: The clinical aspects. Angle Orthod 2002;72(2):180–4.

20. Stuteville OE. Injuries to the teeth and supporting structures caused by various orthodontic appliances and methods fo preventing these injuries. J Am Dent Assoc 1938;24:1494–507.

21. Kvam E. Scanning electron microscopy of human premolars following experimental tooth movement. Trans Eur Orthod Soc 1972:381–91.

22. Reitan K. Initial tissue behavior during apical root resorption. Angle Orthod 1974;44(1):68–82.

23. Brudvik P, Rygh P. Multi-nucleated cells remove the main hyalinized tissue and start resorption of adjacent root surfaces. Eur J Orthod 1994;16(4):265–73.

24. Brudvik P, Rygh P. The initial phase of orthodontic root resorption incident to local compression of the periodontal ligament. Eur J Orthod 1993;15(4): 249–63.

25. Harry MR, Sims MR. Root resorption in bicuspid intrusion. A scanning electron microscope study. Angle Orthod 1982;52(3):235–58.

26. Timms DJ, Moss JP. A histological investigation into the effects of rapid maxillary expansion on the teeth and their supporting tissues. Trans Eur Orthod Soc 1971: 263–71.

27. Malek S, Darendeliler MA, Swain MV. Physical properties of root cementum: Part I. A new method for 3-dimensional evaluation. Am J Orthod Dentofacial Orthop 2001;120(2):198–208.

28. Poolthong S. Determination of the Mechanical Properties of Enamel, Dentine and Cementum by an Ultra Micro-Indentation System. University of Sydney, Sydney, 1998.

29. Chutimanutskul W, Ali Darendeliler M, Shen G, Petocz P, Swain M. Changes in the physical properties of human premolar cementum after application of 4 weeks of controlled orthodontic forces. Eur J Orthod 2006;28(4):313–18.

30. Rex T, Kharbanda OP, Petocz P, Darendeliler MA. Physical properties of root cementum: part 6. A comparative quantitative analysis of the mineral composition of human premolar cementum after the application of orthodontic forces. Am J Orthod Dentofacial Orthop 2006;129(3): 358–67.

31. Harris EF, Kineret SE, Tolley EA. A heritable component for external apical root resorption in patients treated orthodontically. Am J Orthod Dentofacial Orthop 1997;111(3):301–9.

32. Bednar JR, Wise RJ. A practical clinical approach to the treatment and management of patients experiencing root resorption during and after orthodontic therapy. In: Davidovitch Z, Mah J (eds) Biological Mechanisms of Tooth Eruption, Resorption and Replacement by Implants. Harvard Society for the Advancement of Orthodontics, Boston, MA, 1998:425–37.

33. Ngan DC, Kharbanda OP, Byloff FK, Darendeliler MA. The genetic contribution to orthodontic root resorption: a retrospective twin study. Aust Orthod J 2004;20(1):1–9.

34. Sameshima GT, Sinclair PM. Predicting and preventing root resorption: Part I. Diagnostic factors. Am J Orthod Dentofacial Orthop 2001;119(5):505–10.

35. McNab S, Battistutta D, Taverne A, Symons AL. External apical root resorption of posterior teeth in asthmatics after orthodontic treatment. Am J Orthod Dentofacial Orthop 1999;116(5):545–51.

36. Davidovitch Z. The etiology of root resorption. In: McNamara JA, Trotman CA (eds) Orthodontic Treatment: Management of Unfavorable Sequelae. Monograph No 31,

Craniofacial Growth Series. Centre for Human Growth and Development, University of Michigan, Ann Arbor, MI, 1995:93–117.

37. Davidovitch Z. Etiologic factors in force-induced root resorption. In: Davidovitch Z, Norton LA (eds) Biological Mechanisms of Tooth Movement and Craniofacial Adaptation. Harvard Society for the Advancement of Orthodontics, Boston, MA, 1996:349–55.

38. Nishioka M, Ioi H, Nakata S, Nakasima A, Counts A. Root resorption and immune system factors in the Japanese. Angle Orthod 2006;76(1):103–8.

39. Yamane A, Fukui T, Chiba M. In vitro measurement of orthodontic tooth movement in rats given beta-aminopropionitrile or hydrocortisone using a time-lapse videotape recorder. Eur J Orthod 1997;19(1):21–8.

40. Kalia S, Melsen B, Verna C. Tissue reaction to orthodontic tooth movement in acute and chronic corticosteroid treatment. Orthod Craniofac Res 2004;7(1):26–34.

41. Ashcraft MB, Southard KA, Tolley EA. The effect of corticosteroid-induced osteoporosis on orthodontic tooth movement. Am J Orthod Dentofacial Orthop 1992;102(4):310–19.

42. Ong CK, Walsh LJ, Harbrow D, Taverne AA, Symons AL. Orthodontic tooth movement in the prednisolone-treated rat. Angle Orthod 2000;70(2):118–25.

43. Verna C, Hartig LE, Kalia S, Melsen B. Influence of steroid drugs on orthodontically induced root resorption. Orthod Craniofac Res 2006;9(1):57–62.

44. Engstrom C, Granstrom G, Thilander B. Effect of orthodontic force on periodontal tissue metabolism. A histologic and biochemical study in normal and hypocalcemic young rats. Am J Orthod Dentofacial Orthop 1988;93(6):486–95.

45. Smith NHH. Monostotic Paget's disease of the mandible, presenting with progressive resorption of the teeth. Oral Surg Oral Med Oral Pathol 1978;46:246–53.

46. Tangney NJ. Hypophosphotasia: a case report and literature review. J Irish Med Assoc 1979;72:530–1.

47. Goultschin J, Nitzan D, Azaz B. Root resorption. Review and discussion. Oral Surg Oral Med Oral Pathol 1982;54(5):586–90.

48. Becks H. Root resorptions and their relation to pathological bone formation. Part 1. statistical data and roentgenographic aspects. Int J Orthodont Oral Surg 1936;22:445–82.

49. Goldie RS, King GJ. Root resorption and tooth movement in orthodontically treated, calcium-deficient, and lactating rats. Am J Orthod 1984;85(5):424–30.

50. Melsen F, Mosekilde L. Morphometric and dynamic studies of bone changes in hyperthyroidism. Acta Pathol Microbiol Scand (A) 1977;85A(2):141–50.

51. Becks H, Cowden R. Root resorptions and their relationship to pathologic bone formation. Part II. Am J Orthod Oral Surg 1942;28:513–26.

52. Wiebkin OW, Cardaci SC, Heithersay GS, Pierce AM. Therapeutic delivery of calcitonin to inhibit external inflammatory root resorption. I. Diffusion kinetics of calcitonin through the dental root. Endod Dent Traumatol 1996;12(6):265–71.

53. Villa PA, Oberti G, Moncada CA, et al. Pulp dentine complex changes and root resorption during intrusive orthodontic tooth movement in patients prescribed nabumetone. J Endod 2005;31(1):61–6.

54. Kameyama Y, Nakane S, Maeda H, Fujita K, Takesue M, Sato E. Inhibitory effect of aspirin on root resorption induced by mechanical injury of the soft periodontal tissues in rats. J Periodontal Res 1994;29(2):113–17.

55. Reszka AA, Halasy-Nagy JM, Masarachia PJ, Rodan GA. Bisphosphonates act directly on the osteoclast to induce caspase

cleavage of mst1 kinase during apoptosis. A link between inhibition of the mevalonate pathway and regulation of an apoptosis-promoting kinase. J Biol Chem 1999;274(49): 34967–73.

56. Liu L, Igarashi K, Haruyama N, Saeki S, Shinoda H, Mitani H. Effects of local administration of clodronate on orthodontic tooth movement and root resorption in rats. Eur J Orthod 2004;26(5):469–73.

57. Felix R, Bettex JD, Fleisch H. Effect of diphosphonates on the synthesis of prostaglandins in cultured calvaria cells. Calcif Tissue Int 1981;33(5):549–52.

58. Pennanen N, Lapinjoki S, Urtti A, Monkkonen J. Effect of liposomal and free bisphosphonates on the IL-1 beta, IL-6 and TNF alpha secretion from RAW 264 cells in vitro. Pharm Res 1995;12(6):916–22.

59. Makkonen N, Salminen A, Rogers MJ, et al. Contrasting effects of alendronate and clodronate on RAW 264 macrophages: the role of a bisphosphonate metabolite. Eur J Pharm Sci 1999;8(2):109–18.

60. Monkkonen J, Pennanen N, Lapinjoki S, Urtti A. Clodronate (dichloromethylene bisphosphonate) inhibits LPS-stimulated IL-6 and TNF production by RAW 264 cells. Life Sci 1994;54(14):PL229–34.

61. Igarashi K, Hirafuji M, Adachi H, Shinoda H, Mitani H. Effects of bisphosphonates on alkaline phosphatase activity, mineralization, and prostaglandin E2 synthesis in the clonal osteoblast-like cell line MC3T3-E1. Prostaglandins Leukot Essent Fatty Acids 1997;56(2):121–5.

62. Mirabella AD, Artun J. Prevalence and severity of apical root resorption of maxillary anterior teeth in adult orthodontic patients. Eur J Orthod 1995;17(2): 93–9.

63. Linge L, Linge BO. Patient characteristics and treatment variables associated with apical root resorption during orthodontic treatment. Am J Orthod Dentofacial Orthop 1991;99(1):35–43.

64. Harris EF, Baker WC. Loss of root length and crestal bone height before and during treatment in adolescent and adult orthodontic patients. Am J Orthod Dentofacial Orthop 1990;98(5):463–9.

65. Rosenberg HN. An evaluation of the incidence and amount of apical root resorption and dilaceration occurring in orthodontically treated teeth having incompletely formed roots at the beginning of Begg treatment. Am J Orthod 1972; 61:524–25.

66. Rudolph CE. An evaluation of root resorption occuring during orthodontic treatment. J Dent Res 1940;19:367.

67. Linge BO, Linge L. Apical root resorption in upper anterior teeth. Eur J Orthod 1983; 5(3):173–83.

68. Odenrick L, Brattstrom V. Nailbiting: frequency and association with root resorption during orthodontic treatment. Br J Orthod 1985;12(2):78–81.

69. Newman WG. Possible etiologic factors in external root resorption. Am J Orthod 1975;67(5):522–39.

70. Harris EF, Butler ML. Patterns of incisor root resorption before and after orthodontic correction in cases with anterior open bites. Am J Orthod Dentofacial Orthop 1992;101(2):112–19.

71. Andreasen JO. External root resorption: its implication in dental traumatology, paedodontics, periodontics, orthodontics and endodontics. Int Endod J 1985;18(2): 109–18.

72. Malmgren O, Goldson L, Hill C, Orwin A, Petrini L, Lundberg M. Root resorption after orthodontic treatment of traumatized teeth. Am J Orthod 1982;82(6): 487–91.

73. Hines FB Jr. A radiographic evaluation of the response of previously avulsed teeth and partially avulsed teeth to orthodontic movement. Am J Orthod 1979;75(1):1–19.

74. Kjaer I. Morphological characteristics of dentitions developing excessive root

resorption during orthodontic treatment. Eur J Orthod 1995;17(1):25–34.

75. Kaley J, Phillips C. Factors related to root resorption in edgewise practice. Angle Orthod 1991;61(2):125–32.

76. Otis LL, Hong JS, Tuncay OC. Bone structure effect on root resorption. Orthod Craniofac Res 2004;7(3):165–77.

77. Verna C, Dalstra M, Melsen B. Bone turnover rate in rats does not influence root resorption induced by orthodontic treatment. Eur J Orthod 2003;25(4):359–63.

78. Beck BW, Harris EF. Apical root resorption in orthodontically treated subjects: analysis of edgewise and light wire mechanics. Am J Orthod Dentofacial Orthop 1994; 105(4):350–61.

79. Selliseth NJ, Selvig KA. The vasculature of the periodontal ligament: a scanning electron microscopic study using corrosion casts in the rat. J Periodontol 1994;65(11): 1079–87.

80. Cooper SM, Sims MR. Evidence of acute inflammation in the periodontal ligament subsequent to orthodontic tooth movement in rats. Aust Orthod J 1989;11(2):107–9.

81. Sringkarnboriboon S, Matsumoto Y, Soma K. Root resorption related to hypofunctional periodontium in experimental tooth movement. J Dent Res 2003;82(6): 486–90.

82. Brezniak N, Wasserstein A. Root resorption after orthodontic treatment: Part 2. Literature review. Am J Orthod Dentofacial Orthop 1993;103(2):138–46.

83. Brin I, Tulloch JF, Koroluk L, Philips C. External apical root resorption in Class II malocclusion: a retrospective review of 1- versus 2-phase treatment. Am J Orthod Dentofacial Orthop 2003;124(2):151–6.

84. Alexander SA. Levels of root resorption associated with continuous arch and sectional arch mechanics. Am J Orthod Dentofacial Orthop 1996;110(3):321–4.

85. Paetyangkul A, Turk T, Elekdag-Turk S, Jones AS, Petocz P, Darendeliler MA. Physical properties of root cementum: part 14. The amount of root resorption after force application for 12 weeks on maxillary and mandibular premolars: a microcomputed-tomography study. Am J Orthod Dentofacial Orthop 2009;136(4):492 e1–9; discussion 92–3.

86. Thongudomporn U, Freer TJ. Anomalous dental morphology and root resorption during orthodontic treatment: a pilot study. Aust Orthod J 1998;15(3):162–7.

87. Lee RY, Artun J, Alonzo TA. Are dental anomalies risk factors for apical root resorption in orthodontic patients? Am J Orthod Dentofacial Orthop 1999;116(2):187–95.

88. Mavragani M, Apisariyakul J, Brudvik P, Selvig KA. Is mild dental invagination a risk factor for apical root resorption in orthodontic patients? Eur J Orthod 2006; 28(4):307–12.

89. Mavragani M, Boe OE, Wisth PJ, Selvig KA. Changes in root length during orthodontic treatment: advantages for immature teeth. Eur J Orthod 2002;24(1):91–7.

90. Levander E, Bajka R, Malmgren O. Early radiographic diagnosis of apical root resorption during orthodontic treatment: a study of maxillary incisors. Eur J Orthod 1998;20(1):57–63.

91. Levander E, Malmgren O. Evaluation of the risk of root resorption during orthodontic treatment: a study of upper incisors. Eur J Orthod 1988;10(1):30–8.

92. Mirabella AD, Artun J. Risk factors for apical root resorption of maxillary anterior teeth in adult orthodontic patients. Am J Orthod Dentofacial Orthop 1995; 108(1):48–55.

93. Oyama K, Motoyoshi M, Hirabayashi M, Hosoi K, Shimizu N. Effects of root morphology on stress distribution at the root apex. Eur J Orthod 2007;29:113–17.

94. Massler M, Malone AJ. Root resorption in human permanent teeth; a roentgenographic study. Am J Orthod 1954;40: 619–33.

95. Wickwire NA, Mc Neil MH, Norton LA, Duell RC. The effects of tooth movement upon endodontically treated teeth. Angle Orthod 1974;44(3):235–42.

96. Spurrier SW, Hall SH, Joondeph DR, Shapiro PA, Riedel RA. A comparison of apical root resorption during orthodontic treatment in endodontically treated and vital teeth. Am J Orthod Dentofacial Orthop 1990;97(2):130–4.

97. Remington DN, Joondeph DR, Artun J, Riedel RA, Chapko MK. Long-term evaluation of root resorption occurring during orthodontic treatment. Am J Orthod Dentofacial Orthop 1989;96(1):43–6.

98. Horiuchi A, Hotokezaka H, Kobayashi K. Correlation between cortical plate proximity and apical root resorption. Am J Orthod Dentofacial Orthop 1998;114(3):311–18.

99. Parker RJ, Harris EF. Directions of orthodontic tooth movements associated with external apical root resorption of the maxillary central incisor. Am J Orthod Dentofacial Orthop 1998;114(6): 677–83.

100. Taner T, Ciger S, Sencift Y. Evaluation of apical root resorption following extraction therapy in subjects with Class I and Class II malocclusions. Eur J Orthod 1999;21(5): 491–6.

101. Brezniak N, Wasserstein A. Root resorption after orthodontic treatment: Part 1. Literature review. Am J Orthod Dentofacial Orthop 1993;103(1):62–6.

102. Goldin B. Labial root torque: effect on the maxilla and incisor root apex. Am J Orthod Dentofacial Orthop 1989;95(3):208–19.

103. McFadden WM, Engstrom C, Engstrom H, Anholm JM. A study of the relationship between incisor intrusion and root shortening. Am J Orthod Dentofacial Orthop 1989;96(5):390–6.

104. Sameshima GT, Sinclair PM. Predicting and preventing root resorption: Part II. Treatment factors. Am J Orthod Dentofacial Orthop 2001;119(5):511–15.

105. Vlaskalic V, Boyd RL, Baumrind S. Etiology and sequelae of root resorption. Semin Orthod 1998;4(2):124–31.

106. Paetyangkul A, Turk T, Elekdag-Turk S, et al. Comparison of the amount of root resorption and the characteristics of resorption craters after the application of light and heavy continuous and controlled orthodontic forces during 4 versus 8 versus 12 weeks. University of Sydney, Sydney, 2009.

107. Hollender L, Ronnerman A, Thilander B. Root resorption, marginal bone support and clinical crown length in orthodontically treated patients. Eur J Orthod 1980;2(4):197–205.

108. Sharpe W, Reed B, Subtelny JD, Polson A. Orthodontic relapse, apical root resorption, and crestal alveolar bone levels. Am J Orthod Dentofacial Orthop 1987;91(3): 252–8.

109. VonderAhe G. Postretention status of maxillary incisors with root-end resorption. Angle Orthod 1973;43(3):247–55.

110. Dermaut LR, De Munck A. Apical root resorption of upper incisors caused by intrusive tooth movement: a radiographic study. Am J Orthod Dentofacial Orthop 1986;90(4):321–6.

111. Dellinger EL. A histologic and cephalometric investigation of premolar intrusion in the Macaca speciosa monkey. Am J Orthod 1967;53(5):325–55.

112. King GJ, Fischlschweiger W. The effect of force magnitude on extractable bone resorptive activity and cemental cratering in orthodontic tooth movement. J Dent Res 1982;61(6):775–9.

113. Vardimon AD, Graber TM, Voss LR, Lenke J. Determinants controlling iatrogenic external root resorption and repair during and after palatal expansion. Angle Orthod 1991;61(2):113–22; discussion 23–4.

114. Casa MA, Faltin RM, Faltin K, Sander FG, Arana-Chavez VE. Root resorptions in

upper first premolars after application of continuous torque moment. Intra-individual study. J Orofac Orthop 2001; 62(4):285–95.

115. Darendeliler MA, Kharbanda OP, Chan EK, et al. Root resorption and its association with alterations in physical properties, mineral contents and resorption craters in human premolars following application of light and heavy controlled orthodontic forces. Orthod Craniofac Res 2004;7(2):79–97.

116. Faltin RM, Arana-Chavez VE, Faltin K, Sander FG, Wichelhaus A. Root resorptions in upper first premolars after application of continuous intrusive forces. Intra-individual study. J Orofac Orthop 1998;59(4):208–19.

117. Faltin RM, Faltin K, Sander FG, Arana-Chavez VE. Ultrastructure of cementum and periodontal ligament after continuous intrusion in humans: a transmission electron microscopy study. Eur J Orthod 2001;23(1):35–49.

118. Bondevik O. Tissue changes in the rat molar periodontium following application of intrusive forces. Eur J Orthod 1980;2(1):41–9.

119. Chan EK, Darendeliler MA, Petocz P, Jones AS. A new method for volumetric measurement of orthodontically induced root resorption craters. Eur J Oral Sci 2004; 112(2):134–9.

120. Harris DA, Jones AS, Darendeliler MA. Physical properties of root cementum: part 8. Volumetric analysis of root resorption craters after application of controlled intrusive light and heavy orthodontic forces: a microcomputed tomography scan study. Am J Orthod Dentofacial Orthop 2006;130(5):639–47.

121. McNab S, Battistutta D, Taverne A, Symons AL. External apical root resorption following orthodontic treatment. Angle Orthod 2000;70(3):227–32.

122. Blake M, Woodside DG, Pharoah MJ. A radiographic comparison of apical root resorption after orthodontic treatment with the edgewise and Speed appliances. Am J Orthod Dentofacial Orthop 1995;108(1):76–84.

123. Armstrong D, Kharbanda OP, Petocz P, Darendeliler MA. Root resorption after orthodontic treatment. Aust Orthod J 2006;22(2):153–60.

124. Barbagallo LJ, Jones AS, Petocz P, Darendeliler MA. Physical properties of root cementum: Part 10. Comparison of the effects of invisible removable thermoplastic appliances with light and heavy orthodontic forces on premolar cementum. A microcomputed-tomography study. Am J Orthod Dentofacial Orthop 2008; 133(2):218–27.

125. Reitan K. Effects of force magnitude and direction of tooth movement on different alveolar bone types. Angle Orthod 1964;34:244–55.

126. Han G, Huang S, Von den Hoff JW, Zeng X, Kuijpers-Jagtman AM. Root resorption after orthodontic intrusion and extrusion: an intraindividual study. Angle Orthod 2005;75(6):912–18.

127. Weekes WT, Wong PD. Extrusion of root-filled incisors in beagles–a light microscope and scanning electron microscope investigation. Aust Dent J 1995;40(2): 115–20.

128. Neitzert SV, Turk T, Colak C, et al. Physical properties of root cementum: Part 20. A micro CT study of root resorption following orthodontic tip, torque and rotation. Am J Orthod Dentofacial Orthop (in press).

129. Acar A, Canyurek U, Kocaaga M, Erverdi N. Continuous vs. discontinuous force application and root resorption. Angle Orthod 1999;69(2):159–63; discussion 63–4.

130. Levander E, Malmgren O, Eliasson S. Evaluation of root resorption in relation to two orthodontic treatment regimes. A clinical experimental study. Eur J Orthod 1994;16(3):223–8.

131. Maltha JC, Dijkman GE. Discontinous forces cause less extensive root resoprtiion than continuous forces. Eur J Orthod 1996;20:420.

132. Oppenheim A. Human tissue response to orthodontic intervention of short and long duration. Am J Orthod Oral Surg 1942;28:263–301.

133. Weiland F. Constant versus dissipating forces in orthodontics: the effect on initial tooth movement and root resorption. Eur J Orthod 2003;25(4):335–42.

134. Reitan K. Some factors determining the evaluation of forces in orthodontics. Am J Orthod 1957;43:32–45.

135. Reitan K. Evaluation of orthodontic forces as related to histologic and mechanical factors. SSO Schweiz Monatsschr Zahnheilkd 1970;80(5):579–96.

136. Ballard D, Jones AS, Petocz P, Darendeliler MA. Physical properties of root cementum: Part 11. Comparison of the effects of continuous versus intermittent controlled orthodontic forces on the amount of root resorption using Micro CT scan. University of Sydney, Sydney, 2006.

137. Vardimon AD, Graber TM, Pitaru S. Repair process of external root resorption subsequent to palatal expansion treatment. Am J Orthod Dentofacial Orthop 1993; 103(2):120–30.

138. Schwartz AM. Tissue changes incidental to tooth movement. Int J Orthod 1932;18:331–52.

139. Listgarten MA. Electron microscopic study of the junction between surgically denuded root surfaces and regenerated periodontal tissues. J Periodontal Res 1972;7(1):68–90.

140. Andreasen JO. Cementum repair after apicoectomy in humans. Acta Odontol Scand 1973;31(4):211–21.

141. Brice GL, Sampson WJ, Sims MR. An ultrastructural evaluation of the relationship between epithelial rests of Malassez and orthodontic root resorption and repair in man. Aust Orthod J 1991;12(2):90–4.

142. Owman Moll P, Kurol J, Lundgren D. The effects of a four-fold increased orthodontic force magnitude on tooth movement and root resorptions. An intra-individual study in adolescents. Eur J Orthod 1996; 18(3):287–94.

143. Owman Moll P, Kurol J. The early reparative process of orthodontically induced root resorption in adolescents – location and type of tissue. Eur J Orthod 1998;20(6): 727–32.

144. Cheng LL. Repair of root resorption four and eight weeks following the application of continuous light and heavy forces four weeks. University of Sydney, Sydney, 2007.

145. Kalkwarf KL, Krejci RF, Pao YC. Effect of apical root resorption on periodontal support. J Prosthet Dent 1986;56(3): 317–19.

146. Jacobson O. Clinical significance of root resorption. Am J Orthod 1952;38: 687–96.

147. Ghatari JG. Root resorption associated with combined orthodontic treatment and orthognathic surgery: modified definitions of the resorptive process sugested. In: Davidovitch Z (ed.) Biological Mechanisms of Tooth Eruption, Resorption and Replacement by Implants. EBSCO Media, Birmingham, 1994:545–56.

148. Levander E, Malmgren O. Long-term follow-up of maxillary incisors with severe apical root resorption. Eur J Orthod 2000;22(1):85–92.

149. Talic NF, Evans C, Zaki AM. Inhibition of orthodontically induced root resorption with echistatin, an RGD-containing peptide. Am J Orthod Dentofacial Orthop 2006;129(2):252–60.

150. Mavragani M, Brudvik P, Selvig KA. Orthodontically induced root and alveolar bone resorption: inhibitory effect of systemic doxycycline administration in rats. Eur J Orthod 2005;27(3):215–25.

151. Vazquez-Landaverde LA, Rojas-Huidobro R, Alonso Gallegos-Corona M, Aceves C.

Periodontal 5′-deiodination on forced-induced root resorption–the protective effect of thyroid hormone administration. Eur J Orthod 2002;24(4):363–9.

152. Mah J, Prasad N. Dentine phosphoproteins in gingival crevicular fluid during root resorption. Eur J Orthod 2004;26(1): 25–30.

153. Balducci L, Ramachandran A, Hao J, Narayanan K, Evans C, George A. Biological markers for evaluation of root resorption. Arch Oral Biol 2007;52(3): 203–8.

The dento-legal and ethical aspects of orthodontic treatment

14

INTRODUCTION

Orthodontics occupies a very interesting position within the dento-legal landscape, raising some issues that are peculiar to the specialty, and others that are particular manifestations of wider issues that apply throughout dentistry. At one extreme, it shares many of the medico-legal complications of treating children (in areas such as consent and the limitation of commencement of legal proceedings), while at the other extreme, it shares some of the risks that are associated with elective, cosmetic procedures carried out for adults.

This chapter will provide an overview of the dento-legal problems that arise in orthodontic treatment, highlighting areas of particular significance, and will then look a little more closely at some of the key issues.

FACTS AND MYTHS

It is a popular myth that orthodontics rarely results in complaints and litigation, and a further myth that orthodontic specialists encounter virtually no dento-legal problems. It is true that the majority of cases involving orthodontics arise from non-specialist practitioners who have not undergone any recognised formal training in the field but also worth noting that specialists and non-specialists tend to have a different 'mix' of cases and issues arising within them.

While nowhere near the levels of endodontic treatment (responsible for 21–22% of all claims) and crown and bridgework (about 19%), orthodontics sits – perhaps surprisingly to those working in the field – at a level not unlike that of implant dentistry, each accounting for 5–7% of the total number of cases. But this needs to be placed in the context of how much of each of these types of treatment is being carried out, however interesting it might be as a 'headline'.

A further myth is that any orthodontic cases that do arise will generally be low-value in terms of the cost of defending, settling or otherwise resolving the cases. In some jurisdictions, a third of all the highest value claims involve orthodontics in one way or another, and in one or two of them some of the highest value of all dental cases have involved orthodontics. It has featured in many regulatory (Dental Board/Dental Council) cases in many parts of the world, and in quite a few criminal cases (including allegations of fraud arising with claims for orthodontic treatment, fraudulent misrepresentation in terms of claims of special expertise on websites and practice literature, and claims of indecent assault).

WHAT GOES WRONG?

There is a difference between the technical/clinical deficiencies and failures in orthodontic treatment that would be apparent to experienced colleagues working in the same field, and the deficiencies and failures that are more visible to, and more easily understood by patients (or perhaps their parents). Because of this, problems of the latter variety are more likely to result in patient dissatisfaction and therefore have the potential to give rise to complaints and claims. Many studies in medicine and a few in dentistry have demonstrated that the drivers for litigation are much more likely to be human than technical. The work of Hickson et al.,[1,2] Mangels,[3] Beckman et al.[4] and others[5,6] have suggested that they have more to do with *how* the treatment is delivered and the relationship between patient and clinician, than with the technical/clinical quality of the treatment provided. Many of the most technically competent and skilled surgeons have the highest rate of litigation against them, and vice versa.

The more technical the specialty, the less likely it is that patients will be in a position to judge the technical aspects of the treatment and its outcomes. As a result, they will tend to judge the treatment by reference to other criteria and not least, by comparing what is being achieved, against what they had been led to expect (Figure 14.1).

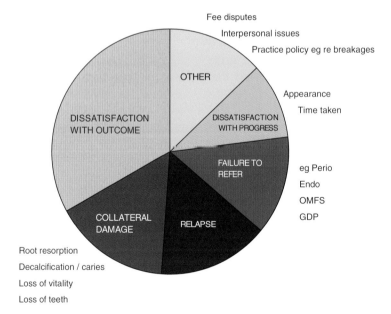

Figure 14.1 Reasons for patient dissatisfaction. OMFS, oral and maxillofacial surgery; GDP, general dental practitioner.

WHEN (AT WHAT STAGE) DOES IT GO WRONG?

Here there is a marked difference between specialist and non-specialist providers of orthodontic treatment. As shown in Figure 14.2, the overwhelming majority of cases are primarily the result of deficiencies in the initial diagnosis, case assessment and treatment plan. This is where the additional knowledge and experience of the specialist pays dividends, and also where the non-specialist can sometimes run into problems which could be said to reflect an underestimation of the complexities of the case, and which treatment approach is most likely to result in the desired outcome.

Specialists have most of their problems in the area(s) of communication and consent – which includes communication with professional colleagues as well as with patients and (in the case of children) their parents. In many instances the problems from this source are compounded by incomplete or inadequate clinical records of the communication and/or consent process. Non-specialists are much more likely than specialists to create problems relating to the technical aspects of the treatment

itself. Much of this relates to the management of expectations both in advance of treatment and as it proceeds, but a high level of specialist knowledge can and does bring its own problems in terms of the consent process. This is often seen where a specialist has a clear and uncompromising view as to what treatment approach should be provided, drawing perhaps from a detailed knowledge of the evidence base, and steers the patient strongly towards this treatment without explaining any alternative approaches or properly involving the patient in the decision-making process.

The evidence base is a crucially important tool in our clinical armamentarium, but it should never be used as a justification for denying a patient their right to autonomy and self-determination.

STANDARDS AND THE LAW

The quality of treatment is a subject that occupies orthodontists every bit as much as other clinicians, but as illustrated above, this can mean different things to different people – not least, the patients themselves. Many aspects of quality are the subject of standards that are specified by others. These can be summarised as:

- Legal standards (e.g. the requirements of national or local legislation)
- Civil standards (e.g. clinical negligence)
- Ethical/professional standards (as specified and enforced by regulatory bodies such as dental councils/boards)
- Voluntary standards (e.g. guidelines issued by bodies such as dental associations, colleges and organisations representing the specialty).

Some of the third parties involved in the above areas may intervene in the relationship between a dentist and a patient, even if the patient is delighted with the quality of care they have received.

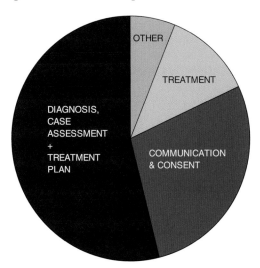

Figure 14.2 Stages when patient management goes wrong.

The principle of negligence arises from the premise that everyone has a duty to act in a reasonable way in order to avoid causing harm, loss or injury to another party. This is often known as the **duty of care** and exists in one form or another in most countries around the world, even though the law operates differently from one country to another. In general, three requirements must be satisfied in order for negligence to be established:

- A duty of care must exist between the dentist and the injured party
- The dentist must have failed in that duty, in one or more respects.
- The patient must have suffered damage, harm or loss as a *direct* result of a specific failure in the dentist's duty of care (so-called 'causation').

The first of these is almost always very easy to satisfy since any dentist who accepts a patient for treatment will have an automatic duty of care to the patient.

The second requirement, i.e. the breach of the duty of care, can be more difficult to establish, and it immediately invites the question of professional standards, and of who decides whether a given treatment is sufficient to discharge the duty of care, or whether it falls below such a standard. In most countries, a dentist is not guilty of negligence if he or she has acted in accordance with a practice which is accepted as being proper by a responsible body of professional (peer) opinion. This remains the case even when it can be shown that there exists one or more other bodies of opinion that take a contrary view. It is sufficient to exercise the ordinary, reasonable skill of someone reasonably competent in your field – an expert level of skill is only necessary if you have professed to be an expert in your field.

These basic principles are sometimes referred to as the 'Bolam test', after a landmark UK case half a century ago,[7] and have since been tested in the English courts at every level up to and including the House of Lords. Around the world, however, there is a progressive tendency to chip away at the edges of the Bolam principle. In Australia, for example, in the defining case of Rogers *v.* Whitaker (1992)[8] the court took the view that it was not sufficient to apply the Bolam test to the question of consent in medical cases, even if there is a body of opinion that would not have given a certain warning to a patient prior to carrying out a medical procedure. The court was free to determine, despite this, whether or not the failure to give such a warning could amount to negligence on the part of the clinician. There is a growing view that the Bolam principle, now over 50 years old, is rather too paternalistic in approach for today's more consumerist society. Rather than leaving it for other doctors and dentists, effectively, to decide what is or is not negligent, new test cases in many jurisdictions are progressively questioning and challenging the Bolam principle, especially in the area of consent.

It is well known that there are strongly held, but entirely divergent, views in a number of areas of orthodontic practice, and the legal background as set out above should remind us that the law will view these differences forensically and objectively and without the emotion that sometimes clouds the debate in professional circles. The challenge for the defendant facing an allegation of negligence is not that of providing that their view is 'right' and any other view is 'wrong' – the law quite properly provides for the existence of many different views. Instead, the defence will succeed if it can be shown to the satisfaction of the court that the clinician has acted in a way that would be considered appropriate, by a responsible body of opinion held among other clinicians working in the same field, providing that this 'responsible body of opinion' is also reasonable, respectable, logical and not of a nature that no reasonable clinician, acting competently, could hold.

ETHICS, DIFFERING VIEWS AND THE REGULATORY ENVIRONMENT

Dental boards, dental councils and other licensing agencies are given the task of regulating the dental profession, that is, setting appropriate ethical and professional standards in various areas of professional practice, and enforcing them. Regulatory bodies will get involved in cases involving poor clinical standards, because in general their primary role is to protect the public, by facilitating high standards and taking steps to ensuring that they are maintained. In general they will adopt something not unlike the 'Bolam' approach (see above) in expecting dentists to follow a reasonable approach to patient care in the light of current professional knowledge, and to maintain appropriate standards in doing so, but they will be concerned when it appears that members of the public are being misled, exploited, or treated unfairly, inappropriately or unprofessionally, and also when the profession is being brought into disrepute. Many high-profile regulatory (disciplinary) cases have been triggered by professional disputes between colleagues with differing views about orthodontic treatment.

Patients who are confused about treatment proposals, or dissatisfied with the progress or results of orthodontic treatment, might consult a second dentist for an opinion. Any second opinion should only be given in a fair, balanced and objective fashion, having taken every opportunity to establish the full facts of the case before providing that opinion. Unfortunately, in the area of 'alternative' orthodontics, patients frequently get caught up in a personal war between two (or more) clinicians who hold diametrically opposing views. Such agreements can take the form of divergent opinion in civil litigation, or, occasionally, criticisms of professional conduct in investigations by dental boards and dental councils. Very often these disagreements extend much more widely than

the individual case(s) under consideration, as both sides seek to defend the fundamental basis of their stance and approach to orthodontics, with a crusading zeal.

While clinicians have the right to hold and express views about the treatment approach that they personally prefer or advocate, this should be done in a way that acknowledges the possibility for other viewpoints to exist. In general, the time and place to conduct these debates is through normal scientific and professional channels such as the literature, or at professional meetings. It is disappointing, and unlikely to promote public confidence in the profession, when patients get stuck in the middle of these conflicts.

Strongly held views (on both sides of the debate) and personality clashes have a habit of creating intolerance and emotive professional conflicts surrounding alternative approaches to orthodontics. The mostly specialist 'mainstream' lobby criticises the 'alternative' lobby, on the grounds of insufficient training and the lack of an authoritative evidence base for the treatment being undertaken. The 'alternative' lobby, in turn, criticises the orthodontic establishment for being too dogmatic, and in refusing to look at alternative treatment approaches with an open mind.

It is always much easier to justify and defend treatment that has been provided in accordance with widely held, established opinion. There is no shortage of expert professional opinion which will be only too willing to spring to the defence of any clinician providing such treatment. This does not mean, however, that there is no room for alternative views, but rather that such views should be based on the same rigorous scientific discipline and scrutiny that one would expect of any professional person claiming to hold any particular skill or expertise.

'Alternative' orthodontists face particular challenges, in dento-legal terms, but there is much that they can do to strengthen their ability to withstand the kind of challenge and criticism that they might encounter during a professional career. Engaging constructively with others in the specialty, contributing to the scientific/evidence base, and paying particular attention to issues of consent and record keeping, is a sensible starting point.

TREATING CHILDREN

Treatment of children carries all the dento-legal risk of treating adults, but is further complicated by a number of other factors. Treatment is generally being provided in an ever-changing environment as the child continues to grow and develop; as a result, clinical decisions tend to have immediate short-term consequences and also some broader and longer-term implications. Sometimes, this impacts upon a case in the sense that it is asked how things might have developed if a specific event had not happened, or if a certain treatment which was not provided, had been provided.

These cases can often be fraught with conflicts and hidden agendas. Parents are invariably involved in treatment decisions and not uncommonly, responses are clouded by feelings of guilt, or natural parental protectiveness (or on occasions, over-protectiveness), of anger and sometimes a single-minded determination to see a dentist 'punished' for some actual or perceived act or omission towards the child.

Consent can be a medicolegal minefield. While this is generally obtained from a parent, the legal situation varies from one country to another. A useful general principle to bear in mind is that while the needs and best interests of the child should always be the paramount consideration, the child's wishes must also be taken into account. This can lead to difficult judgements on the part of a clinician, who must assess the child's capacity to understand the nature and purpose of the treatment being proposed for them.

In older children who may not yet have reached the legal age of adulthood/majority but who are perfectly capable of understanding the issues surrounding a proposed dental procedure, this can create some very difficult situations. This is particularly likely when the child and the parents do not agree as to what treatment should be provided. If in doubt, it is always wiser to postpone treatment than to proceed against the wishes of either the child, or the parent(s).

When negligence claims do arise, another problem is the extended limitation period in which legal proceedings can be brought. In many countries, legal proceedings in child cases can be brought at any time up to (and for a short period after) the time when the child reaches the age of adulthood. Throughout this extended period, legal costs can continue to accrue. Because of this, solicitors acting for child patients and their parents are under no pressure to act quickly. This, coupled with the natural wish to make a measured assessment of the eventual consequences in the context of the child's subsequent development, means that progress can be painfully slow. This can be an added burden for clinicians who can have a case hanging over their head for many years.

ADULT ORTHODONTICS

Here, while the special complications of treating children are no longer present, a number of different considerations apply. First, there may be a number of other treatment options, including that of simply accepting a situation that has probably been present for many years, and doing nothing. The patient may impose constraints on how the treatment is to be carried out (especially in terms of the type of appliance and its visibility), and the treatment plan may be complicated by previous orthodontic treatment, missing teeth, the presence of restorations or periodontal disease. On the other hand, adult patients who are prepared to commit themselves to orthodontics, will generally not do so lightly and may be highly compliant and cooperative with the treatment.

One type of adult orthodontics that has particular medicolegal significance is the combined orthognathic surgery/orthodontic approach. These cases require very careful pre-operative assessment, using a multidisciplinary approach, a meticulous and well-documented consent process and excellent communication between all the clinicians involved. Managing the psychological aspects of treatment of this kind is crucial to a successful outcome, and in many cases where the patient ends up dissatisfied with the outcome, clinicians will often observe that they would never have undertaken the treatment had they known more at the time about the patient's background and psychological status.

RETIREMENT

Orthodontics presents a particular challenge in terms of the length of time that patients can be under active treatment or review. Just like any other practitioner, an orthodontist's personal and professional circumstances will change, whether through ill health, or domestic/personal issues, or simply reaching retirement age.

Some, but not all, of these situations can be anticipated, planned for and managed, but there is always the potential for patients to be on a waiting list, or in mid-treatment or at a critical stage in their development, at the time when it becomes obvious that it will not be possible for the treating orthodontist to see the patient through to the completion of their orthodontic care and treatment. Where a practice is sold as a going concern, and/or where other suitably trained and experienced colleagues are willing and able to take over the patient's care, problems at the point of transfer are likely to be minimal. But in some situations a suitable purchaser cannot be found for an orthodontic practice, and in some areas local colleagues are not in a position to accept more than a small minority (or any) of the patients under active treatment or review.

In these cases retiring orthodontists must use their best endeavours to discharge their duty of care to the patients, perhaps 'triaging' them to give greatest priority to those patients who stand to be the most disadvantaged (or harmed) by the break in the continuity of care. Keeping patients and their parents informed, and communicating with them in a caring and supportive way is the key to minimising problems. Individual advice can be sought from one's protection/defence organisation.

CONSENT

Patients are entitled to receive accurate and balanced information about what treatment is being proposed for them, and why, and what other treatment options are available. Patients should be given all relevant information that could be material to their decision as to whether or not to proceed with the proposed treatment. A fact or a piece of information is material if it could influence the patient's decision. Included here is the possibility of a different kind of treatment being available – if necessary, from a different clinician if such treatment is not being offered by the present clinician. Patients have a right to be made aware of the difference between specialist and non-specialist treatment, especially in fields such as orthodontics where there is a recognised specialty and a recognised training pathway. But it does not follow from this that all patients must always be referred for specialist treatment, for the reasons outlined above.

Not unnaturally, a patient who has been on the receiving end of orthodontics that has not been successful, will maintain that they would never have agreed to undertake the treatment at all if they had been properly informed about the skill, training and experience – or the lack of it – of the dentist carrying out the treatment, or had been made aware of other (perhaps quicker or more widely accepted) forms of treatment that might have been available from other clinicians.

The widely used term 'informed consent' is unfortunate and misleading and indeed, in UK law the term 'informed consent' is not formally recognised. Its use tends to perpetuate the perception that it is up to the clinician to decide when the patient has been given all the information they need in order to decide whether or not to proceed with the proposed treatment. Yet however much information you impart, there will always be one more piece of information, which the patient will be in a position to maintain would have made all the difference to the decision they took.

It is more helpful to focus on the patient's *understanding* of the information provided, and to ensure that they are given the opportunity to have their questions answered, and to have any areas of uncertainty clarified in terms that they can understand and relate to. It is easy for us to forget that orthodontics can be a highly technical and unfamiliar concept for patients to fully grasp.

Assess the patient's competence to consent, bearing in mind their age and their ability to understand:

- The nature of the proposed treatment – exactly what it involves and how long it is likely to take
- What any appliances would look and feel like
- What the treatment is designed to achieve and why it is being carried out
- Any risks and limitations (e.g. any extractions, how likely is the treatment to achieved the desired outcome, are there any factors present that might compromise the outcome in any way?)
- Comparisons with any alternative treatment options which are available (including that of doing no treatment at all).

Satisfy yourself regarding the authority of the patient (or that of anyone else acting on the patient's behalf) to give consent to the proposed treatment, and also that consent has been given voluntarily. Keep good and careful records of all discussions concerning the question of consent.

SPECIALISTS AND GENERALISTS

The issue of consent is more complicated than it might appear at first sight. Many dento-legal cases arise after an initial course of orthodontic treatment has proved unsuccessful in some way. Faced with starting a new course of orthodontic treatment after investing much time, effort (and perhaps, money) into the original (unsuccessful) treatment, the patient may well feel angry. They might, for example, argue that they would never have allowed a general dental practitioner to carry out the original treatment had it been fully explained that their orthodontic problem was more appropriate for treatment by an experienced specialist. If the general dental practitioner did not make it clear that he (or she) was not a specialist, and had not offered the option of a specialist referral for an initial opinion and/or for the treatment itself, the practitioner might be vulnerable on the question of consent. This would apply even though the patient happily proceeded with the treatment without asking for any such referral.

Patients cannot be expected to understand the significance of orthodontic training, or to appreciate the complexity of their own malocclusion; they must be given a balanced and fair explanation of their options (including that of a referral) and allowed to decide for themselves. But this is not to suggest that a general dental practitioner should never be undertaking orthodontic treatment within the limits of their training, skill and competence – this would clearly be nonsense. When these considerations become central to a claim or complaint, as they often do, the allegation that is frequently made is that the practitioner failed to assess the case adequately, or perhaps through inexperience, failed to recognise the complexities of a case and to take them into account in the treatment plan.

This begs the question of whether an experienced orthodontist, who had undergone specialist training, would have assessed the case differently, would have recognised the problems and would have been able to overcome them successfully. Unless this can be shown to be the case, then the all-important question of causation (see 'Standards and the Law' above) is not established and the case against the practitioner becomes easier to defend.

It is in the nature of dento-legal proceedings that experts are called on to review a patient's treatment, with the help of clinical records, photographs, models, X-rays, etc. Two recurring problems are commonly encountered:

- The clinician appears not to have identified and taken account of certain complicating factors
  The clinician was not slow to realise that treatment was not progressing as planned, and failed to take steps to reassess the case personally, or with the help of an appropriately trained colleague.

CLINICAL RECORDS

In medicine and dentistry, our professional world is becoming increasingly litigious and good record keeping can provide vital evidence of the proper level of skill, care and attention that a patient has received. Sometimes there will be a conflict of evidence between the versions of events given by the patient and the dentist respectively. In such situations, the patient's version is often preferred unless the records can provide clear evidence to support the dentist's account of events.

Adequate records will allow a clinician to reconstruct the details of a patient's dental care, without having to rely upon memory alone. Chapter 8 addresses the question of the appro-

priate records that should be kept in relation to orthodontic care. Excellent records go further than this, because they provide contemporaneous (i.e. made at the time) evidence of the thought processes which lie behind the decisions that were made, the conversations that took place and the information, explanations and warnings given. They will also provide a lot more useful detail and because of this, they can anticipate and answer all the key questions that might arise in the future, arising from the treatment provided (or sometimes, not provided). Detailed records of all contacts between different clinicians involved in a patient's care can also be crucially important.

References

1. Hickson GB, Clayton EW, Entman SS, et al. Obstetricians; prior malpractice experience and patients' satisfaction with care. JAMA 1994;272:1583 7.
2. Hickson G B, Federspiel C F, Pichert J W, Miller C S, Gauld-Jaeger J, Bost P. Patient complaints and malpractice risk. JAMA 2002;287:2951–7.
3. Mangels LS. Tips from doctors who've never been sued. Med Econ 1991;68(4):56–8, 60–4.
4. Beckman HB, Markakis KM, Suchman AL, Frankel RM. The doctor-patient relationship and malpractice: lessons from plaintiff depositions. Arch Int Med 1994;154:1365–70.
5. Vincent C, Young M, Phillips A. Why do people sue doctors? A study of patients and relatives taking legal action. Lancet 1994;343:1609–13.
6. Shapiro RS, Simpson DE, Lawrence SL, Talsky AM, Sobocinski KA, Schiedermayer DL. A survey of sued and nonsued physicians and suing patients. Arch Int Med 1989;149:2190–6.
7. Bolam v. Friern Barnet Hospital Management Committee [1957] 1 WLR 582.
8. Rogers v. Whitaker (1992) 109 ALR 625–631 [1993] 4 med LR79–82 (High Court of Australia).

Further Reading

Schloendorff v. Society of New York Hospital. 105 NE 92 [NY 1914].

Department of Health. A Guide to Consent for Examination or Treatment. acc. HC(90)22. London, Department of Health, 1990.

Gillick v. West Norfolk and Wisbech Area Health Authority [1986] AC 112.

Bunting RF Jr, Benton J, Morgan WD. Practical risk management for physicians. J Health Risk Manag 1998;18(4):29–53.

Dental Protection, UK. Orthodontics (Risk Management Module 6). Available at: www.dentalprotection.org (accessed 9th June 2011).

Dental Protection, UK. Alternative Orthodontics (Risk Management Module 29). Available at: www.dentalprotection.org (accessed 9th June 2011).

Dental Protection, UK. Duty of Care (Ethics Module 4). Available at: www.dental protection.org (accessed 9th June 2011).

Dental Protection, UK. Patient Autonomy and Consent (Ethics Module 8) Available at: www.dentalprotection.org (accessed 9th June 2011)

Dental Protection, UK. Relating to Colleagues (Ethics Module 11). Available at: www.dentalprotection.org (accessed 9th June 2011).

The Management of Malocclusion

3

15

Class I malocclusion

Class I malocclusion is defined as that malocclusion in which the lower incisors occlude on or directly beneath the cingulum plateau of the upper incisors (Figure 2.1). The upper incisor inclination is average and the overjet is 2–3 mm. The anteroposterior relationship is normal, but there may be vertical or transverse malrelationships of the jaws or teeth.

Houston et al.[1] quoting Foster and Day (1974) give the percentages of the various malocclusions in a UK population as follows:

- Class I malocclusions – 44%
- Class II division 1 – 27%
- Class II division 2 – 17%
- Class III – 3%
- Indeterminate – 9%.

FEATURES OF CLASS I MALOCCLUSION

Occlusal Features

The incisor relationship is classed as normal (overjet 2–3 mm) although there may be localised transverse discrepancies. The commonest occlusal feature of Class I malocclusion is crowding, while spacing is less common. The canine relationship may be normal or it may be Class II or Class III. The molar relationship may be normal, Class II or Class III.

The vertical relationship may be normal or increased, and marked increase in the vertical dimension may result in an anterior open bite; if the incisor overbite is increased this, by definition, makes it a Class II incisor relationship: sometimes this may be referred to as a 'deep bite Class I occlusion'. Transversely, there may be a unilateral or bilateral crossbite, which may be dentally related or due to a true transverse skeletal problem. Bimaxillary protrusion (where both cephalometric angles SNA and SNB are increased but ANB is within the normal range) can occur in Class I malocclusion. Bimaxillary proclination is where both the upper and lower incisors are proclined, and the proclined upper incisors will automatically have an increased overjet even if the lower incisors occlude with the middle third of the palatal surface of the upper incisors.

Orthodontics: Principles and Practice, First Edition. Edited by Daljit S. Gill, Farhad B. Naini.
© 2011 Daljit S. Gill, Farhad B. Naini and Dental Update. Published 2011 by Blackwell Publishing Ltd.

Skeletal Features

A Class I skeletal pattern shows upper and lower jaws of approximately the same size, with a SNA of 80°, SNB of 78°, and an ANB difference of 2°. The maxillo-mandibular planes angle (MMPA) may be increased or average (27°). If the MMPA is decreased there may an increased overbite and a tendency towards a Class II skeletal pattern.

Soft Tissues

If the jaws are the same size, and there is a normal eruptive mechanism, with a normal soft tissue behaviour pattern, the upper and lower incisors will tend to erupt into a Class I relationship. If there is any change in the vertical or anteroposterior skeletal pattern, the soft tissues may compensate for this, but the dentoalveolar compensatory mechanism can compensate for mild to moderate degrees of skeletal discrepancy in order to achieve a Class I incisal relationship (Figure 15.1).[2]

Growth

Growth of the jaws is usually favourable, with the incisor relationship being maintained. There is a tendency for the mandible to become slightly more prognathic with age, and a mild Class II relationship will tend to improve with time.

Path of Closure

The path of closure is usually direct and unless there are premature occlusal contacts, there will be no deviations or displacements. However, these should be checked for during the clinical examination of the patient, as an apparent Class I malocclusion in centric occlusion may be very different to that in centric relation (which is the maximum retruded contact position of the teeth).

PRINCIPLES OF TREATMENT IN CLASS I MALOCCLUSIONS

The principles of treatment in class I malocclusions are:

- Relief of crowding
- Correction of canine relationships
- Alignment of the incisors
- Space closure
- Detailing of the occlusion.

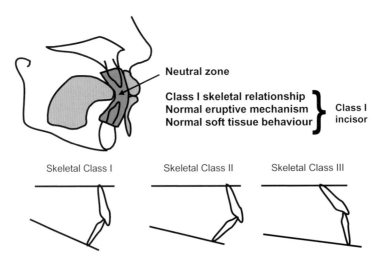

Neutral zone

Class I skeletal relationship
Normal eruptive mechanism } Class I
Normal soft tissue behaviour } incisor

Skeletal Class I   Skeletal Class II   Skeletal Class III

Figure 15.1 The dentoalveolar compensatory mechanism (after Solow[2]).

Relief of Crowding

The commonest way of relieving crowding is by extraction of teeth. In Class I malocclusions, the commonest problem is crowding, and the commonest extraction pattern has traditionally involved the upper and lower first premolars. The reason for this is because these teeth are close to the site of anterior crowding, allowing easier alignment of the canines and incisors. In the past the extraction of the four first premolars (sometimes as part of a serial extraction procedure) was popular where no appliance therapy was contemplated. Spaces will close if the extractions are undertaken at an early age (say around 9–12 years) (Figure 15.2).

The extraction of second premolars was undertaken in the past when the anterior crowding was mild, and such an extraction site was not as visible as the first premolar extraction site. However, the tendency for the first permanent molars to tip and rotate mesiolingually afterwards confines second premolar extractions to cases where fixed appliance treatment is to be undertaken, unless these teeth are totally excluded from the arch.

Another way of achieving space is to distalise the buccal segments. This can be undertaken with a removable appliance to the upper molars (Figure 15.3). Often headgear will be needed to reinforce the anchorage. Mild crowding can be relieved by expansion of the arch in the transverse dimension again using either removable appliances (Figure 15.4) or fixed appliances as described in the next section.

Fixed Appliances to Expand the Upper Arch

Fixed appliances that can be used to expand the upper arch include the quadhelix appliance, which uses bands cemented to the molars and

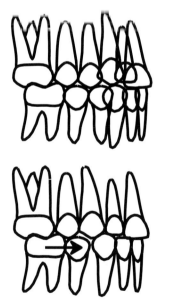
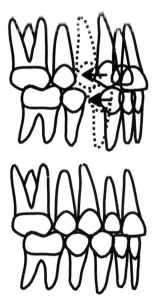

Figure 15.2 Class I malocclusion with upper and lower arch crowding. Upper and lower first premolars are extracted. With orthodontic treatment, canine relationships are then corrected, space closure accomplished, and molars should be in Class I relationship at the end of treatment. In a serial extraction procedure, a similar extraction pattern would take place but one would rely on spontaneous tooth movements to close space and align the teeth. However, complete success in extraction-only cases cannot be predicted or guaranteed.

palatal arms to the buccal teeth. An example is shown in Figure 15.5.

Another method of expanding the upper arch is rapid maxillary expansion (Figures 15.6, 15.7). In this case the buccal teeth are covered with metal (or acrylic) cap splints connected in the centre of the palate by a midline screw. The patient turns the key once or twice a day and a midline diastema appears, indicating expansion in the transverse dimension. This form of expansion separates the maxillary bones in the midline suture. New bone is formed in the gap and the diastema closes spontaneously over a period of some weeks due to the influence of the transseptal fibres.

EXTRACTIONS OTHER THAN PREMOLARS

Upper Central Incisors

The extraction of upper central incisors is undertaken only if these teeth are involved in some pathology, for example, severe root resorption by impacted maxillary canines or other causes, severe fractures, gross caries, etc. If these teeth are extracted, a decision must be made to:

- Maintain the space and provide a restorative solution later (bridge or implant)
- Bring the lateral incisor into the space and then disguise it as a central incisor by restorative means
- Transplant a tooth from another part of the arch (usually a lower premolar).

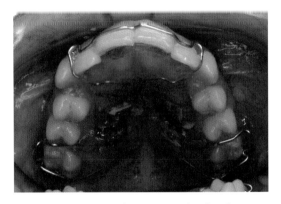

Figure 15.3 Screw plate in situ to distalise the upper molars.

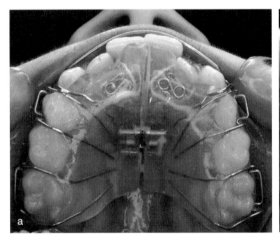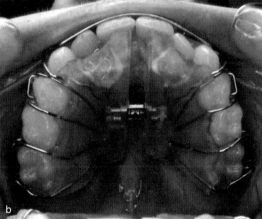

Figure 15.4 (a) Upper removable appliance to expand the upper arch (note midline screw and z-springs to the upper lateral incisors). (b) After expansion, the arch length has increased and the lateral incisors are aligning.

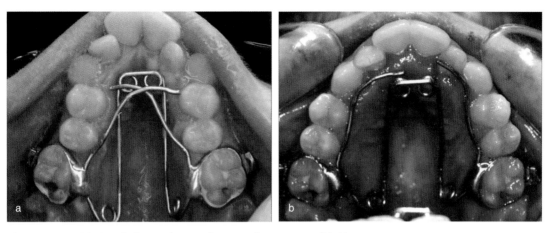

Figure 15.5 (a) Quadhelix in place at the start of expansion. (b) After expansion.

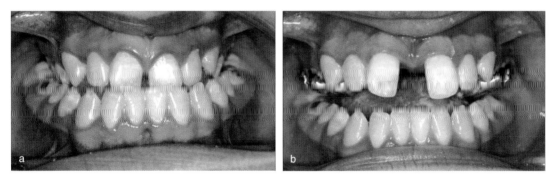

Figure 15.6 (a) Narrow upper arch prior to rapid maxillary expansion. (b) Arch after rapid maxillary expansion.

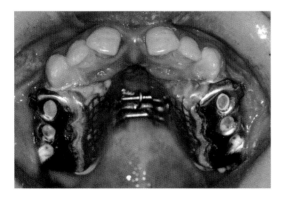

Figure 15.7 Occlusal view of a rapid maxillary expansion splint.

Upper Lateral Incisors

Lateral incisors may be considered for extraction if:

• They are carious
• They have undergone severe root resorption (e.g. by unerupted canines)
• There is a dens in dente and prognosis is poor
• They are totally excluded from the arch
• They are peg shaped and restoration is not possible.

Lateral incisors may also be congenitally absent. If they are absent, or have to be extracted, the canines may be brought forward orthodontically into contact with the central incisors. In these cases, the canines may need to be reshaped and built up with composite or ceramic to make them appear more like lateral incisors.

Canines

Canines may be removed if they are:

- Carious or involved in some other pathology
- Totally excluded from the arch and if the lateral incisor-premolar contact has resulted in a good appearance
- Severely impacted or grossly displaced from their eruptive path.

The lateral incisor-first premolar contact point that results in these cases is often satisfactory or it can be aligned with fixed appliances. With good oral hygiene, it should provide for a stable and long-lasting result.

First Permanent Molars

The extraction of first permanent molars as a general interceptive measure was advocated by Wilkinson[3] at a time when caries was widespread. Later articles by Crabb and Rock[4] and Mackie et al.[5] give more contemporary guidance on first permanent molar extractions. Where no appliance therapy is contemplated and the patient has a Class I malocclusion, with little or no crowding, the ideal age for extraction of first permanent molars is between the ages of 8.5 and 10 years, when the interradicular crescent of the second molars are just forming on radiographic examination (Figure 15.8). Extraction after this age will result in tipping of the second molars and residual spacing. Severe crowding will require active

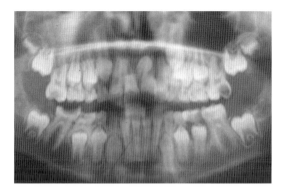

Figure 15.8 Upper and lower first molars are grossly carious. Interradicular crescent of the second molars is just forming. This would be an appropriate stage to extract the upper and lower first permanent molars as an interceptive measure.

treatment, possibly with fixed appliances or space maintainers to prevent the second molars from drifting too far mesially.

Second molar extraction benefits can include eruption of the third molars and avoidance of hospitalisation for removal of impacted wisdom teeth. The third molars should be at the interradicular crescent-forming stage and not tipped more than 30° to the occlusal plane when the second molars are extracted.[6]

CORRECTION OF CANINE RELATIONSHIPS

The relationships of the upper and lower canines is the key to successful treatment. The canines should be in a Class I relationship to the lower canines at the end of treatment (the tip of the upper canine should occlude in the embrasure between the lower canine and first premolar). Where the crowding is mild, distal movement of the canines can be done quite simply, either by tipping with a removable appliance or by independent retraction with a fixed appliance, allowing alignment of the incisors. Where the crowding is more severe, or

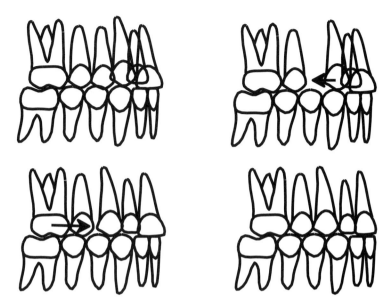

Figure 15.9 Correction of Class I crowding by extraction of the upper first premolars only. Note correction of canine relationship to Class I and mesial movement of the upper molar to a slightly more than Class II relationship (a premolar is slightly wider mesiodistally than a molar mesiobuccal cusp).

where the canine is distally tipped, and there is a risk of the posterior segments moving forward due to loss of anchorage, augmentation of anchorage may be necessary. Figure 15.9 shows an example of upper first premolar extractions only performed to relieve crowding in the upper arch when there is a well-aligned lower arch. The molar relationship is Class II and remains so at the end of treatment, while the canines and incisors are in a Class I relationship.

INCISOR ALIGNMENT

Once the upper canines are in a Class I relationship with the lower canines, the incisors can be aligned and crossbites and rotations eliminated. Care should be taken when aligning the lower incisors that excessive proclination does not occur, as this may be unstable due to lower lip pressure.[7]

SPACE CLOSURE

Space closure can be passive, either by 'drift-odontics',[8] whereby the space closes naturally after extractions or space creation (such as distalisation of buccal segments), or active, using fixed appliances. The end result of treatment should be a normal incisor and canine relationship, with the molars in Class I, Class II or (occasionally) Class III relationship, and well-aligned, coordinated arches.

LOCAL FACTORS AND MALOCCLUSIONS

The treatment of Class I malocclusions, apart from crowding, may involve any combination of the following:

- Tooth size/alveolar bone discrepancy
- Variations in tooth numbers (congenitally absent, supernumeraries, supplemental)

- Variation in tooth size, shape and position:
  - Macro-/microdont teeth
  - Accessory cusps
  - Dens in dente
  - Fusion
  - Gemination
  - Concrescence
  - Morphological problems (e.g. dilacerations)
  - Impactions
  - Crossbites
  - Transpositions
- Early loss of deciduous teeth (space loss, centreline shifts)
- Retained deciduous teeth (submergence, ankylosis, ectopic eruption of successors)
- Premature loss of permanent teeth
- Eruption anomalies (variation in eruption sequence).

References

1. Houston WJB, Stephens CD, Tulley J. A Textbook of Orthodontics, 2nd edn. Wright, Oxford, 1992.

2. Solow B. The dento-alveolar compensatory mechanism: background and clinical applications. Br J Orthod 1980;7:145–61.

3. Wilkinson AA. The early extraction of the first permanent molar as the best method of preserving the dentition as a whole. Dent Rec 1944;64:1–8.

4. Crabb JJ, Rock WP. Treatment planning in relation to the first permanent molar. Br Dent J 1971;131:396–401.

5. Mackie IC, Blinkhorn AS, Davies PHJ. The extraction of permanent first molars during the mixed-dentition period – a guide to treatment planning. J Paediatr Dent 1989;5: 85–92.

6. Dacre JT. The criteria for lower second molar extraction. Br J Orthod 1987;14:1–9.

7. Mills JR. The stability of the lower labial segment. A cephalometric survey. Dent Pract Dent Rec 1968;18(8):2930–306.

8. Stephens CD. The use of spontaneous tooth movements in treatment of malocclusion. Dent Update 1989;16:337–42.

Class II division 1 malocclusion

A Class II division 1 malocclusion presents when the lower incisor edges are posterior to the cingulum plateau of the upper incisors, there is an increase in overjet, and the upper central incisors are normally inclined or proclined (British Standards Classification, Figure 16.1).[1] The prevalence in a Caucasian population has been reported to be as high as 27%.[2] An increased overjet is associated with an increased risk of traumatic dental injuries especially if there is poor coverage of the upper incisors by the lower lip (incompetent lips).

AETIOLOGY

Skeletal Pattern

Class II division 1 malocclusion is normally associated with a Class II skeletal pattern, often as a result of mandibular retrognathia (Figure 16.2). In contrast to Class III malocclusion, there are less hereditary influences on the development of Class II malocclusion. A Class I, or even Class III, skeletal pattern may exist if the presence of a soft tissue factor, or habit, results in proclination of the upper incisors and/or retroclination of the lower incisors. The presence of a vertical skeletal discrepancy, with either an increase, or decrease, in the Frankfort mandibular planes angle and lower anterior facial height proportion, will make management of the mal occlusion more difficult.

Soft Tissues

Soft tissues play a more important role in Class II malocclusion in comparison with Class III malocclusion. The position of the soft tissues at rest is dictated by the anteroposterior and vertical skeletal pattern, and their activity is of particular relevance. A Class II division 1 incisor relationship is typically associated with a lip apart posture. An anterior oral seal can be achieved in a variety of ways.

- *Mandibular posture to allow the lips to meet.* In these circumstances the soft tissues promote dentoalveolar compensation and reduce the influence of the Class II skeletal pattern.

Orthodontics: Principles and Practice, First Edition. Edited by Daljit S. Gill, Farhad B. Naini.
© 2011 Daljit S. Gill, Farhad B. Naini and Dental Update. Published 2011 by Blackwell Publishing Ltd.

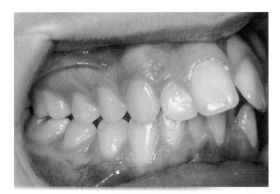

Figure 16.1 Class II division 1 incisor relationship.

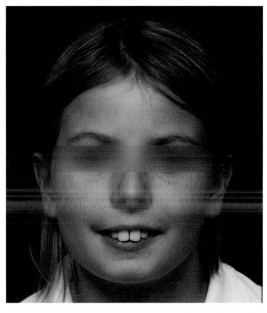

Figure 16.3 Lip apart posture with the lower lip functioning palatal to the upper incisors.

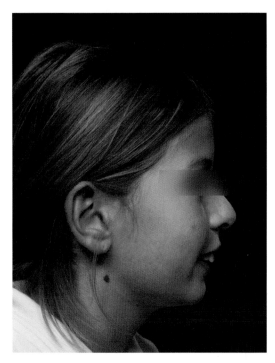

Figure 16.2 Typical facial profile associated with Class II skeletal pattern.

• *The lower lip functions palatal to the upper incisors in the presence of an increased and complete overbite.* This is a more common presentation and is associated with retroclination of the lower incisors and/or proclination of the upper incisors (Figure 16.3). A larger overjet

than would be expected as a result of the skeletal relationship is observed.

• *The tongue is pushed forward to contact the lower lip and the overbite is incomplete.* The lower incisors are often proclined and the overbite just incomplete. This forward tongue posture can be described as an adaptive tongue thrust. A true endogenous tongue thrust is a rare presentation where the tongue is pushed forcibly forward during swallowing as a result of a neuromuscular defect.

In certain individuals, hyperactive lower lip musculature will exacerbate an increased overjet, and these patients are described as having a strap-like lower lip. The prognosis for stable overjet reduction in these circumstances is poor.

Dental Factors

Maxillary arch crowding can predispose to an increased overjet as a result of labial exclusion of one or both of the central incisors. An increase in overjet can also present as pathological tooth migration as a result of periodontal attachment loss affecting the upper incisors in adult patients.

Habits

Digit sucking of sufficient duration and intensity is associated with an increased overjet and reduced overbite. The effect on the incisor relationship may be asymmetrical, and this appearance can help in diagnosis especially if there is a skin callus seen on the digit that is used as part of the habit (see Figure 4.6, Chapter 4).

ASSESSMENT AND DIAGNOSIS

With Class II division 1 malocclusion, the patient's principal concern will usually be related to the increased overjet and there may have been a previous history of traumatic dental injuries. Individuals with a significant Class II skeletal discrepancy may also be aware of their jaw malrelationship and, if so, should be asked in more detail what concern they have about their overall dentofacial appearance.

The skeletal pattern should be recorded in the anteroposterior, vertical and transverse dimensions. An assessment of facial profile is important, together with a careful examination of the lip position both at rest, and during swallowing and expressive behaviour. A detailed occlusal examination will include:

- Presence/absence of teeth
- Arch alignment (crowding/spacing and the presence of rotations)
- Maxillary and mandibular incisor inclinations (normal, proclined or retroclined)
- Measurement of overjet and overbite
- Buccal segment relationships.

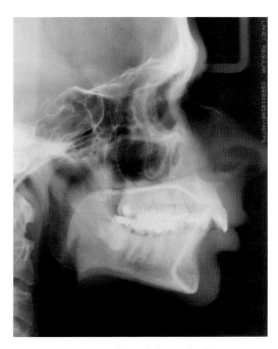

Figure 16.4 lateral cephalograph demonstrating Class II anteroposterior and the vertical skeletal base relationship

Radiographs are often required to complete the diagnosis.[3] Information from a lateral cephalograph can be helpful in determining the extent of a significant malrelationship between the maxilla and mandible. This will assist in deciding whether orthodontic camouflage can be suitably undertaken, or if orthognathic surgery would be required to treat the malocclusion[4] (Figure 16.4). The soft tissues are a major determinant of stability following overjet reduction. Ideally, the lower lip should act on the incisal third of the labial surface of the upper incisors with a competent lip seal.[5]

TREATMENT (TABLE 16.1)

Deciduous Dentition

Orthodontic treatment during the deciduous dentition does not prevent the development of

Table 16.1 Overview of treatment approaches for Class II division 1 malocclusions

Presentation	Management
Mixed dentition	
Upper incisors at risk of damage due to increased overjet	Consider early treatment with a removable or functional appliance to reduce overjet
Dental appearance promoting teasing	Retain until comprehensive later treatment
Late mixed/early permanent dentition	
Mild/moderate skeletal discrepancy	Functional appliance therapy (if appropriate) maximising effect of any favourable skeletal growth
Severe skeletal discrepancy or a concern about facial appearance	Fixed appliance therapy with premolar extractions to relieve crowding or distal movement of upper posterior teeth
	Accept malocclusion will require a combination of orthodontic treatment and orthognathic surgery at maturity
Adult treatment	
Mild/moderate skeletal discrepancy – no concern about facial appearance	Camouflage skeletal pattern using fixed appliances – premolar extractions may be required for relief of crowding and to allow upper incisor retraction
Severe skeletal discrepancy or a concern about facial appearance	Orthognathic surgery required necessitating fixed appliance treatment to align and coordinate arches with correction of incisor inclinations (decompensation)

a Class II division 1 malocclusion in the permanent dentition, or reduce the complexity of later management. Appliance therapy is not, therefore, indicated at this stage of dental development. Digit sucking habits should be discouraged particularly just before eruption of the permanent maxillary central incisors.

Mixed Dentition Treatment

Children presenting with a significantly increased overjet, and also inadequate lip coverage, have an increased risk of trauma to the permanent upper incisor teeth.[6] These patients may also have been teased by other children and, if cooperation with appliance wear can be achieved, early treatment can be worthwhile to reduce the psychological impact of the malocclusion.[7] Any digit sucking habits should stop before treatment. If treatment is not undertaken

at this stage, a mouthguard should be prescribed for wear during sport.

Growth modification with functional appliance therapy has an important place in the management of Class II division 1 malocclusion. Class II functional appliances produce their effects by a combination of the following:

- Small amount of restraint of maxillary skeletal growth
- Small amount of mandibular growth with increase in condylar length and remodelling in the glenoid fossae
- Distal translation of the upper teeth
- Mesial translation of the lower teeth
- Retroclination of the upper incisors and proclination of the lower incisors.

If appliance treatment is carried out when little growth is occurring, relatively more dental than skeletal changes are observed.[8] These dental changes may be more likely to relapse at the end of treatment. Functional appliance treatment can, therefore, successfully reduce an increased overjet during the mixed dentition. The disadvantage of this approach is the necessity to then await eruption of the premolar and permanent canine teeth before comprehensive orthodontic treatment can be completed with fixed appliances. Either the functional appliance or a removable retainer will be needed to maintain overjet reduction, and continued compliance with appliance wear can be a problem. There is little evidence to support the benefit of early treatment in terms of final treatment outcome when compared with undertaking definitive treatment in the late mixed/early permanent dentition.[9]

Late Mixed/Early Permanent Dentition

The majority of treatment for Class II division 1 malocclusion is undertaken at this stage of dental development and ideally coincides with peak skeletal growth with relatively greater forward and downward growth of the mandible, compared with the maxilla, within the facial skeleton. Any improvement in the skeletal pattern will generally be favourable, whether or not this can be attributed to appliance therapy. Appliance treatment aims to produce a Class I incisor relationship with the upper incisors brought under the control of the lower lip to ensure stability of overjet reduction. This is of particular importance when the lower lip has previously functioned palatal to the upper incisors.

Non-crowded Arches

The absence of significant crowding will dictate a non-extraction approach to treatment. If the molar relationship is Class I, the upper incisors are frequently spaced and proclined. Contemporary management will involve the use of a fixed appliance to close space with

retraction of the upper incisors using appropriate anchorage reinforcement to prevent forward movement of the molar teeth. Cases that present with mild crowding (less than 4 mm) can usually be treated with a combination of arch expansion and distal movement of the upper posterior teeth with extraoral traction provided by headgear (Figure 16.5).

Rapid correction of a Class II division 1 malocclusion can be achieved when functional appliance therapy is prescribed at the time of peak skeletal growth. Popularity of the twin block appliance in the UK has been reported,[10] and this two-part appliance is possibly the easiest for a patient to wear (Figure 16.6). However, other types of functional appliance, such as the activator, more readily allow posterior tooth eruption.[11] This can be advantageous in reducing an increased overbite that is

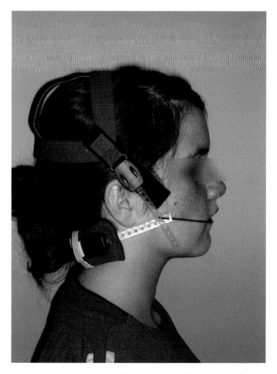

Figure 16.5 Extraoral traction (headgear) to achieve distal movement of the upper posterior teeth prior to overjet correction. (Reproduced with permission from Daljit Gill.)

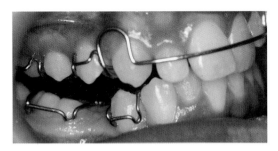

Figure 16.6 Twin block functional appliance therapy.

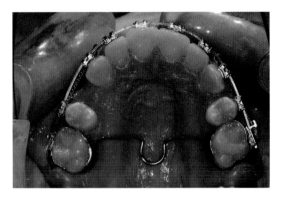

Figure 16.8 Overjet reduction using a fixed appliance and transpalatal arch to reinforce anchorage.

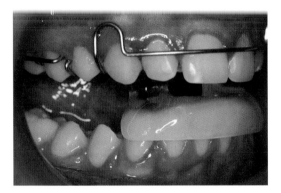

Figure 16.7 Activator-style functional appliance therapy.

frequently associated with Class II division 1 malocclusion (Figure 16.7). Full records including study models, photographs and a lateral cephalogram should be taken at the end of the functional phase in order to assess the change in the lower incisor position and degree of crowding within the arches. This will indicate the space required (see Chapter 10) before prescribing fixed appliances. Detailing of the occlusion, and ideal tooth positioning, necessitates the use of a fixed appliance in the majority of cases.

Crowded Arches

If significant crowding and/or bimaxillary proclination is present, space will be required to level and align the arches, and also to provide

space for overjet reduction with fixed appliance therapy. A common extraction pattern would be removal of all four first premolars if space requirements are large (see Chapter 10). However, if the molar relationship is Class II, and space requirements permit, the removal of lower second premolars can be considered, as this will help correction of the posterior occlusion to a Class I relationship by facilitating mesial movement of the lower molars. The available anchorage should be assessed with particular regard to mesial movement of the upper posterior teeth while the overjet is reduced. Anchorage can be reinforced for the upper molars with either headgear or intraoral devices, and final correction assisted by use of Class II intermaxillary traction (Figures 16.8, 16.9). An initial phase of functional appliance treatment to correct a Class II molar relationship to Class I, with simultaneous reduction of the increased overjet and overbite, can be beneficial in reducing anchorage requirements but increases the overall duration of treatment.

Adult Treatment

A Class II camouflage treatment can be successful in specific cases where the anteroposterior

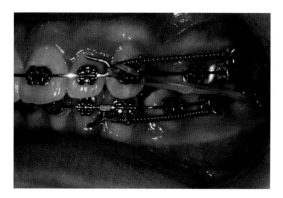

Figure 16.9 Class II intermaxillary traction applied to fixed appliances.

skeletal discrepancy is not severe and facial profile is potentially acceptable. Additional factors that can complicate treatment for adults include lack of growth, the effect of previous orthodontic treatment, missing teeth, periodontal disease and the presence of restorations. Therefore, treatment aims may be limited to achieving a Class I incisor relationship with alignment of the anterior teeth, accepting the best possible posterior occlusion. Orthognathic surgery (see Chapter 25) will be required for those with significant skeletal discrepancies.

Stability

The stability of overjet correction is reliant upon ensuring that the upper incisors are retracted sufficiently to be in control of the lower lip. Future mandibular growth is also important for the stability of overjet correction. A significant backwards (clockwise) mandibular growth rotation can lead to an increase in overjet as the lower incisors are also rotated downwards and backwards. The resultant increase in vertical facial dimension with this type of growth rotation also reduces lip competency, which predisposes to relapse. Factors influencing the stability of deep overbite correction are considered in Chapter 23.

References

1. British Standards Institute. British Standards Institute Glossary of Dental Terms (BS EN 21942). BSI, London, 1992.
2. Foster TD, Day AJ. A survey of malocclusion and the need for orthodontic treatment in a Shropshire school population. Br J Orthod 1974;1:73–8.
3. Issacson KG, Thom AR, Horner K, Waites E. Guidelines for the Use of Radiographs in Clinical Orthodontics, 3rd edn. British Orthodontic Society, London, 2008.
4. Proffit WR, Fields HW, Sarver DM. Contemporary Orthodontics, 4th edn. Mosby/Elsevier, St Louis, 2007:689–93.
5. Mitchell L. An Introduction to Orthodontics, 3rd edn. Oxford University Press, Oxford, 2007.
6. Burden DJ. An investigation of the association between overjet size, lip coverage, and traumatic injury to maxillary incisors. Eur J Orthod 1995;17:513–17.
7. O'Brien K, Wright J, Conboy F, et al. Effectiveness of early orthodontic treatment with the twin-block appliance: a multicenter, randomised controlled trial. Part 2: Psychosocial effects. Am J Orthod Dentofacial Orthop 2003;124:128–37.
8. O'Brien K, Wright J, Conboy F, et al. Effectiveness of early orthodontic treatment with the twin-block appliance: a multicenter, randomised controlled trial. Part 1: Dental and skeletal effects. Am J Orthod Dentofacial Orthop 2003;124:234–43.
9. Tulloch CJF, Proffit WR, Phillips C. Outcomes in a 2-phase randomised clinical trial of early Class II treatment. Am J Orthod Dentofacial Orthop 2004;125:657–67.
10. Chadwick SM, Banks P, Wright JL. Use of myofunctional appliances in the UK: A survey of British orthodontists. Dent Update 1998;25:302–8.
11. Orton HS. Functional Appliances in Orthodontic Treatment. Quintessence, London, 1990.

Class II division 2 malocclusion

17

INTRODUCTION

The British Standards Classification defines Class II division 2 malocclusion as follows: the lower incisor edges occlude posterior to the cingulum plateau of the upper incisors; the upper central incisors are retroclined, the overjet is usually minimal but may be increased. Among Caucasians, the prevalence is reported to be about 10%.[1]

AETIOLOGY

This malocclusion has a strong genetic component[2] with most resulting from the interplay of skeletal and soft tissue factors.

Skeletal Factors

Usually the skeletal pattern is mildly Class II, due to mandibular retrognathia, but it may be Class I or even mildly Class III.[3,4] A reduced lower facial height is typical,[5] in association with an anterior (anticlockwise) mandibular

growth rotation, which tends to increase the overbite and lead to forward projection of the chin[2,5] (Figure 17.1a). Due to the relatively wide maxillary base, and narrower lower intercanine width,[6] the first premolars may be in lingual crossbite (scissors bite).

Soft Tissue Factors

As the lower facial height is reduced, the lower lip line is high on the upper incisors, covering more that one-third of the labial surface, and is the predominant cause of their retroclination[7] (Figure 17.1b). Increased resting lower lip pressure (~2.5 times as high as the upper lip resting pressure) is a complementary factor.[8] Upper and lower lips are also thicker compared with Class 1 malocclusion.[9] Depending on the lower lip level, the relatively shorter maxillary lateral incisor crowns may either be retroclined along with the central incisors or escape lower lip control and be of average inclination but mesio-labially rotated, a manifestation of inherent crowding (Figure 17.1c). The reduced lower

Orthodontics: Principles and Practice, First Edition. Edited by Daljit S. Gill, Farhad B. Naini.
© 2011 Daljit S. Gill, Farhad B. Naini and Dental Update. Published 2011 by Blackwell Publishing Ltd.

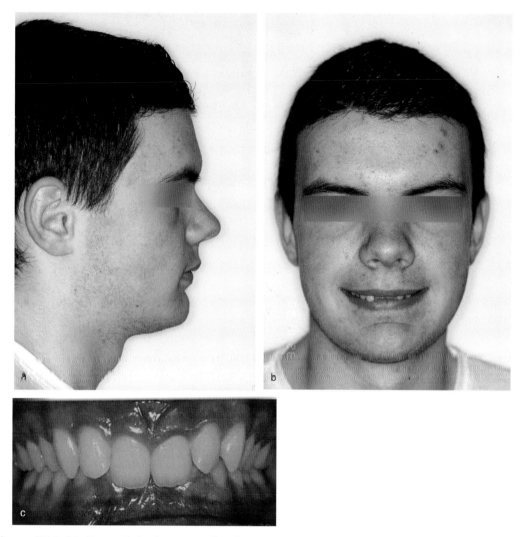

Figure 17.1 (a) Class II skeletal pattern with reduced FMPA, deep labiomental fold and relatively prominent chin point; (b) associated high lower lip line evident on smiling; and (c) typical Class II division 2 malocclusion.

facial height also leads to a relative soft tissue excess of the lower lip, reflected in the commonly observed deep labio-mental fold. Where the lips are strap-like regardless of the skeletal pattern, the upper and lower incisors may be retroclined (bimaxillary retroclination; Figure 17.2); this is sometimes associated with a gummy smile and may be aggravated by upper incisor overeruption.

Dental Factors

The cingulum on the upper incisors may be reduced or absent, thereby allowing overeruption

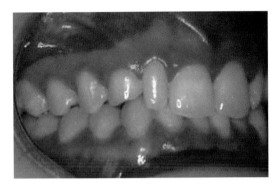

Figure 17.2 Bimaxillary retroclination; peg shaped lateral incisor; retained primary canine (the permanent canine was palatally displaced).

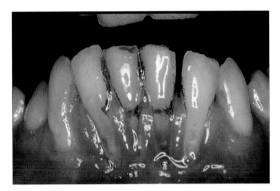

Figure 17.3 Traumatic overbite due to markedly retroclined upper incisors; note also attrition of the incisal and labial aspects of the lower incisors. (Reproduced with permission from Elsevier.)

of the lower incisors to increase the interincisal angle and deepen the overbite.[10] The latter may be exacerbated by a Class II skeletal pattern and retroclination of upper and lower incisors. Relative to other malocclusion types, a more acute upper incisor crown–root angulation[10] and smaller mesiodistal width of the upper and lower incisors have been identified.[2] There is also a higher incidence of palatally impacted maxillary canines[11] and of peg-shaped or absent maxillary lateral incisors[12] (Figure 17.2). Retroclination of the upper incisors, and possibly of the lower incisors, worsens pre-existing crowding.

TREATMENT PLANNING

The factors which should be considered, in particular, with regard to treatment planning are given in Table 17.1. Two principal decisions have to be made with regard to treatment in relation to the incisor relationship and crowding: to accept or correct the incisor relationship; to extract or not for relief of crowding and incisor alignment.

Treatment

Mild cases are best accepted. Where the overbite is onto tooth tissue and the retroclination of the upper incisors is acceptably mild, treat-ment may be confined to relief of upper arch crowding sufficient for alignment of the lateral incisors.

Where the incisor relationship is to be corrected, this may be undertaken by:

• Functional appliance followed by fixed appliances
• Fixed appliances
• Surgical-orthodontic treatment.

Dentofacial aesthetics will be improved by these means. A traumatic overbite, if present, will also be corrected.

The overbite *and* the interincisal angle must be corrected for the best prospect of stability[13] (Figure 17.4). Methods of overbite reduction and means of interincisal angle correction are given in Table 17.2. Intrusion of the upper incisors should be included in treatment to eliminate the high lower lip pressure.[7,8]

Functional Appliance Treatment

Functional appliance treatment is indicated in a growing child with a mild to moderate Class II skeletal pattern, reduced lower facial height, deep overbite and Class II molar relationship. To allow mandibular posturing for the construction bite and to ensure favourable arch

Table 17.1 Factors to consider in treatment planning of Class II division 2 malocclusions

Factor	Implications for management
Underlying anteroposterior and vertical skeletal discrepancy	In general, the more Class II the skeletal pattern and the more reduced the Frankfort-mandibular planes angle (FMPA), the more difficult to achieve optimal dentofacial correction by orthodontic means alone. Consider along with growth potential and profile (see below)
Growth potential and pattern of facial growth	Skeletal II deep bite correction is facilitated by favourable facial growth. Inherent forward mandibular growth rotation tendency (anticlockwise) aids skeletal Class II correction but tends to increase overbite unless the interincisal angle is altered and a cingulum stop created. In an adult, overbite reduction by incisor intrusion rather than molar extrusion is advisable as the latter is unlikely to be stable
Profile considerations	Little objective difference exists in lip fullness between extraction and non-extraction treatment, but the latter is favoured, particularly with bimaxillary retroclination. For an unfavourable profile (marked skeletal Class II and very reduced FMPA) in an adult, a combined surgical orthodontic approach is required
Lower lip level	Inferior lower lip movement away from the upper incisor crowns is essential to promote stability. Where the lower lip covers the full crown height of the upper incisors, permanent retention is likely
Presence and degree of crowding	Avoid lower arch extractions as may encourage overbite increase by retroclination of the labial segment. Because it is often trapped lingually by the upper incisors, proclination of the lower incisors and mild intercanine expansion is possible to relieve crowding and may be reasonably stable
Depth of overbite and incisor inclinations	Overbite depth and *upper* incisor inclination determine the treatment approach: accepting or correcting the incisor relationship (Table 17.2). Traumatic overbite (palatal to upper incisors/labial to lower incisors with/without attrition; Figure 17.3) may require joint restorative/orthodontic management (Table 17.2)
Local factors	Impacted maxillary canines/absent or small upper lateral incisors will require orthodontic-oral surgical, orthodontic-restorative planning as appropriate

coordination following treatment, the upper incisors are proclined and where necessary the upper arch expanded slightly. A removable appliance or an anterior sectional fixed appliance may be required for the requisite movements. Where a twin block appliance is being used, springs may be included in the upper appliance, with step-wise mandibular advancement, thereby avoiding a separate preparatory phase.[14] Following correction of the incisor and molar relationships, detailing of the occlusion may be undertaken with fixed appliances, often on a non-extraction basis (Figure 17.5).

Retention, at least, until growth is complete is then advisable but indefinite lower labial segment retention may be warranted if any doubt exists about stability. Bonded retention may also be required to prevent rotational relapse of the maxillary lateral incisors.

Fixed Appliance Treatment

Where the skeletal pattern is milder, fixed appliances may be used to effect palatal/lingual root torque and/or proclination of the lower labial segment.[13] The latter is indicated,

Table 17.2 Methods of overbite reduction and means of altering the interincisal angle

Methods of overbite reduction	Means of altering the interincisal angle
Incisor intrusion by fixed appliances *(more 'relative' than actual intrusion as incisors held while vertical facial growth continues and molars are extruded)*. Utility arches produce some actual intrusion but also extrude molars	Incisor root torque *(palatal for uppers; lingual for lowers)* by fixed appliances
Lower incisor proclination by fixed appliances – requires careful planning *(upper removable appliance [URA] with a flat anterior bite plane allows some spontaneous lower incisor proclination if trapped behind upper labial segment)*	Lower labial segment proclination *(provided held lingually by upper labial segment)*
Molar eruption *(in a growing patient, flat anterior bite plane on URA or incisor capping on functional appliance retards lower incisor eruption and facilitates molar eruption; facial growth accommodates facial height increase)*	Upper labial segment proclination followed by functional appliance to correct overjet and buccal segment relationship
Molar extrusion *(by cervical pull headgear to upper molars; or intermaxillary elastics to upper/lower molars with a fixed appliance)*	Combination of any of above
Orthognathic surgery *(by mandibular advancement or lower labial segment set-down)*	Orthognathic surgery *(severe Class II with/ without reduced Frankfort-mandibular planes angle [FMPA])*
Restorative management *(if loss of posterior occlusal support: increase posterior occlusal vertical dimension; occlusal splint may be needed to reduce nocturnal bruxism; Dahl appliance for intrusion of lower incisors/lower molar eruption followed by palatal surface restorations of upper incisors)*	

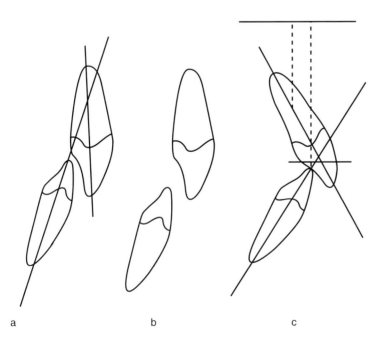

a   b   c

Figure 17.4 Diagrammatic representation of overbite reduction (a, b) and alteration of interincisal angle (c) required for correction of (a) Class II division 2 incisor relationship. (b) will revert to (a) after treatment as it is unstable. For maximal chances of overbite stability, the interincisal angle and the overbite must be reduced (c); the lower incisor edge to upper incisor centroid (midpoint of long axis of root) relationship should be corrected so that the centroid is at least 2 mm behind the lower incisor edge (c).

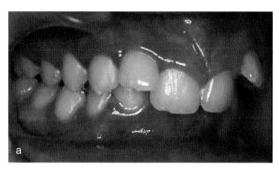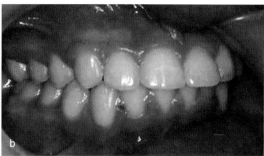

Figures 17.5 (a) Pretreatment intraoral photograph and (b) after treatment with functional appliances followed by non-extraction fixed appliance treatment.

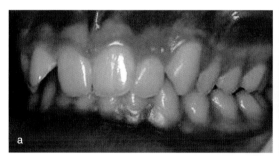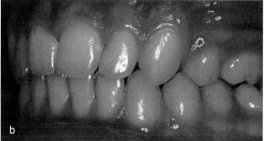

Figures 17.6 (a) Pretreatment intraoral photograph and (b) after fixed appliance treatment with extraction of upper first premolars.

sometimes in conjunction with interproximal stripping, where the lower arch exhibits mild to moderate crowding. Space required in the upper arch, for relief of crowding and correction of the incisor relationship, may be created by moving the buccal segments distally, with headgear, or with the aid of temporary anchorage devices (see Chapter 30); alternatively extraction of upper first premolars only with anchorage reinforcement may suffice accepting a full unit Class II molar relationship (Figure 17.6). Where crowding is more marked, extraction of upper first and lower second premolars, will is some, but not all cases be necessary. This extraction pattern favours mesial movement of lower molars, with minimal lower incisor retroclination, and upper incisor retraction with less mesial movement of upper molars (anchorage loss).

Currently, evidence is lacking as to the most effective means of treatment (by functional or fixed appliances).[15]

Surgical-orthodontic Treatment

In a non-growing patient, where the facial profile is poor due to a marked anteroposterior and/or vertical skeletal discrepancy, a combined surgical-orthodontic approach is best. Presurgically, a Class II division 1 malocclusion is created with the arches aligned and coordinated; the increased curve of Spee is maintained.[16] Following mandibular advancement for overjet correction, the lower buccal segment teeth are extruded to level the arch and close the lateral open bites. This approach, with molar extrusion, maximises the increase in the lower anterior face height. On occasion a reduction genioplasty may also be required to optimise the profile. Where the lower facial height is average or mildly increased, the overbite may be reduced by a lower labial segment set-down at the time of surgery.

RETENTION AND STABILITY

Rotational correction of the maxillary lateral incisors is prone to relapse.[17] Pericision (severing of the interdental and dentogingival fibres) prior to fixed appliance removal may help prevent this[18] but, as stability is not guaranteed, bonded palatal retention is advisable although this can be problematic if the overbite has not been fully reduced.

For the best prospect of stable overbite reduction, the interincisal angle must be reduced favourably (close to 135°) and the upper incisor centroid positioned at least 2 mm behind the lower incisor edge (see Figure 17.4) with a cingulum stop created on the upper incisors. The high lower lip line must also be eliminated to prevent relapse.[7] Post-treatment vertical facial growth contributes to stability of overbite correction[19] although the incisors tend to upright post retention.[17,19,20] To combat the forward (anticlockwise) pattern of mandibular growth rotation which tends to increase overbite, night-time wear of an upper removable retainer incorporating a flat anterior biteplane (to fit over the bonded retainer) is advised until growth has reduced to adult levels.

Excessive proclination of the lower incisors should be avoided during treatment as this is inherently unstable. Where the lower incisors have been proclined, long-term retention is likely to be required.[13]

ACKNOWLEDGEMENTS

The author thanks Mr John Brown and Ms Sadie Scott for their assistance with photographic material.

References

1. Foster TD, Day AJ. A survey of malocclusion and the need for orthodontic treatment in a Shropshire school population. Br J Orthod 1974;1:73–8.
2. Peck S, Peck L, Kataja M. Class II division 2 malocclusion: a heritable pattern of small teeth in well-developed jaws. Angle Orthod 1998;68:9–20.
3. Brezniak N, Arad A, Heller M, Dinbar A, Dinte A, Wasserstein A. Pathognomonic cephalometric characteristics of Angle Class II Division 2 malocclusion. Angle Orthod 2002;72:251–7.
4. Pancherz H, Zieber K, Hoyer B. Cephalometric characteristics of Class II division 1 and Class II division 2 malocclusions: a comparative study in children. Angle Orthod 1997;67:111–20.
5. Karlsen AT. Craniofacial characteristics in children with Angle Class II div.2 malocclusion combined with extreme deep bite. Angle Orthod 1994;64:123–30.
6. Isik F, Nalbantgil D, Sayinsu K, Arun T. A comparative study of cephalometric and arch width characteristics of Class II division 1 and division 2 malocclusions. Eur J Orthod 2006;28:179–83.
7. Lapatki BG, Klatt A, Schulte-Moenting J, Jonas IE. Dentofacial parameters explaining variability in retroclination of the maxillary central incisors. J Orofac Orthop 2007;68:109–23.
8. Lapatki BG, Mager AS, Schulte-Moenting J, Jonas IE. The importance of the level of the lip line and resting lip pressure in Class II division 2 malocclusion. J Dent Res 2002;81:323–8.
9. McIntyre GT, Millett DT. Lip shape and position in Class II division 2 malocclusion. Angle Orthod 2006;76:739–44.
10. McIntyre GT, Millett DT. Crown-root shape of the permanent maxillary central incisor. Angle Orthod 2003;73:710–15.
11. Al-Nimri K, Gharaibeh T. Space conditions and dental and occlusal features in patients

with palatally impacted maxillary canines: an aetiological study. Eur J Orthod 2005;27: 461–5.

12. Basdra EK, Kiokpasoglou M, Stellzig A. The Class II division 2 craniofacial type is associated with numerous congenital tooth anomalies. Eur J Orthod 2000;22: 529–35.

13. Selwyn-Barnett BJ. Class II division 2 malocclusion: a method of planning and treatment. Br J Orthod 1996;23:29–36.

14. Dyer FM, McKeown HF, Sandler PJ. The modified twin block appliance in the treatment of Class II division 2 malocclusions. J Orthod 2001;28:271–80.

15. Millett DT, Cunningham SJ, O'Brien KD, Benson P, Williams A, de Oliviera CM. Orthodontic treatment for deep bite and retroclined upper front teeth in children. Cochrane Database Syst Rev 2006;(4): CD005972.

16. Proffit WR, Sarver DM. Combined surgical and orthodontic treatment. In: Proffit WR,

Fields HW, Sarver DM. Contemporary Orthodontics. Mosby/Elsevier, St Louis, 2007:686–718.

17. Canut JA, Arias S. A long-term evaluation of treated Class II division 2 malocclusions: a retrospective study model analysis. Eur J Orthod 1999;21:377–86.

18. Edwards JG. A long-term prospective evaluation of the circumferential supracrestal fiberotomy in alleviating orthodontic relapse. Am J Orthod Dentofacial Orthop 1988;93:380–7.

19. Kim TW, Little RM. Postretention assessment of deep overbite in Class II division 2 malocclusion. Angle Orthod 1999;69: 175–86.

20. Devreese H, De Pauw G, van Maele G, Kuijpers-Jagtman AM, Dermaut L. Stability of upper incisor changes in Class II division 2 patients. Eur J Orthod 2007;29:314–20.

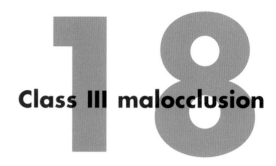

Class III malocclusion

INTRODUCTION

A Class III incisor relationship exists when the lower incisor edges occlude anterior to the cingulum plateau of the palatal surface of the upper incisors (Figure 18.1a; British Standards Classification). The overjet is reduced and may be reversed. The prevalence of Class III malocclusion in the UK is 3.2%.[1]

AETIOLOGY

Class III malocclusion can have a strong genetic predisposition and hence may run in families. Usually an anteroposterior Class III skeletal base relationship, due to maxillary retrusion and/or mandibular protrusion, accompanies a Class III malocclusion with a reduced or negative ANB angle (Figure 18.1b). Cases with increased Frankfort-mandibular planes angle (FMPA) and anterior open bite require more complex management than those with decreased vertical proportions, while bilateral buccal crossbites usually reflect a transverse maxillary deficiency.

The soft tissues encourage dentoalveolar compensation. The tongue proclines the maxillary incisors, while a strong lower lip retroclines the mandibular incisors to try to achieve incisor contact. Rarely, a Class III malocclusion may result from retroclined upper and lower incisors on a Class I skeletal base.[2]

ASSESSMENT

In addition to detailing the patient's concerns, it is important to question both the patient and their parents about the presence of skeletal disharmonies in any relatives as the patient may also exhibit the same at the completion of growth.

A comprehensive clinical examination should include extra- and intraoral components. The anteroposterior skeletal base relationship and the vertical facial proportions should be assessed with the patient in natural head position. Profile disharmonies (Figure 18.2) and any facial/dental asymmetries should be noted. To supplement the clinical examination, a lateral cephalogram should be analysed

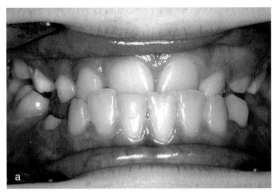
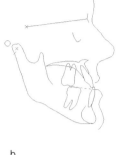

SKELETAL			SOFT TISSUES		
SNA	°	79.5	Lip Sep	mm	5.5
SNB	°	86.0	Exp UI	mm	4.0
ANB	°	-6.5	LS-E	mm	-10.0
SN/MxP	°	-0.5	LI-E	mm	-4.5
MxP/MnP	°	30.0	NLA	°	144.5
LAFH	mm	54.5	LLA	°	139.0
UAFH	mm	35.5	Holdaway	°	0.5
LAFH/TAFH	%	60.5			
LPFH	mm	30.0	NOSE PROMINENCE		
UPFH	mm	38.0	Nose tip	mm	20.0
PFH	mm	60.0	Nose angle	°	38.0
Wits	mm	-11.5			
TEETH			CHIN PROMINENCE		
Overjet	mm	-1.5	Chin tip	mm	10.5
Overbite	mm	0.5	B-NPo	mm	-2.5
UI/MxP	°	110.5	LADH	mm	31.5
LI/MnP	°	82.5			
IIangle	°	137.0			
LI-APo	mm	4.0			
LI-NPo	mm	0.5			

Figure 18.1 (a) Class III incisor relationship. (b) Lateral cephalometric analysis demonstrating Class III skeletal base relationship.

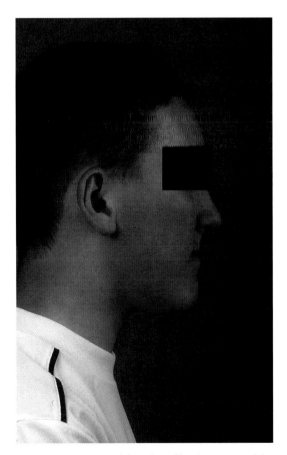

Figure 18.2 Typical facial profile characterised by a retrusive maxilla in a severe Class III malocclusion.

(Figure 18.1b),[3] which may support whether the case can be treated by orthodontics, or where orthognathic surgery is required.

Minimal or no overbite is a poor prognostic factor for orthodontic success. Conversely, a deep overbite is helpful in the retention of the corrected incisor relationship.

TREATMENT (TABLE 18.1)

Primary Dentition

There is no evidence to suggest that orthodontic intervention during the primary dentition avoids, or reduces, the complexity of later orthodontic treatment.

Early Mixed Dentition Treatment

Where permanent incisors erupt palatally to their predecessors, the retained primary teeth should be removed. Class III incisor relationships resulting from a premature contact and subsequent mandibular shift should also be treated early due to the association between childhood crossbites and adult temporomandibular joint dysfunction.[4] Frequently, the primary canines are the prematurely contacting

Table 18.1 Management of Class III malocclusion

Clinically	Management
Early mixed dentition	
Incisor crossbites	
Retained primary incisors	Extract retained primary teeth
Premature contact and mandibular displacement	Extract or grind cusp tips (usually primary canines)
	Procline maxillary permanent incisor(s) using an upper removable appliance (URA) or a fixed appliance
Late mixed dentition	
Proclined lower incisors	URA incorporating inverted labial bow
Class III incisors with deep overbite and mild/moderate skeletal Class III	Protraction headgear and rapid maxillary expansion
Early permanent dentition	
Mild/moderate skeletal discrepancy	Procline maxillary permanent incisors using URA/fixed appliance
– no concern about facial appearance	Camouflage skeletal pattern using fixed appliances
	Postpone treatment decision until skeletal growth completed
Severe skeletal discrepancy or a concern about facial appearance	Accept malocclusion will require combined orthodontic treatment/orthognathic surgery in adulthood
	Align maxillary arch with fixed appliance and relieve crowding, accepting Class III incisor relationship will require orthognathic surgery in adulthood
Adult treatment	
Mild/moderate skeletal discrepancy	Procline maxillary permanent incisors using URA/fixed appliance
– no concern about facial appearance	Camouflage skeletal pattern using fixed appliances
Severe skeletal discrepancy or a concern about facial appearance	Combined orthodontic treatment/orthognathic surgery

teeth requiring cuspal grinding or extraction. If the prematurely contacting teeth are permanent incisors, wear facets may occur. In this situation, the maxillary incisors should be proclined using an upper removable appliance (URA) incorporating 'Z'-springs (double coiled cantilever springs) or a screw-section if there is insufficient anterior retention (Figure 18.3). Posterior bite planes are required if the overbite is deep.

An alternative compliance-free solution useful for incisor rotations, is to use the '2 by 4' appliance.[2] Brackets are placed on the incisors and molars. Neighbouring primary teeth may need to be extracted for crowding. The teeth are levelled and aligned using nickel-titanium alloy wires. A stainless steel wire should then be placed with coil spring compressed buccally to procline the maxillary incisors (Figure 18.4). Success depends on the presence of an overbite

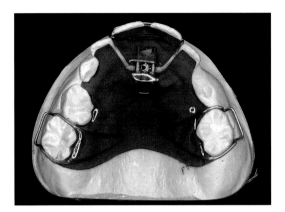

Figure 18.3 Upper removable appliance design commonly used to procline the maxillary incisors. A screw section has been used as there is insufficient anterior retention without clasping the permanent incisors.

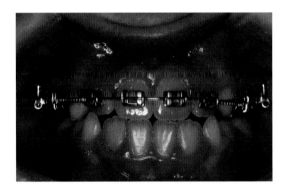

Figure 18.4 Mixed dentition Class III fixed appliance treatment.

for retention. A bonded retainer will be required for pretreatment rotations or spacing.

Mid-late Mixed Dentition Treatment

In Class III incisor relationships with retroclined maxillary and proclined mandibular incisors (no appreciable skeletal discrepancy), a URA incorporating an inverted labial bow will procline the maxillary incisors and retrocline the mandibular incisors (Figure 18.5). Retention

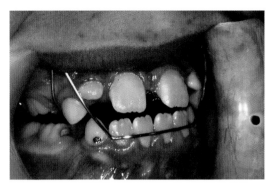

Figure 18.5 Inverted labial bow appliance.

must be excellent. Composite resin 'undercuts' may be required on the primary teeth. The inverted labial bow becomes active as the patient occludes. Retention may be necessary following correction of the incisor relationship. Treatment in cases with a reduced overbite or rotations should be postponed until the permanent dentition has established.

Growth modification in Class III malocclusion is unpredictable, particularly where mandibular and/or vertical excess is present.[5] The Functional Regulator III and chin-cup appliances were historically used in the pubertal Class III patient. However, their long-term results have been disappointing.[6] More recently the Class III twin block appliance has been proposed.[7]

It is currently accepted that the most appropriate treatment for patients with a retrusive maxilla in the late mixed dentition stage involves protraction headgear (Figure 18.6) to apply orthopaedic forces.[8] To maximise the skeletal change, simultaneous rapid maxillary expansion (RME) has been suggested.[9]

Orthodontic Treatment in the Permanent Dentition

Comprehensive orthodontic treatment in the permanent dentition aims to camouflage the underlying skeletal discrepancy with dental movements. Several prognostic factors will

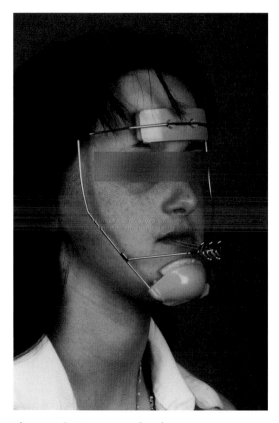

Figure 18.6 Protraction headgear.

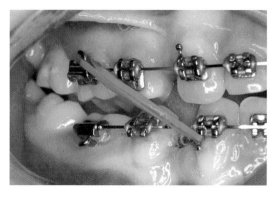

Figure 18.7 Class III intermaxillary traction applied to fixed appliances

> **Box 18.1** Favourable prognostic factors for Class III orthodontic camouflage
>
> • Patient past peak skeletal growth
> • No pre-existing dentoalveolar compensation
> • The ability to achieve an edge-to-edge incisor relationship
> • Adequate overbite with a normal or slightly reduced lower facial height.
> • Mild/moderate skeletal Class III relationship: ANB angle greater than 0°
> • Once crowding and mandibular displacements corrected, molar relationship less than half unit Class III

influence the success or failure of Class III camouflage treatment (Box 18.1).

The clinician should identify severe underlying skeletal discrepancies where orthodontic camouflage would fail. Moreover, the clinician must be confident that any expected skeletal growth (principally mandibular) will not affect treatment. Pretreatment dentoalveolar compensation limits this although anterior mandibular displacements arising from premature contacts are favourable. Mild Class III skeletal discrepancies can be treated by proclination of the maxillary incisors using removable or fixed appliances (described above). A positive overbite usually provides adequate retention. In moderate skeletal Class III discrepancies, proclination of the upper incisors produces an unstable result. Active lower incisor retroclination is required necessitating a lower fixed appliance. Where crowding is present, mandibular arch extractions are usually required – frequently the first premolars (Figure 18.7). In the maxillary arch, proclination of the incisors may give sufficient space to relieve the crowding and where transverse arch expansion is required for the correction of crossbites, this will also produce space for relief of crowding (see Chapter 10). However, crowding may necessitate the extraction of maxillary premolars – commonly the second premolars but the first premolars may be extracted if crowding is severe (e.g. excluded canines). Class III inter-maxillary elastics (Figure 18.7) are usually required to retrocline the mandibular incisors and maintain the position of the upper incisors during space closure. Removable retainers may need to be augmented with bonded retainers for teeth with pretreatment rotations/spacing.

For moderate Class III skeletal discrepancies, particularly where the lower face height is reduced, the outcome of camouflage treatment will result in compromised aesthetics. Conversely, where the overbite is reduced or an anterior open bite is present, long-term stability is doubtful. Cases with vertical skeletal discrepancies are best treated using a combination of orthodontic treatment and orthognathic surgery (see Chapter 25).

If orthognathic surgery is planned later to correct the underlying Class III discrepancy, the maxillary arch can be aligned during adolescence if the patient is sufficiently concerned about crowding at this stage. Extractions may be required for the relief of crowding.

Borderline Camouflage/ Orthognathic Surgery Patients

These patients present treatment planning challenges because of the difficulties in determining when patients cease facial growth. A single cephalometric image is of little use in the prediction of facial growth.[10] Hand-wrist radiographs to assess 'bone age' are not justified in growth prediction[11] since they are no more accurate than the patient's chronological age. Information such as a change in height and shoe size over a year can aid decision-making as can the magnitude of skeletal discrepancy present in parents or older siblings. For patients approaching the limits of Class III camouflage treatment, orthodontic camouflage should be deferred until the remaining skeletal growth has been expressed.

Combined Orthodontic/ Orthognathic Surgery Treatment

In cases with moderate or severe Class III anteroposterior skeletal discrepancies, and where a vertical or transverse skeletal discrepancy is present, a combination of orthodontic treatment and orthognathic surgery at the completion of skeletal growth will be required. Planning should involve the patient, orthodontist and surgeon integrating the findings from the clinical examination, study model analysis and cephalometric prediction. Presurgical orthodontic treatment usually involves fixed appliances to align the maxillary and mandibular arches, in order that they subsequently coordinate (see Chapter 25). This necessitates both alignment and 'decompensation' of the axial inclination of the incisors (Figure 18.8). Thus the maxillary incisors are retroclined and the mandibular incisors are proclined to approximately 109° and 90° to the maxillary and mandibular planes respectively. A period of orthodontic finishing is usually required after surgery to detail the occlusion.

Patients present for combined orthodontic/ orthognathic treatment in adulthood, where adolescent management failed to account

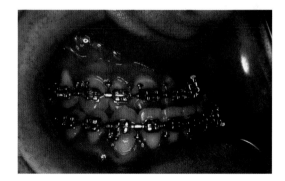

Figure 18.8 Decompensated incisors in preparation for orthognathic surgery – note the interdental hooks that have been placed in preparation for the operation.

adequately for the underlying skeletal discrepancy, or where late growth was particularly unfavourable. Where mandibular arch extractions have been undertaken during previous orthodontic treatment, orthodontic decompensation is more difficult, and it is seldom possible to fully decompensate the mandibular arch without reopening of the extraction space. This is why lower arch extractions should be undertaken with extreme caution if treatment is attempted during adolescence.

Adult Treatment

A pseudo-Class III malocclusion may result from loss of posterior tooth support and mandibular overclosure. The primary treatment objective in these patients is prosthodontic rehabilitation to prevent the overclosure.

Class III adult camouflage can be successful where the skeletal discrepancy is mild and an adequate overbite exists. Although adult patients are often more committed to orthodontic treatment than adolescents, their tolerance with appliance therapy is reduced. Previous orthodontic treatment, the presence of restorations, and missing teeth also complicate adult orthodontic treatment (Figure 18.9).

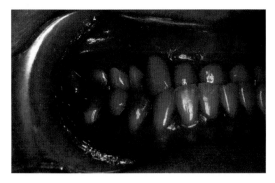

Figure 18.9 Pretreatment view of an adult Class III malocclusion. Treatment will be complicated by the number and type of restorations.

Stability

The stability of anterior crossbite correction is greatly facilitated by achieving a positive overbite at the completion of orthodontic treatment. Continuing mandibular growth in adolescence may also be a significant factor contributing to relapse.

ACKNOWLEDGEMENT

The cephalometric analysis in Figure 18.1b was produced using Opal (Orthognathic Planning and Analysis, www.cix.co.uk/~felix/Opal/).

References

1. Foster TD, Day AJ. A survey of malocclusion and the need for orthodontic treatment in a Shropshire school population. Br J Orthod 1974;1:73–8.
2. Skeggs RM, Sandler PJ. Rapid correction of anterior crossbite using a fixed appliance: a case report. Dent Update 2002;29:299–302.
3. Isaacson KG, Thom AR (eds) Orthodontic Radiographs: Guidelines, 3rd edn. British Orthodontic Society, London, 2008:13.
4. Thilander B, Rubio G, Pena L, de Mayorga C. Prevalence of temporomandibular dysfunction and its association with malocclusion in children and adolescents: an epidemiologic study related to specified stages of dental development. Angle Orthod 2002;72:146–54.
5. Kluemper GT, Spalding PM. Realities of craniofacial growth modification. Atlas Oral Maxillofac Surg Clin North Am 2001;9:23–51.
6. Sugawara J, Mitani H. Facial growth of skeletal Class III malocclusion and the effects, limitations, and long-term dentofacial adaptations to chincap therapy. Semin Orthod 1997;3:244–54.
7. Kidner G, DiBiase A, DiBiase D. Class III twin blocks: a case series. J Orthod 2003;30:197–201.

8. Macey-Dare LV. The early management of Class III malocclusions using protraction headgear. Dent Update 2000;27:508–13.
9. Kim JH, Viana MA, Graber TM, Omerza FF, BeGole EA. The effectiveness of protraction face mask therapy: a meta-analysis. Am J Orthod Dentofacial Orthop 1999;115: 675–85.
10. Houston WJ. The current status of facial growth predictions: a review. Br J Orthod 1979;6:11–17.
11. Houston WJ, Miller JC, Tanner JM. Prediction of the timing of the adolescent growth spurt from ossification events in hand-wrist films. Br J Orthod 1979;6: 145–52.

19
Facial asymmetry

INTRODUCTION

Symmetry is defined as correspondence in size, shape and relative position of parts on opposite sides of a dividing line or median plane. Asymmetry is described as a lack or absence of symmetry. The facial midline is usually taken as the dividing line of the face and is a line passing through soft tissue nasion and the midpoint of the upper lip.

A degree of facial asymmetry is normal and acceptable within the face.[1] It can be caused by an asymmetry in the facial skeleton and/or overlying soft tissue drape. The point at which an asymmetry becomes unacceptable is when an individual begins to experience aesthetic concerns and/or functional limitations. Although asymmetries can occur at many levels of the face, this chapter will focus on developmental asymmetries affecting the mandible and maxilla as these are most relevant to the dental profession. Table 19.1 provides a classification of facial asymmetries.

DEVELOPMENTAL CAUSES

Hemi-mandibular Elongation and Hyperplasia

Hemi-mandibular elongation was first described by Obwegeser and Makek[2] and is a developmental deformity of unknown aetiology affecting the mandible. It presents with a progressively increasing transverse displacement of the chin, away from the affected side, which usually becomes apparent during or after the adolescent growth spurt (Figure 19.1a,b). The mandibular dentition follows the skeletal displacement which predisposes to buccal crossbite and centreline displacement away from the affected side and a scissor bite on the affected side. Since there is a *minimal* vertical component to the abnormal growth pattern, there is typically no overeruption of the maxillary dentition on the affected side. Radiographically, there is clear elongation of the affected side of the mandible, principally located in the condylar region and the body of the mandible (Figure 19.1b).

Orthodontics: Principles and Practice, First Edition. Edited by Daljit S. Gill, Farhad B. Naini.
© 2011 Daljit S. Gill, Farhad B. Naini and Dental Update. Published 2011 by Blackwell Publishing Ltd.

Table 19.1 A classification of facial asymmetry

Cause	Examples
Developmental	Hemi-mandibular elongation
	Hemi-mandibular hyperplasia
	Hemifacial microsomia
	Hemifacial hypertrophy
	Torticollis
	Hemifacial atrophy (Parry–Romberg syndrome)
Pathological	Tumours and cysts
	Infection
	Condylar resorption
	Condylar fractures
Traumatic	Post irradiation
Functional	Mandibular displacement

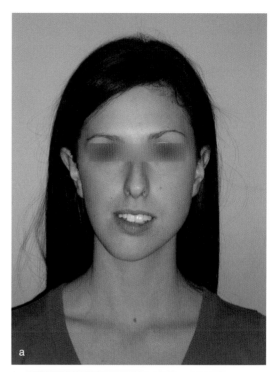

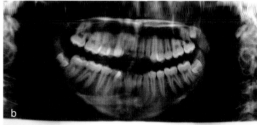

Figure 19.1a,b A case of left-sided hemi-mandibular elongation with the corresponding dental panoramic tomograph.

In contrast, hemi-mandibular hyperplasia presents with a three-dimensional enlargement of one side of the mandible during adolescence (Figure 19.2). As a consequence of the vertical component of abnormal growth, there is an increase in height on the affected side of the face, the dentition on that side overerupts to maintain occlusal contact, with a resultant cant in the maxillary occlusal plane and an increase in alveolar height above the inferior dental canal, and the face develops a twisted appearance. If abnormal growth is rapid, a lateral open bite may develop on the affected side as the rate of eruption is outpaced by the rate of vertical skeletal growth. Radiographically, a panoramic tomogram will show that the ascending ramus is elongated vertically with enlargement of the condyle (Figure 19.2b). There is also an elongation and thickening of the condylar neck. The angle of the mandible is rounded, while the lower border is bowed downwards to a lower level compared with the opposite side. There is an increase in the height of the mandibular body, which appears to increase the distance between the molar roots and the mandibular canal. The unaffected side appears to have a normal height. This growth defect is clearly demarcated by the symphysis (Figure 19.2b).

Hybrid forms of hemi-mandibular elongation and hyperplasia exist where the patient exhibits features of both conditions. The

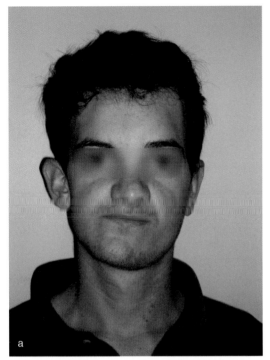

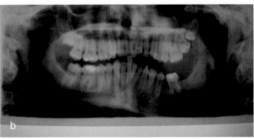

Figure 19.2a,b A case of left-sided hemi-mandibular hyperplasia with the corresponding dental panoramic tomograph.

differences between the two conditions are summarised in Table 19.2.

Hemifacial Microsomia

Hemifacial microsomia is a congenital disorder, with a prevalence of 1 in 5000 births, that occurs unilaterally in the majority (80%) of cases. The condition is caused by a defect in proliferation and migration of neural crest cells and results

Table 19.2 Comparison of hemi-mandibular elongation and hyperplasia

Hemi-mandibular elongation	Hemi-mandibular hyperplasia
Unilateral horizontal enlargement of mandible	Unilateral three-dimensional enlargement of mandible
Transverse displacement of chin point	Vertical displacement of chin and mandible. Chin may be rotated
No transverse canting of maxillary occlusal plane	Transverse canting of maxillary occlusal plane
Normal alveolar bone height above inferior dental canal on affected side	Increased alveolar bone height above the inferior dental canal on affected side

in a deficiency of hard and soft tissue structures derived from the first and second branchial arches, however, the first branchial arch structures are primarily affected (Table 19.3).

There is commonly under-development of the temporomandibular joint, mandibular ramus, masticatory muscles and ears on the affected side(s) (Figure 19.3). In severe cases, the mandibular condyles and ramus may completely fail to develop. Because of reduced vertical growth, there is often undereruption on the affected side with a resultant cant in the maxillary occlusal plane. Owing to the association of the specific cranial nerves with the branchial arches, varying degrees of nerve palsy (especially in the facial nerve [cranial nerve VII]) may be exhibited. Numerous classification systems have been proposed for hemifacial microsomia but the Pruzansky and OMENS classifications appear to be the most popular.[3]

PATHOLOGICAL CAUSES

A number of pathological conditions can result in facial asymmetry, but these are out of the scope of this book (the reader is referred to

Table 19.3 The derivatives of the first and second branchial arches

Branchial arch	Derivatives
First branchial arch	Meckel's cartilage (malleus, anterior ligament of malleus, sphenomandibular ligament), mandible, incus
	From the pouch: auditory tube, middle ear cavity, tympanic membrane and external auditory meatus
	Maxillary and mandibular divisions of the trigeminal nerve (V)
Second branchial arch	Reichert's cartilage (stapes, styloid process, stylohyoid ligament, lesser cornu and body of the hyoid bone)
	Facial cranial nerve (VII)

textbooks of oral pathology). A rare pathologi cal cause of particular interest to orthodontists is condylar resorption. Condylar resorption can occur following traumatic injuries, use of steroids, in connective tissue diseases (e.g. rheumatoid arthritis, scleroderma, systemic lupus erythematosus) and following orthognathic surgery.[4] If one condyle is affected more than the other, there is often a unilateral shift of the chin point to the side of greater resorption. If both condyles are affected, the patient may present with a progressively increasing anterior open bite ± asymmetry. Treatment should only be considered once the primary pathology has been stabilised and should avoid ramus surgery as there is a risk of retriggering the primary pathology. Treatment can often be undertaken with genioplasty alone ± maxillary surgery.

FUNCTIONAL CAUSES

A lateral mandibular displacement, due to an occlusal interference, can be the cause of a mandibular dental centreline shift and displace-

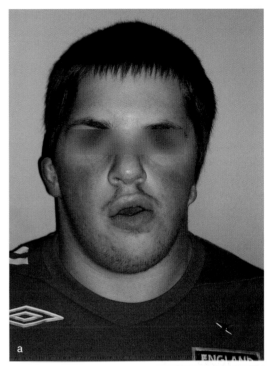
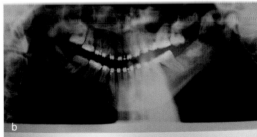

Figure 19,3a,b A case of left-sided hemifacial microsomia with the corresponding dental panoramic tomograph.

ment of the chin point. Treatment in such cases should be directed at removing the occlusal interference.

MANAGEMENT OF ASYMMETRIES

Before treating asymmetries of developmental origin it is important to ensure that the abnormal growth pattern has ceased. This can be achieved by comparing serial study models (with accurate bite registrations), sequential photographs and three-dimensional soft tissue facial scans. Some clinicians undertake technetium 90m isotope scans to determine if the condyle is actively growing but the results can be unreliable. Ideally, there should be no change between serial records taken at least 6 months apart before commencing treatment. Imaging techniques used to assess asymmetries include conventional radiographs (panoramic tomogram, lateral/posteroanterior cephalogram), three-dimensional computed tomography (CT) and laser scanning or stereophotogrammetry.

The panoramic radiograph allows a comparison of the shape of the mandibular rami and condyles bilaterally. It also provides an overview of the dental and bony structures of the mandible, providing information regarding pathology, the number of teeth and any other hard tissue anomalies. However, there can be distortions in different areas of the image.[5] Three-dimensional CT overcomes these problems but is associated with increased radiation doses. Cone-beam CT may be a useful alternative technique as radiation doses are reduced compared with conventional CT scanning.[6] Surface soft tissue laser scanning (Figure 19.4) or stereophotogrammetry can provide a useful technique for comparing sequential scans for growth changes and these techniques allow quantitative assessment of facial asymmetry by techniques such as flip registration.[7]

Treatment planning should involve a joint orthodontic-orthognathic team approach (see Chapter 25). Patients with hemifacial microsomia, or any other craniofacial abnormalities, should be managed by dedicated craniofacial teams. Currently within the UK there are such centres at Great Ormond Street Hospital (children's services) and University College London (UCL) Eastman Dental Hospital (adult services), Oxford, Birmingham and Liverpool. These services are centrally funded through the

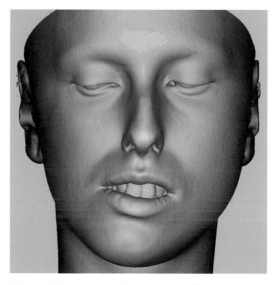

Figure 19.4 A three-dimensional surface laser scan used to monitor facial growth.

National Commissioning Group (NCG) of the Department of Health.

Where a developmental asymmetry is identified at a young age that is due to undergrowth of one side (e.g. hemifacial microsomia), a hybrid functional appliance can be used to maximise growth on the affected side (Figure 19.5). Such appliances may create a more favourable environment to encourage growth of the deficient condyle, although there is no strong evidence to support this, and also help to level any maxillary cant by selective molar eruption. This can simplify later surgical treatment but requires considerable compliance.

Patients with severe asymmetries (e.g. hemifacial microsomia) who are experiencing aesthetic and functional problems may be treated at a young age (5–8 years) with distraction osteogenesis or a costochondral bone graft if there is complete absence of a condyle (e.g. hemifacial microsomia). This will provide a temporary measure, as the abnormal growth pattern will continue, and finite correction can be undertaken at the completion of growth.

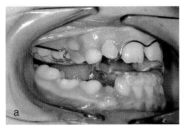 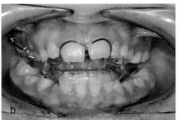 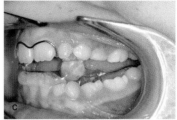

Figure 19.5a–c An example of a hybrid functional appliance used to maximise the growth potential of the deficient side. Photographs courtesy of Catherine Campbell, John Radcliffe Hospital, Oxford.

In severe cases of hemi-mandibular elongation and hyperplasia, it may be necessary to consider abolishing the abnormal growth pattern during adolescence.[8] This will involve condylar shaving where the abnormal cartilaginous growth site is removed. Patients may require later surgery for finite correction. Final treatment is undertaken at the end of growth using a comprehensive orthodontic-orthognathic approach. After joint planning, this will involve orthodontic decompensation followed by surgery to correct the underlying skeletal asymmetry. Surgery will often involve a bilateral sagittal split osteotomy with asymmetrical moves ± a Le Fort 1 maxillary procedure to correct any cant in the maxillary occlusal plane.

Often patients with an asymmetry in the chin point will also have asymmetries in other regions of the face (e.g. nose). In such cases it is important for informed consent purposes to make the patient aware that their attention may be diverted towards these once the primary focus, the chin point, has been normalised. It is important that patients understand that a degree of facial asymmetry is normal and that it is not possible to make the face completely symmetrical.

Once the underlying skeletal asymmetry has been treated it may be necessary to undertake secondary surgical procedures to further correct any underlying hard or soft tissue deficiency/ excesses. Mild soft tissue deficiencies can be masked by autologous fat transfer[9] whereas more major defects may require free flap transfer. In cases of hemi-mandibular hyperplasia, it may be necessary to undertake lower mandibular border recontouring to help compensate for excessive vertical growth of the mandible.

CONCLUSION

A degree of asymmetry is normal in most individuals. There are numerous causes of severe facial asymmetry. The origin of the asymmetry may lie in undergrowth/overgrowth of the facial skeletal and/or soft tissue drape. Treatment should only commence once the abnormal growth pattern has stabilised in the majority of cases and should occur within a multidisciplinary setting. Patients should be made aware at the outset that it is not possible to make the face completely symmetrical. A general principle of the management of complex facial asymmetry is correction of the underlying skeletal asymmetry first followed by reassessment and correction of the soft tissue asymmetry.

References

1. Haraguchi S, Iguchi Y, Takada K. Asymmetry of the facia in orthodontic patients. Angle Orthod 2008;78(3):421–6.
2. Obwegeser HL, Makek MS. Hemimandibular hyperplasia – hemimandibular elongation. J Maxillofac Surg 1986;14:183–208.

3. Rodgers SF, Eppley BL, Nelson CL, Sadove AM. Hemifacial microsomia: assessment of classification systems. J Craniofac Surg 1991; 2(3):114–26.

4. Gill DS, El Maaytah M, Naini FB. Risk factors for post-orthognathic condylar resorption: a review. World J Orthod 2008;9(1):21–5.

5. Van Elslande DC, Russett SJ, Major PW, Flores-Mir C. Mandibular asymmetry diagnosis with panoramic imaging. Am J Orthod Dentofacial Orthop 2008;134(2):183–92.

6. Schulze D, Heiland M, Thurmann H, Adam C. Radiation exposure during midfacial imaging using 4- and 16-slice computed tomography, cone beam computed tomogra-phy systems and conventional radiography. Dentomaxillofac Radiol 2004;33(2):83–6.

7. Yu Z, Mu X, Feng S, Han J, Chang T. Flip-registration procedure of three-dimensional laser surface scanning images on quantita-tive evaluation of facial asymmetries. J Craniofac Surg 2009;20(1):157–60.

8. Wolford LM, Mehra P, Reiche-Fischel O, Morales-Ryan CA, García-Morales P. Efficacy of high condylectomy for management of condylar hyperplasia. Am J Orthod Dentofacial Orthop 2002;121(2):136–50; dis-cussion 150–1.

9. Coleman SR. Facial recontouring with lipo-structure. Clin Plast Surg 1997;24(2):347–67.

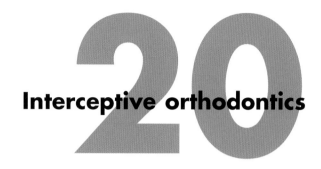

Interceptive orthodontics

INTRODUCTION

A pleasing smile is extremely important for psychological well-being. There are a number of goals that we should be aiming for when we consider dental attractiveness such as symmetry, alignment, the smile line, dental arch shape and gingival contour as well as the quality and the morphology of the dental tissue itself.

Orthodontic management of the developing dentition is important to ensure that the established dentition is in the most functional and aesthetic position. Orthodontics requires great understanding of facial and dental growth and the effects of occlusal guidance. It has been commonplace for patients to be referred to an orthodontist once the secondary dentition has established. This practice has allowed many mild problems to become significantly worse and ultimately more difficult to correct. For these reasons general dental practitioners must consider early referral to a specialist orthodontist.

This chapter aims to outline some interceptive measures that will reduce or eliminate malocclusion in the growing patient that can be carried out in the primary care setting under the guidance of an orthodontist.

WHAT DO WE KNOW ABOUT GROWTH?

We know that there is continued facial growth from birth to adulthood and we have an understanding of the average rate and direction of growth and the presence of growth rotations (Figure 20.1).[1,2] We have some understanding of the role of the facial muscles and the influence environmental factors have on the dentition but cannot reliably predict the timing of growth or the ultimate amount of growth for any individual until it is almost at an end. In addition we are aware that the soft tissue balance between the tongue and the lips and cheeks changes over time but again cannot rely on prediction to accurately inform us of the influences that these may have on the dental arch.

THUMB/FINGER SUCKING

Thumb/finger sucking can cause significant distortion of the dental arches (Figure 20.2).

Orthodontics: Principles and Practice, First Edition. Edited by Daljit S. Gill, Farhad B. Naini.
© 2011 Daljit S. Gill, Farhad B. Naini and Dental Update. Published 2011 by Blackwell Publishing Ltd.

Many 7 year olds suck their thumb and although dental displacement is not present in all cases it is important to review the dental development, particularly of the upper incisors.[3,4] There are a number of options to intercept the distortion effects of a digit habit but young children are rarely able to cope with appliance treatment

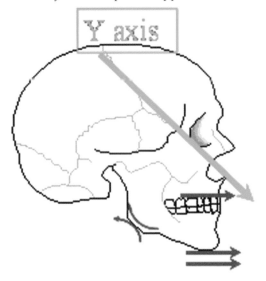

Figure 20.1 There is downwards and forwards growth of the facial skeleton, in relationship to the cranial base, with normal facial growth and development. The mandible, in particular, also rotates during this translation.

before the age of 6 years. Cognitive behavioural management with reward charts is effective at rewarding 'good' behaviour and is the interceptive measure of choice in the younger patient. Appliances or simple measures such as nail paint or putting gloves on can be used to deter the habit in the older patient, although it must be remembered that anything removable can easily be removed at times when the urge to suck a digit is at its greatest and is therefore best used for those who actively want to give up. Appliance wear can not only deter the habit but also have adjunctive effects such as arch expansion or overbite control.

The only true deterrent appliance, however, is the fixed thumb guard (Figures 20.3, 20.4). These appliances ensure full compliance (as they cannot be removed) and are well tolerated. They should be left *in situ* for at least 6 months to ensure the habit is broken. Fixed orthodontic expansion appliances such as a quadhelix can also be used so that arch expansion can be incorporated, but these are not as effective as a thumb guard as they are less obstructive to a thumb or digit being placed into the mouth. For patients who have a significant sagittal discrepancy a functional appliance, such as the twin block appliance, can be used to combine a deterrent with Class II correction.

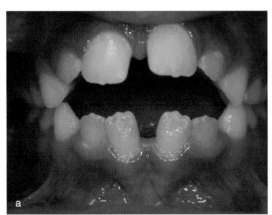
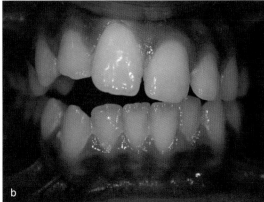

Figure 20.2a,b Examples of the effects of digit sucking on the developing occlusion.

CROSSBITES

Anterior crossbites (Figure 20.5a) should be treated early to avoid periodontal damage such as fenestration of the lower labial plate due to incisor displacement, toothwear due to abnor-

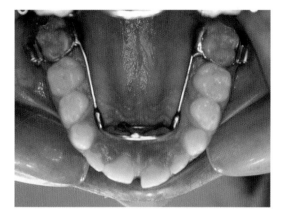

Figure 20.3 A fixed thumb guard *in situ*.

mal contact or mandibular displacement and the potential for temporomandibular joint (TMJ) dysfunction. An increase in arch circumference can also help to increase space within the arch for the developing dentition. It is important to remember that the correction of anterior crossbites needs bite opening to avoid compensatory movement of the opposing teeth.

Posterior expansion, for the correction of a posterior crossbite (Figure 20.5b) is a more contentious subject. There is little evidence to confirm that early expansion in the absence of a crossbite will create an environment for the permanent teeth to develop into an improved arch form with greater stability. However, if there is a mandibular displacement with the crossbite, expansion is indicated and can have the added potential (in cases with mild crowding) of eliminating the need for extractions in the permanent dentition by producing a symmetrical and correct arch form (Figure 20.6).

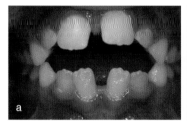
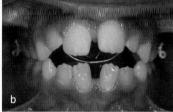
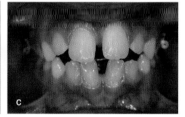

Figure 20.4 Spontaneous improvement of an anterior open bite after fitting a fixed thumb guard appliance. (a) Start; (b) 3 months; (c) 6 months.

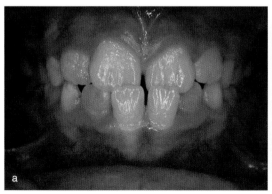
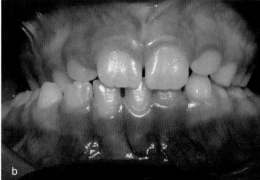

Figure 20.5 An example of (a) anterior and (b) posterior crossbite.

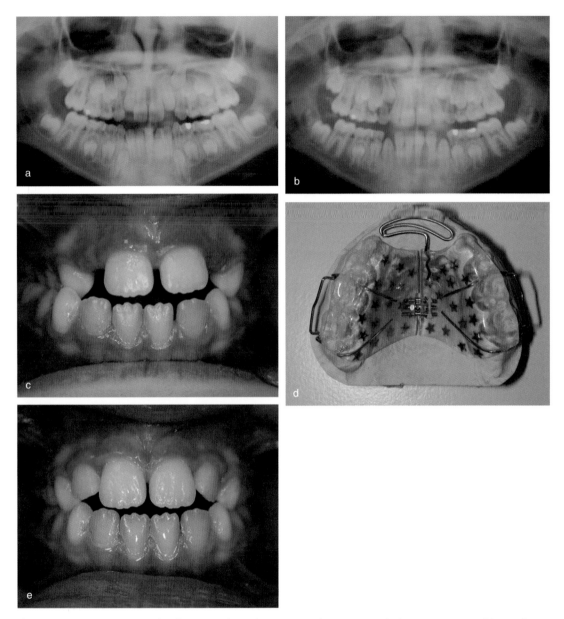

Figure 20.6a–e An example of a case where the upper arch was expanded, using a removable appliance (shown), to correct a posterior crossbite, associated with a mandibular displacement, and to create space for the relief of mild maxillary crowding.

ANTERIOR CROWDING

Early extraction of the primary canines to create space to guide the eruption of the permanent incisors has also been the source of much debate with little evidence base. In cases where the permanent lateral incisors are short of space and are either rotated or displaced palatally there are a number of benefits to the extraction of the primary canines (Figure 20.7). Space is

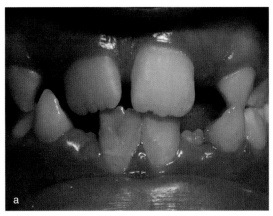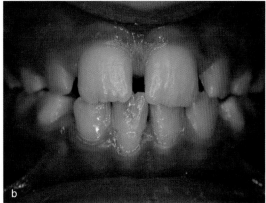

Figure 20.7 (a) There is a potential lack of space for eruption of the maxillary lateral incisors. (b) Early loss of the maxillary primary canines has provided the required space to allow the lateral incisors to erupt into a good position.

created for the permanent incisors to erupt without rotations, leading to better aesthetics and the potential for less post-orthodontic relapse as it can be postulated that if the incisors are not rotated at the start of treatment the periodontal fibres will not need to realign at the end of orthodontic tooth movement.

Early extraction of primary canines is also indicated if one primary canine is lost early, to prevent a centreline shift (balancing extractions). For the best outcome the teeth should be removed before the permanent lateral incisors have erupted to avoid any unwanted displacement.

SERIAL EXTRACTION – A MODERN APPROACH

Serial extraction was introduced in the 1940s to guide the developing dentition at a time when orthodontic appliances did not easily allow precise control of tooth movement. Its practice fell out of favour with the introduction of sophisticated fixed appliance systems in the 1970s. More recently due to the demand for higher aesthetic standards, particularly during the developing dentition phase, and as our understanding of interceptive tooth guidance improves it has been reintroduced by some clinicians.

The modern approach includes the removal of the primary canines to allow the incisors to align as the lateral incisors are erupting (7/8 years) followed by a period of occlusal monitoring (Figures 20.8, 20.9). As the first premolars erupt (10 years) the position of the permanent canines is assessed and if crowding is present the first premolars should be removed to allow the unimpeded development of the canines and second premolars into the line of the dental arch (Figure 20.10). The occlusion can be reassessed once the permanent dentition has established and fixed appliances can be used to idealise the alignment (Figure 20.11). This approach uses the natural eruptive potential of the teeth to improve tooth position rather than allowing teeth to move ectopically before orthodontic treatment. This can significantly shorten the active orthodontic treatment time. In cases where there is a skeletal element to the malocclusion, serial extraction can be combined with sagittal correction with headgear of functional appliances.

THE UNERUPTED CENTRAL INCISOR

If the eruption of one central incisor is more than 6 months delayed with respect to the

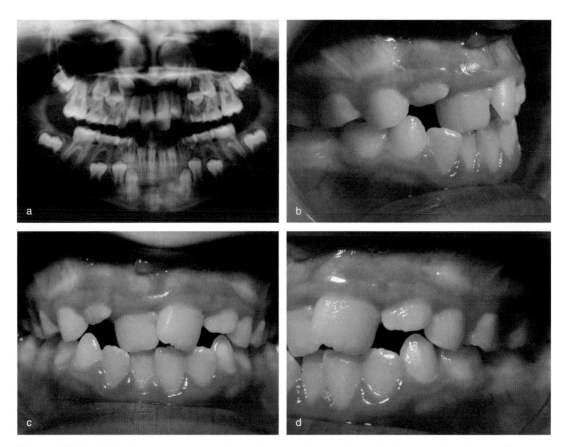

Figure 20.8a–d Serial extraction start: A class I case with crowding developing within the maxillary arch.

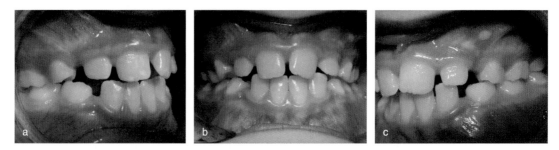

Figure 20.9a–c Serial extraction: 6 months after canine extraction. The primary maxillary canines were extracted to allow spontaneous alignment of the maxillary incisors.

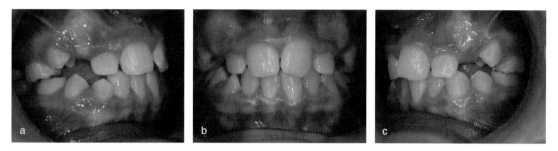

Figure 20.10a–c Serial extraction: first premolars erupted and ready for extraction. During follow-up it was noted that there was a lack of space for the developing maxillary canines. The decision was made to extract the first premolars to allow the canines to erupt into a good position.

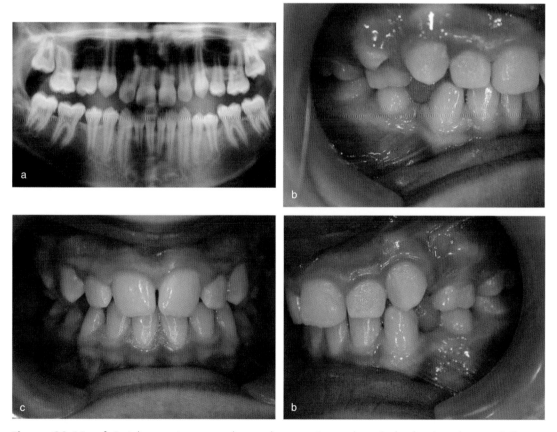

Figure 20.11a–d Serial extraction: second premolars erupting and ready for fixed appliances. Following eruption of the permanent dentition it was decided that a fixed appliance could be used to detail tooth position.

other, or the maxillary lateral incisor has erupted before the central incisor, it is important to take radiographs to assess the position of the missing central incisor.[5] The most common cause of delayed eruption is the presence of a supernumerary tooth (Figure 20.12).[6] After removal of the obstruction, 68% of incisors have been shown to erupt spontaneously (if there is sufficient space in the arch) within 12 months.[7] It is common practice, however, to bond a gold chain to the unerupted tooth at the time of the surgical intervention to ensure a second procedure is avoided if there is not spontaneous eruption. A number of clinicians have employed autotransplantation as a way of restoring the tooth, as moving a lateral incisor into a central incisor space is not aesthetic due to the difficulty of gaining good gingival margin aesthetics.[8] Nowadays, due to the success of single tooth implants, however, this practice is not so popular.

INFRAOCCLUSION OF PRIMARY LOWER SECOND MOLARS

Infraocclusion occurs as a result of ankylosis where there is fusion between cementum and alveolar bone (Figure 20.13). This results in a failure of eruption of an ankylosed tooth giving rise to infraocclusion as neighbouring teeth continue to develop vertically. The evidence for the management of infraoccluded teeth is limited. Ericson and Kurol's guidance is that if there is a successor they usually exfoliate naturally although with some delay. However, the teeth should be extracted if there is space loss or if they are below the gingival level, to avoid periodontal problems.[9–11]

FUSION, GEMINATION AND MORPHOLOGY ISSUES

Gemination is an incomplete splitting of a dental germ resulting in a wide tooth, and

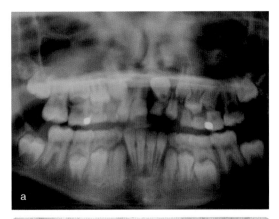

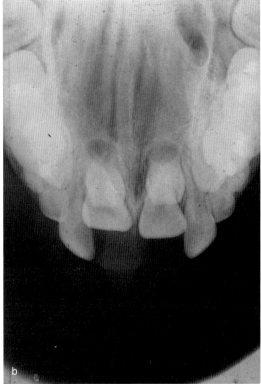

Figure 20.12a,b Radiographic examples of impacted incisors associated with supernumerary teeth.

fusion is merger of two germs that produces a large tooth (Figure 20.14). These anomalies are best managed early if possible to ensure that there is as little disruption of the developing dentition as possible. Reducing the width of

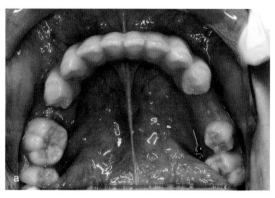

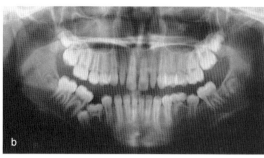

Figure 20.13a,b An example of significant infraocclusion of the lower right second primary molar.

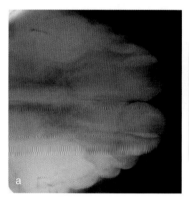

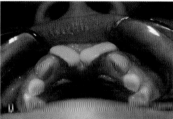

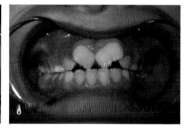

Figure 20.14a,b An example of gemination of the upper left permanent central incisor.

teeth should be attempted only if a limited amount of reduction is needed. The size of the root and pulp chamber is critical in deciding if the tooth will eventually be kept. Fused or geminated teeth often cause space inadequacy and rarely do well if they are sectioned as the periodontal tissues are compromised. Careful planning considering the malocclusion as a whole must be undertaken and if a tooth is removed early the dental centreline and space maintenance must be considered.

SOFT TISSUES

A large upper labial frenum can cause a median diastema and can be traumatised with tooth brushing or eating. As part of a long-term orthodontic plan a prominent labial frenum is often removed if large or if there are attachments of the fibres into the incisive foramen. There is little agreement whether it is better to remove the frenum before or after orthodontic treatment. On one hand it is difficult to remove all the tissue if the upper incisors are together but if the frenum is removed early with the incisors apart it is suggested that scar tissue makes diastema closure and retention difficult. In most cases the decision is left to the individual clinician or the demand of the malocclusion.

Lip traps (Figure 20.15) can cause displacement of the teeth and are often signs of an underlying skeletal discrepancy. They can

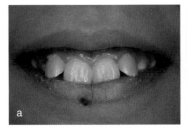
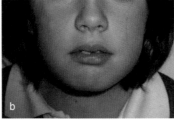
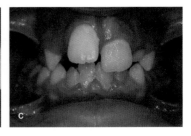

Figure 20.15 Example of a lip trap on the (a) upper lateral incisors, (b) the upper right central incisor, and (c) dental effects of a lip trap with proclination of the upper right central incisor.

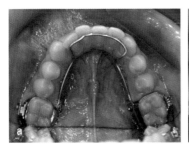
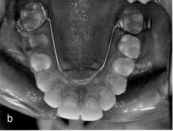
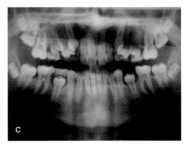

Figure 20.16a–c A lingual arch and a Nance palatal arch.

be treated early to avoid unwanted tooth movement. Care must be taken to ensure that unwanted effects, such as converting a Class II division 1 incisor relationship into a Class II division 2 relationship (due to the underlying skeletal discrepancy), are not induced.

LEEWAY SPACE AND THE USE OF INTRAORAL ANCHORAGE ARCHES

Leeway space is the size differential between the primary posterior teeth (canine, first and second molars) and the permanent successors. Usually the sum of the primary tooth widths is greater than that of their permanent successors. So when these primary teeth fall out, there is usually a small amount of space (about 2.5 mm per side in the lower arch and 1.5 mm per side in the upper arch) available for the correction of crowding. If nothing is done to preserve this space, the permanent first molars almost always drift forward to close it. If there is mild crowding evident within the dental arch it is possible to utilize the Leeway space for its correction.[12] By placing a lingual or palatal arch (Figure 20.16) before the exfoliation of the primary molar the first permanent molar is prevented in its natural mesial migration and the space can be used with fixed appliances to distalise the buccal segment teeth and canines.[13,14] This allows the elimination of anterior incisor crowding without the use of extractions or interdental stripping in milder cases.

SAGITTAL PROBLEMS – CLASS II

A great deal of research has been undertaken into the effects of sagittal Class II correction

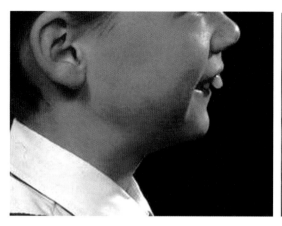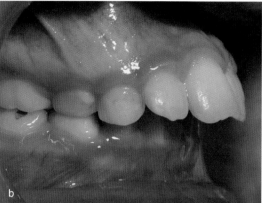

Figure 20.17 A Class II case demonstrating (a) upper incisor protrusion and (b) an increased overjet, which results in the incisors being prone to traumatic injuries.

either by functional or fixed appliances. The majority of the evidence shows that there is often minimal skeletal change combined with a much larger dental and alveolar change as a response to treatment. Studies have shown that the rate of change with treatment may be quicker during the pubertal growth spurt but no study has been able to answer the question of how stable the changes are in the long term and whether or not the skeletal growth would have achieved the same position (even if the dental relationship would not) at the end of the growth period.[15,16] As a result of this it is important for a clinician to look at more than the growth evidence when choosing the ideal time for introducing treatment.

More than 40% of children with an overjet of more than 8 mm will traumatise their incisors (Figure 20.17) and although the peak incidence of trauma to the incisors is 2–4 years of age there is a second peak at 7–9 years when the permanent successors are present. This trauma can lead to permanent injury to the incisors.

This fact combined with an improvement in aesthetics should be the driving force for early treatment. At 8/9 years, compliance with appli-

ances is often excellent as the challenges of adolescence have yet to become apparent. Bringing the incisors out of danger will reduce the likelihood of injury and may improve social contact and reduce bullying even if it does not correct the overall malocclusion. Psychological factors have been found and significant benefit from treatment in terms of increased self-concept scores and reduced negative social experiences with improved self-esteem and improved facial profile.[17,18] A second phase of treatment with fixed appliance alignment of the teeth once the permanent dentition has established can be used to manage long-term occlusal needs.[19]

SAGITTAL PROBLEMS – CLASS III

It is important with Class III patients to monitor the growth of the maxilla and mandible carefully. Early protraction headgear or chin-cup therapy can be useful although if the skeletal discrepancy is large it may be difficult to achieve good facial aesthetics. Dentoalveolar camouflage of a Class III incisor relationship will depend on the severity of the discrepancy

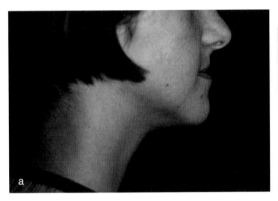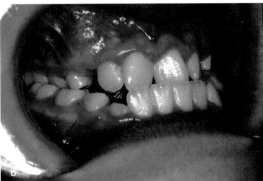

Figure 20.18 A severe Class III case demonstrating (a) a Class III skeletal pattern and (b) a reverse overjet.

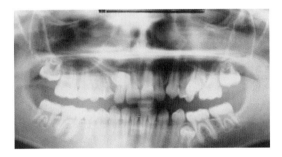

Figure 20.19 A panoramic radiograph showing an impacted upper right canine and lower left second premolar.

in the skeletal bases but may be worth undertaking for aesthetic reasons even if complete correction cannot be achieved. Interceptive alignment of a crowded upper arch in a severe skeletal Class III patient is often important during adolescence for social acceptance even if the ultimate treatment plan is orthognathic surgery at the completion of facial growth (Figure 20.18).[20–22]

ECTOPIC TEETH

The commonest ectopic tooth within the developing child is the upper canine (Figure 20.19). Guidance with early extraction of the primary canines is a common management protocol.[23–25] Its use, however, is based on weak scientific evidence and careful assessment of the position of the canine vertically and towards the mid-line is important to ensure the effectiveness of this intervention. All children should be assessed clinically at the age of 9 years and if the canine bulge cannot be palpated a panoramic radiograph and upper standard occlusal radiographs should be taken to identify the position of the tooth. If the canine is palatally positioned, consideration should be given to loss of the primary canine.

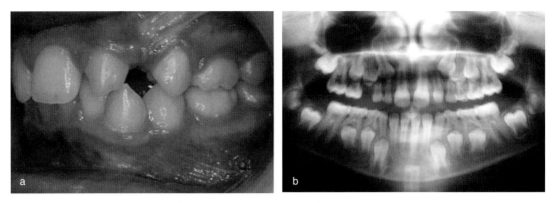

Figure 20.20a,b An example of a patient with missing maxillary lateral incisors.

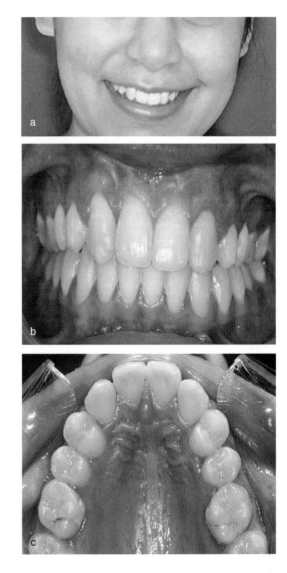

Figure 20.21a–c An example where the maxillary canines have been masked to serve as the lateral incisors.

MISSING TEETH

Where the upper lateral incisors are missing (Figure 20.20) the dilemma is whether to close or open the space. This decision should be based on the malocclusion as a whole as well as the wishes of the patient. There are considerable advantages in having a healthy dentition with no prosthetic placement. On the one hand, if the canine teeth are of good size, shape and colour they can make an excellent replacement for the lateral incisor with some composite additions and cusp tip trimming (Figure 20.21). On the other hand, the single tooth implant has also made the management of anterior spacing predictable and effective. The decision as to which is the better option in the long term is often based on the wishes of the patient and the underlying skeletal relationship. If implants are contemplated it is important to ensure that there is adequate alveolar bone and it is often helpful to allow the upper canine to erupt into the lateral incisor space, and encourage bone development within the area, before retracting it to leave a broad ridge in the lateral incisor position (orthodontic implant site development). This also provides improved aesthetics during the younger years.

Where there are missing second premolars assessment of the malocclusion may lead to the decision to extract the second deciduous molars early to allow the first permanent molars to drift forward thus aiding space closure physiologically. If the malocclusion dictates that the space should be maintained, consideration should be given to interproximal reduction of the second deciduous molar to the size of a permanent second premolar in order that the malocclusion during orthodontic treatment can be treated comprehensively with good buccal segment interdigitation. This tooth can then be left in place until it naturally exfoliates and then immediately replaced with an implant or bridge.

CONCLUSION

This chapter has tried to assess a number of the common developmental problems and their orthodontic management. Until there is enough evidence base to lead us to the ideal treatment plan, we must rely on the experience and training of the orthodontist to form a cohesive strategy. Nature is not always our friend but common sense and critical thinking based on sound academic principles often is. In the twenty-first century our approach must rely not only on the available evidence but also on patients' wishes and their informed consent.

References

1. Bjork A, Skieller V. Normal and abnormal growth of the mandible. A synthesis of longitudinal cephalometric implant studies overt a period of 25 years. Eur J Orthod 1983;5:1–46.
2. Bjork A. Facial growth in man, studied with the aid of metallic implants. Acta Odontol Scand 1955;13(1):9–34.
3. Patel A. The prevalence of digit sucking amongst primary school children in Kettering. MSc Thesis, University of London, 2006.
4. Larsson E. The effect of finger-sucking on the occlusion: a review. Eur J Orthod 1987; 9:279–82.
5. DiBiase DD. Midline supernumeries and euption of maxillary central incisors. Transactions of the BSSO 1968;69:83–8.
6. Mitchell L, Bennett TG. Supernumerary teeth causing delayed eruption – A retrospective study. Br J Orthod 1992;19:41–6.
7. Witsenberg B, Boering G. Eruption of impacted permanent incisors after removal of supernumerary teeth. Int J Oral Surg 1981;10:423–31.
8. Kristensen L. Auto-transplantation of human teeth: a clinical and radiological study of 100 teeth. Int J Oral Surg 1985; 14:200–13.

9. Bjerklin K, Al-Najjar M, Kårestedtand H, Andrén A. Agenesis of mandibular second premolars with retained primary molars. A longitudinal radiographic study of 99 subjects from 12 years of age to adulthood. Eur J Orthod 2008;30:254–61.

10. Bjerklin K, Bennett J. The long-term survival of lower second primary molars in subjects with agenesis of the premolars. Eur J Orthod 2000;22(3):245–55.

11. Kurol J, Koch G. The effect of extraction of infraoccluded deciduous molars: A longitudinal study. Am J Orthod 1985;87(1):46–55.

12. Ngan P, Alkire RG, Fields H Jr. Management of space problems in the primary and mixed dentitions. J Am Dent Assoc 2000;131(1):16, 18.

13. Zablocki HL, McNamara JA Jr, Franchi L, Baccetti T. Effect of the transpalatal arch during extraction treatment. Am J Orthod Dentofacial Orthop 2008;133(6):852–60.

14. Brennan MM, Cianelly AA. The use of the lingual arch in the mixed dentition to resolve incisor crowding. Am J Orthod Dentofacial Orthop 2000;117(1):81–5.

15. Tulloch JF, Phillips C, Proffit WR. Preadolescent children with overjet greater than 7 mm were random. Benefit of early Class II treatment: progress report of a two-phase randomized clinical trial. Am J Orthod Dentofacial Orthop 1998;113(1):62–72.

16. O'Brien K, Wright J, Conboy F, et al. Early treatment for Class II Division 1 malocclusion with the twin-block appliance: a multicenter, randomized, controlled trial. Am J Orthod Dentofacial Orthop 2009;135(5):573–9.

17. O'Brien K, Macfarlane T, Wright J, et al. Early treatment for Class II malocclusion and perceived improvements in facial profile. Am J Orthod Dentofacial Orthop 2009;135(5):580–5.

18. Koroluk LD, Tulloch JF, Phillips C. Incisor trauma and early treatment for Class II Division 1 malocclusion. Am J Orthod Dentofacial Orthop 2003;123(2):117–25; discussion 125–6.

19. Livieratos FA, Johnston LE Jr. A comparison of one-stage and two-stage nonextraction alternatives in matched Class II samples. Am J Orthod Dentofacial Orthop 1995;108(2):118–31.

20. Delaire J. Maxillary development revisited: relevance to the orthopaedic treatment of malocclusions. Eur J Orthod 1997;19:289–311.

21. Baccetti T, Tollaro I. A retrospective comparison of functional appliance treatment of Class III malocclusion in the deciduous and mixed dentitions. Eur J Orthod 1998;20:309–17.

22. Baccetti T, Franchi L, McNamara J. Treatment and post treatment craniofacial changes after rapid maxillary expansion and facemask therapy. Am J Orthod Dentofacial Orthop 2000;118:404–13.

23. Baccetti T, Leonardi M, Armi P. A randomized clinical study of two interceptive approaches to palatally displaced canines. Eur J Orthod 2008;30(4):381–5.

24. Erikson S, Kurol J. Early treatment of palatally erupting maxillary canines by extraction of the primary canines. Eur J Orthod 1988;10:283–95.

25. Power S, Short M. An investigation into the response of palatally displaced canines to the removal of deciduous canines and an assessment of factors contributing to favourable eruption. Br J Orthod 1993;20:215–23.

Impacted teeth and their orthodontic management

INTRODUCTION

When we look at the intraoral photographs of an untreated malocclusion of a patient under our care, we can often identify the patient by name, because of features of the malocclusion peculiar to that patient. We see erupted teeth in malalignment, we know the perfect result we wish to emulate and the movements needed to attain this – the rotations, uprighting and torque that will be necessary – and we plan the biomechanics accordingly. By contrast, looking at the post-treatment intraoral photographs of a finished case, 'it could be anybody'! The precision with which we are able to treat these cases, with a high degree of predictability and level of excellence, is the envy of the dental and medical professions. Nevertheless, when it comes to the treatment of impacted teeth, that is another story – our professional confidence receives a nasty jolt. The reason for this is that several additional factors become involved when treating impacted teeth, factors over which we may not have total control and which do not need to be considered in routine orthodontics. To find out why, we need to start from basic principles.

Teeth of the permanent series normally erupt when their root development is approximately two thirds of its final length,[1] with the apical third completing 2.5–3 years later.[2] It is during this time period that the eruptive potential of the tooth is at its greatest. This innate eruptive force is reduced when less than half the root is developed and similarly when the root apex has been completed. Nevertheless, when deeply carious deciduous molar teeth are extracted before their due time, particularly when bone-destroying periapical lesions are present, the permanent successors will often erupt prematurely, with relatively underdeveloped roots. A permanent tooth which remains unerupted when its root has developed beyond two thirds of its final length might be labelled as having delayed eruption, in contrast with an impacted tooth, which may be defined as a similarly developed tooth which is not expected to erupt in a reasonable time.[3] It is this latter category of teeth which will be discussed in this chapter.

Orthodontics: Principles and Practice, First Edition. Edited by Daljit S. Gill, Farhad B. Naini.
© 2011 Daljit S. Gill, Farhad B. Naini and Dental Update. Published 2011 by Blackwell Publishing Ltd.

PREVALENCE

The tooth most frequently impacted is the mandibular third molar, and its treatment usually involves extraction, although there is a small but significant number of cases in which a conservative, orthodontic resolution of the impaction may be wholly worthwhile.

Impaction of the maxillary canine may be a distant second in terms of frequency but, because of its location, it is the most important tooth to be affected, with potentially serious implications in terms of damage to the roots of adjacent teeth and difficulty in orthodontic and surgical resolution of the problem. However, its existence may be a chance finding in a routine visit to the dentist since, with an over-retained deciduous canine in place, appearance may not be adversely affected and detection of the condition can be missed. It is variously described as occurring in 1–2% of a given population,[4,5] with females affected more than twice as frequently as males[6,7] and Oriental populations less vulnerable than those from the West.[8]

Maxillary central incisor impaction is less prevalent, but its abnormal presentation is the most obvious symptom and is the likely reason that parents will bring a high proportion of these children to the dentist, most frequently at the age of 8–9 years. Other teeth do become impacted from time to time, but these are largely due to local conditions which are not necessarily specific to one tooth type or another. There are also general conditions and syndromes that cause multiple impactions in an individual and which are beyond the scope of this work. The reader is referred to a comprehensive text on the various aspects relating to the treatment of impacted teeth.[3]

DIAGNOSIS

The first diagnostic steps to be taken in any orthodontic case should always include a history, specifically a record of trauma that may have occurred in the recent or in the distant past. This should be followed by a careful clinical examination. The key for suspecting the existence and discovering the location of impacted teeth lies in the search for incongruities. A young person may have a single deciduous tooth, retained well over its normal shedding time, when all other deciduous teeth have shed and their successional teeth are fully erupted. A single, erupted, permanent tooth may have an unusual orientation of its long axis, with the root displaced mesiodistally and/or buccolingually and for no obvious reason. An unerupted central incisor may be palpable labially, if displaced by a supernumerary tooth or odontome, or very high in the labial sulcus if it is dilacerated. An unerupted canine may be palpable on the buccal side of the ridge or in the palate, behind the incisors, depending on its location. Certain anomalies are often associated with impacted canines, notably small teeth, spaced dentitions, anomalous lateral incisors and several other associated phenomena.[9]

In order to gather more evidence, it becomes necessary to commission a simple radiographic examination. This should always begin with one or more periapical views, from which two basic questions need to be answered.

- *Question 1: Why has this tooth not erupted?* A history of trauma to the face may have adversely influenced the development of an unerupted anterior permanent tooth. Perhaps there is an impediment to the eruption, which may take the form of a hard tissue structure (supernumerary tooth or odontoma) or a soft tissue lesion (apical pathology of a non-vital deciduous incisor or follicle abnormality of the impacted tooth itself). Root resorption of the lateral incisor associated with an impacted canine could also be present, although it is more likely to be the result than the cause of the phenomenon. There may be a primary displacement and orientation of a canine or incisor tooth germ *ab initio*, which gives rise to a deviated eruptive path that is unfruitful. Pursuant to a history of very early trauma, the impacted incisor may develop an abnormal form (dilaceration), expressing its eruptive potential in an upward rotating direction and its crown tip completing its course close to the root of the nose.[3] These conditions can all be revealed by careful examination of a good-quality periapical radiograph. Ankylosis or cervical root resorption in an unerupted tooth will undoubtedly prevent a tooth erupting, although both conditions are rare in untreated subjects and are likely to escape discovery by radiography, particularly in their earlier stages.

- *Question 2: What is the exact location of this tooth, its apex–crown tip orientation in the three planes of space and its proximity to the roots of adjacent teeth?* It is clear that, for any proposed full course of routine orthodontic treatment, certain radiographs will be performed as standard and these classically include an intraoral periapical survey or a panoramic view and a lateral cephalogram. Although not their primary purpose, much information will be obtainable from them regarding the location and orientation of an impacted tooth. Combining these two-dimensional plane films can usually provide considerable three-dimensional information, which may be adequate in defining the position of the tooth in space. Methods such as the tube-shift technique[10] or the combination of a periapical film or a panoramic film with the lateral cephalogram (see Figure 21.1d,e), may be used in determining whether a canine is palatally or buccally displaced.

In some situations, information regarding the locale of an impacted tooth in the buccolingual plane, using plane film radiography alone, may be insufficient. An unerupted labial or palatal maxillary canine will have to have caused severe, oblique resorption of the labial or palatal surface of the root of the lateral incisor before it will be discovered on any of these films. The lesion will only become visible when the resorption has reached the advanced stage where it actually causes alteration in the continuity of the mesial or distal profile of the root anatomy. Furthermore, buccolingual proximity of the two adjacent teeth will be impossible to assess and this has orthodontic implications insofar as it affects the direction that traction must be applied to avoid a collision course with the adjacent root. It also has surgical implications, since the surgeon must expose the tooth from an appropriate aspect to minimise tissue trauma and to avoid damaging neighbouring teeth.

So, when more information is needed to achieve comprehensive success in the overall treatment endeavour, more sophisticated diagnostic measures need to be used. Computed tomography (CT) has been used in medicine for several decades and, while its efficacy in the present context is obvious, the level of ionising radiation that it emits is too high to justify its use on a routine basis, in this context. Over the past few years, however, with the introduction of cone-beam volumetric CT, excellent resolution and all the advantages of the traditional spiral CT has been gained, while reducing the radiation dosage by around 90%, to within the same range as that for panoramic and lateral skull films. From a single revolution of the beam around the patient's head, cone-beam CT is able to provide parallel 'slices' in any direction and at varying intervals and views of the surface of the bony anatomy. Added contrast can 'strip' away the bone from the picture to leave only teeth in their three-dimensional inter-relationships and, with some cone-beam CT machines, this can be animated into a video film rotating the head in any direction. Guesswork is eliminated and replaced with accurate positional diagnosis while, at the same time, displaying root resorption on any surface, with great clarity.[11,12]

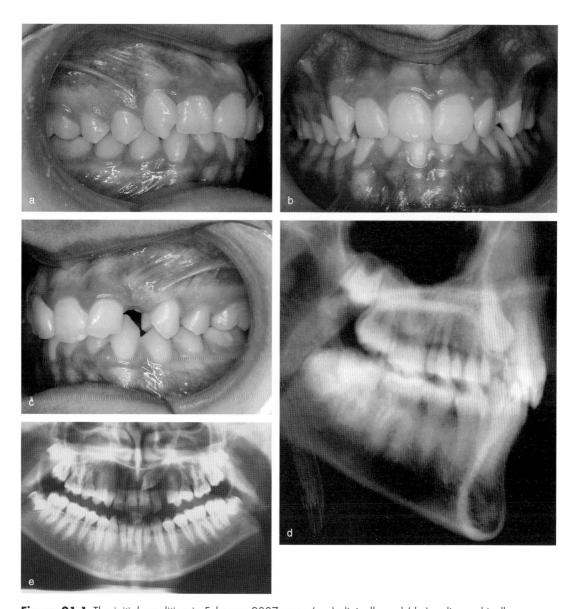

Figure 21.1 The initial condition in February 2007, seen (a–c) clinically and (d,e) radiographically.

TREATMENT PLANNING

Following confirmation of the exact location of the impacted tooth and its relationship to the other teeth, a definitive strategy for directional traction needs to be planned, aimed at bringing the tooth into the arch. But first, a full case analysis must be undertaken, in which resolution of the impaction is just one part of the treatment as a whole. In general, appliance therapy begins with levelling and alignment of the teeth and space is created at the

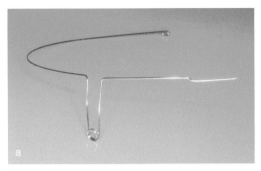
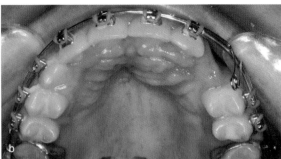
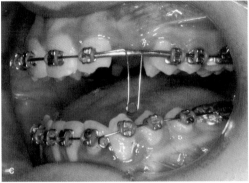

Figure 21.2 Intraoral views following alignment, levelling and space opening. (a) An auxiliary labial arch. (b,c) The arch placed piggy-back over the base arch in its passive mode, immediately prior to surgery.

appropriate site in the arch (see Figure 21.2 below). A majority of impacted teeth are situated close to the line of the arch and will often improve their positions spontaneously during the space opening procedure. Some may even erupt unaided and, in the case of impacted second premolars, this is a frequent occurrence.

Up to this point, actual treatment of the unerupted tooth is largely ignored. With its accurate positional diagnosis established, the safest unencumbered and most desirable route which the tooth must follow is strategized. In preparation for a surgical exposure and active eruption phase, a special auxiliary must be devised, whose function is to apply the planned directional traction. In its simplest form, this may consist of elastic thread that will be tied directly between the tooth and the labial arch-

wire. If, however, the root of an adjacent tooth lies in that direct path, then a custom-designed auxiliary spring will need to be made to circumvent the obstacle. At the same time, a heavy, passive, base arch should be ligated into all the brackets to provide a composite anchorage unit encompassing all the teeth in the arch, against which light traction forces will be applied to erupt the impacted tooth. During this phase, meticulous maintenance of the prepared space must be incorporated into the appliance (see Figure 21.2).

SURGICAL EXPOSURE AND ATTACHMENT BONDING

Essentially there are two principal approaches to the surgical episode, both of which have been modified over the years. The open eruption procedure in its simplest form has been termed the 'window' technique and simply involves removing that section of palatal or labial mucosa, together with any overlying bone, actually covering the tooth. This leaves a circular hole bound by freshly cut soft tissue and the tooth exposed to the oral environment. In order to ensure that the tissues do not re-heal over the tooth during the subsequent weeks, the edges of the excised area may be widened and/or a surgical pack placed during the healing period.

Since the palatal mucosa is completely bound to the underlying bone, the window technique has been advocated for palatally displaced canines, followed by a latent period in which unaided eruption of the canines is expected to occur.[13,14] However, it would seem that, while the health of the periodontal tissues is generally good at the completion of treatment, the attachment of the gingiva to the tooth is at or apically beyond the cementoenamel junction, particularly on the palatal side of the tooth, leaving an elongated clinical crown and, often, some exposed root surface. This is probably related to the amount of gingival tissue that has to be removed to reduce the possibility of the tissues healing over the tooth again and/or to the pressure of the surgical pack. Objectively, crestal bone support has been shown to be significantly reduced in the long term.[15,16]

The method is also suitable for a buccally displaced tooth which is only mildly buccal to the line of the arch, immediately opposite the prepared space in the arch and low down in the alveolar process. In this situation and in the presence of a fairly wide band of attached gingiva, the window may be incised in such a way as to leave a small part of the attached gingiva still covering the more cervical area of the crown of the impacted tooth. This ensures that the finally aligned tooth will be invested with attached gingiva. If the method were to be employed with an impaction at a higher

level, above the attached gingival, it would leave the treated tooth with a poor attachment of mobile, delicate and easily damaged oral mucosa – and a potential periodontal hazard.[13] In this situation, therefore, an apically repositioned flap has been advocated,[17] in which attached gingiva is raised as part of the flap and sutured to the crown of the newly uncovered tooth. There is some argument as to whether this may be done for a buccally/labially displaced tooth which is also mesially or distally displaced from its normal place,[13] since the procedure inevitably leaves a wide area of exposed bone that needs to be covered with a suitable pack during the healing stage. The tooth is then brought down and aligned in its place in the arch, drawing its attached labial gingiva with it.

In the closed eruption technique,[18,19] a wide soft tissue flap is raised and the thin shell of bone and follicle are carefully removed over an area limited to the most superficial side of the unerupted tooth (see Figure 21.3). The opening into the crypt should be small, only made large enough to allow a small eyelet attachment to be immediately bonded under conditions of good haemostasis. No attempt is made to remove more soft or hard tissue. A twisted steel ligature or gold chain is drawn from the eyelet to the exterior, through the sutured edges or elsewhere on the fully replaced flap. The tooth is lost from view and the ligature (or chain) is now used for force application to the tooth.

In the open eruption technique the attachment may be placed at a later appointment, although there is often difficulty in achieving adequate isolation of the tooth surface from the haemorrhagic and swollen tissues which are likely to have encroached on the opening. It has been shown that bonding at the time of surgery is much more reliable than when performed subsequently.[20]

If the attachment to be placed on the tooth is of the same type as the other brackets of the particular appliance system favoured by the

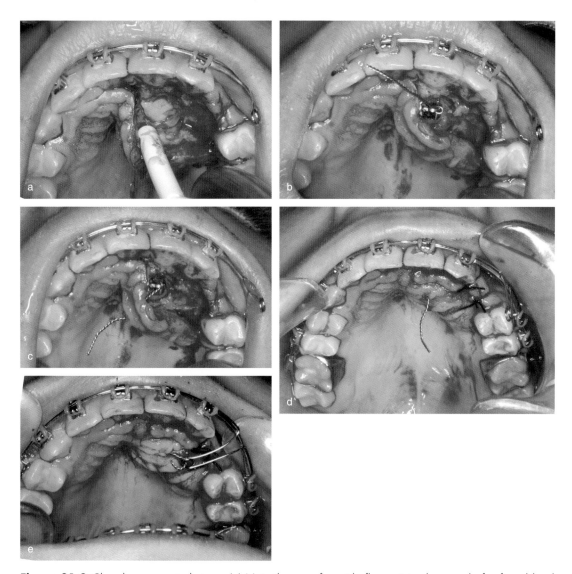

Figure 21.3 Closed exposure technique. (a) Note the use of a wide flap, minimal removal of soft and hard tissues and (b) eyelet bonding. (c) The ligature wire exits through flap opposite impacted tooth. (d) Full flap closure and (e) immediate application of traction.

practitioner, it cannot usually be placed in its ideal mid-buccal position on the crown of the tooth, due to bracket size and to the proximity to the roots of other teeth or because the tooth is rotated. The initial part of the resolu-

tion of the impaction involves the application of extrusive and tipping forces to the tooth only and none of the programmed root moving elements for which a sophisticated orthodontic bracket has been designed. Furthermore, the prescription bracket is bulky and possesses sharp corners, which will make it very irritant during the mechanotherapy, as it passes through the gingival tissues to emerge into the oral cavity, or along an open pathway that was provided by an open exposure and which is inevitably partially closed by swollen gingival tissue. For these reasons, the significantly smaller and rounded eyelet is to be preferred initially and until the tooth has been fully erupted. It is much less prone to accidental debonding,[20] it will offer a much more modest profile than any conventional bracket and will thus be much kinder to the tissues. Because of its size, it may be placed on the tooth crown in the ideal mid-labial/buccal location much more frequently than is the case with a prescription bracket.

There is considerable benefit to be gained by activating the auxiliary traction mechanism at the time of surgery, since the area is anaesthetised and may then be left untouched for several weeks. During this time much healing will have occurred to minimise the discomfort that will accompany further activations as they become necessary. An activation of good range may minimise or even eliminate the need for subsequent adjustments for several weeks.

While most orthodontists absent themselves from the surgical procedure, it is the view of the present authors that the surgical episode is critical, insofar as it offers the opportunity to view the impacted tooth for the first time, to confirm its three-dimensional location, to place the attachment and to apply appropriate force and direction to the activation. For these crucial functions, the orthodontist is far more skilled than the surgeon and is, after all, the person responsible for a successful outcome. Thus, the patient's best interests are served if the orthodontist is present and involved.

Studies over the past 30 years have shown a superior periodontal prognosis of teeth treated with a closed eruption technique than with an open one.[21] Open procedures are more radical in terms of surgical removal of soft and hard tissues and are often associated with long clinical crowns and a poorer appearance. In the post-treatment follow-up with the apically repositioned flap technique, there is additionally a modicum of post-treatment vertical relapse of the tooth position and a poor gingival contour and a long clinical crown, when compared with its untreated antimere.[22] In the final analysis, the ability to identify, after the treatment, which tooth had been affected is usually easier following an open exposure. Closed eruption procedures are more conservative and the outcome of the final bony support of the affected tooth is favourable, when compared with that on the untreated side.[15,21] Postsurgical pain and discomfort are also markedly reduced with the wound fully closed by the original flap.[23] For a more comprehensive description of the various methods of surgical exposure and their outcomes, the reader is referred elsewhere.[3,13,24,25]

The success rate in the treatment of young patients using this approach is very high,[26] provided that:

- The location of the tooth and its orientation are properly assessed
- A large anchor unit comprising as many teeth as possible is set up, with heavy passive base wire to hold the space in the arch and the alignment of the teeth
- Careful conservative exposure is performed with respect for the soft tissues
- Attachment bonding has been performed under appropriate conditions of isolation from moisture control
- Traction is applied in the appropriate direction using a customised auxiliary and, where necessary, is made in two distinct directional movements, to avoid the root of an adjacent tooth.

Success of the orthodontic/surgical modality is measured in four distinct contexts: **radiologically**, it involves accurately determining the three-dimensional location and orientation of the tooth and its relations with adjacent structures; **surgically**, in the ability to provide access to the tooth; **orthodontically**, in achieving its eruption and alignment in the arch and **periodontally** in the long-term prognosis and aesthetic outcome of the result.

When a closed eruption procedure is performed for an impacted maxillary canine, a rapidly progressing resolution of the impaction produces a large and prominent bulge of the thick palatal mucosa, which may sometimes require a soft tissue 'circumcision' to facilitate eruption.

Advancing age has been shown to be a negative factor and a maxillary canine in the over 30-year age group will sometimes fail to respond to mechanotherapy.[27] In adults, therefore, there is merit in testing the canine for movement before placing orthodontic appliances. This may be done by placing a small screw temporary anchorage device (TAD) in the molar region of the palate and applying traction from the attachment on the canine to the TAD, using an elastic chain.[3] In the event that the tooth does not respond, it should be extracted. If the tooth begins to move, an orthodontic appliance may be placed to complete the resolution of the impaction and the malocclusion, in the normal way.

MANAGEMENT

The management of these cases will now be illustrated with a representative case, which has already been referred to in the text.

The young female patient was aged 14 years at the time she presented for treatment. She exhibited a Class 1 malocclusion with lingually inclined maxillary and mandibular incisors accompanied by a mild degree of crowding.

The maxillary left deciduous canine had been extracted, while its successor was unerupted, in an otherwise full permanent dentition, excepting third molars. The permanent maxillary canine was palpable high and close to the midline of the palate. Good three-dimensional positional and orientational diagnosis was achieved with a combination of the lateral cephalogram and the panoramic view, while a periapical view revealed no observable pathology (Figure 21.1).

The initial stage of orthodontic treatment, using Tip-Edge Plus appliances, was concerned with alignment of the teeth in both jaws and the creation of space in the left canine area. A base arch of 0.020 inch round steel wire was placed, with a length of steel tubing threaded on the wire to hold the space between lateral incisor and first premolar brackets. An auxiliary 0.016 inch steel archwire was prepared for ligation into the brackets, overlying the base arch, with a vertical loop and terminal helix formed in the canine area.[3,28] The length of this vertical loop was marginally less than the distance between the palatally palpable canine crown to the labial archwire (Figure 21.2). This auxiliary archwire was tied into place at the surgeon's chairside immediately prior to surgical exposure of the impacted tooth.

At surgery (Figure 21.3), the tooth was uncovered by reflection of a large palatal flap and minimal removal of the thin bone and follicular tissue covering the tooth. The eyelet attachment, carrying a twisted soft steel ligature was bonded by the orthodontist, at its most superficial surface and through a small opening into the follicle – small enough to accept the eyelet and for the surgeon to maintain haemostasis. Because of the height differential between the tooth in the palatal vault and the labial archwire and because of potential interference by incisor roots, the tooth needed to be brought down vertically, before moving it laterally into the arch. A closed procedure was performed, with the palatal flap fully replaced and the twisted ligature wire

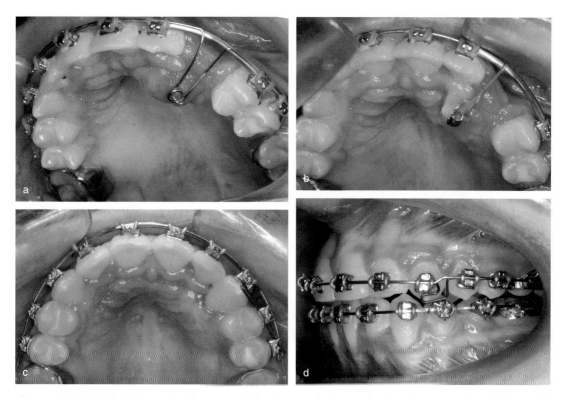

Figure 21.4 (a) Vertical traction has caused the tissue to bulge markedly, prior to eruption of the tooth. (b) Following eruption, labial traction direct to the archwire is applied to a new labial eyelet. (c,d) Following alignment, buccal root torque has been applied.

passed though the flap immediately opposite the eyelet, which was now re-covered by the fully resutured flap.

Before the patient was released from the chair, the vertical loop of the auxiliary archwire was turned palatally and superiorly, with light finger pressure, to be ensnared by the turned, shortened end of the twisted ligature, thereby creating light and controllable, vertically directed traction of good range.

Over the next 2 months, the palatal tissue bulged more and more until the tooth finally emerged with a generous rim of alveolar bone surrounding it. At that point, a new eyelet was placed in the mid-buccal position of the crown and the tooth drawn laterally to its place in the

arch, with its rotation correcting as it proceeded. Once in the line of the arch, a Tip-Edge Plus bracket was substituted for the eyelet, to achieve the final uprighting and torquing movements (Figure 21.4).

At the completion of treatment (Figure 21.5), the case shows good alignment and finishing, with the clinical crown of the previously impacted canine notably shorter than its untreated antimere, which has been present 4 years longer. This is typical for this surgical technique and is usually indistinguishable from that seen with any normal and recently erupted tooth. Following an open exposure procedure, one should expect to see a much longer clinical crown.

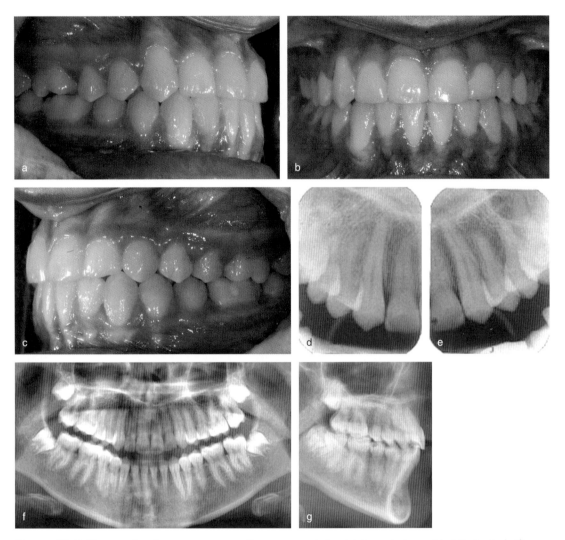

Figure 21.5 The completed case seen at appliance removal. (a–c) Intraoral views. (d,e) Periapical, (f) panoramic and (f) lateral skull radiographic views.

References

1. Demerjian A, Goldstein H, Tanner JM. A new system of dental age assessment. Hum Biol 1973;45:211–27.
2. Nolla CM. The development of permanent teeth. J Dent Child 1960;27:254–66.
3. Becker A. The Orthodontic Treatment of Impacted Teeth, 2nd ed. Informa Healthcare Publishers, Abingdon, 2007.
4. Brin I, Becker A, Shalhav M. Position of the maxillary permanent canine in relation to anomalous or missing lateral incisors: A population study. Eur J Orthod 1986;8:12–16.
5. Thilander B, Jacobson SO. Local factors in impaction of maxillary canines. Acta Odont Scand 1968;26:145–68.
6. Becker A, Smith, P, Behar R. The incidence of anomalous lateral incisors in relation to

palatally-displaced cuspids. Angle Orthod 1981;51:24–9.

7. Sacerdoti R, Baccetti T. Dentoskeletal features associated with unilateral or bilateral palatal displacement of maxillary canines. Angle Orthod 2004;74:725–32.

8. Oliver RG, Mannion JE, Robinson JM. Morphology of the maxillary lateral incisor in cases of unilateral impaction of the maxillary canine. Br J Orthod 1989;16:9–16.

9. Becker A, Gillis I, Shpack N. The etiology of palatal displacement of maxillary canines. Clin Orthod Res 1999;2:62–6.

10. Clark CA. A method of ascertaining the relative position of unerupted teeth by means of film radiographs. Proc R Soc Med (Odontological Section) 1910;3: 87–90.

11. Walker L, Enciso R, Mah J. Three-dimensional localization of maxillary canines with cone beam computed tomography. Am J Orthod Dentofacial Orthop 2005;128:418–23.

12. Chaushu S, Chaushu G, Becker A. The role of digital volume tomography in the imaging of impacted teeth. World J Orthod 2004;5:120–32.

13. Kokich VG. Surgical and orthodontic management of impacted maxillary canines. Am J Orthod Dentofacial Orthop 2004;126: 278–83.

14. Schmidt AD, Kokich VG. Periodontal response to early uncovering autonomous eruption and orthodontic alignment of palatally impacted maxillary canines. Am J Orthod Dentofacial Orthop 2007;131: 449–55.

15. Kohavi D, Becker A, Zilberman Y. Surgical exposure, orthodontic movement and final tooth position as factors in periodontal breakdown of treated palatally impacted canines. Am J Orthod 1984;85:72–7.

16. Chaushu S, Brin I, Ben-Bassat Y, Zilberman Y, Becker A. Periodontal status following surgical-orthodontic alignment of impacted central incisors by an open-

eruption technique. Eur J Orthod 2003;25: 579–84.

17. Vanarsdall RL, Corn H. Soft tissue management of labially positioned unerupted teeth. Am J Orthod Dentofacial Orthop 1977;72:53–64.

18. McBride, LJ. Traction- a surgical/ orthodontic procedure. Am J Orthod 1979; 76:287–99.

19. Hunt NP. Direct traction applied to unerupted teeth using the acid-etch technique. Br J Orthod 1977;4:211–12.

20. Becker A, Shpack N, Shteyer A. Attachment bonding to impacted teeth at the time of surgical exposure. Eur J Orthod 1996;18: 457–63.

21. Chaushu S, Dykstein N, Ben-Bassat Y, Becker A. Periodontal status of impacted maxillary incisors uncovered by two different surgical techniques. J Oral Maxillofac Surg 2009;67:120–4.

22. Vermette ME, Kokich VG, Kennedy DB. Uncovering labially impacted teeth: apically positioned flap and closed-eruption technique. Angle Orthod 1995;65: 23–32.

23. Chaushu S, Becker A, Zeltser R, Branski S, Vasker N, Chaushu G. Patients' perception of recovery after exposure of impacted teeth: A comparison of closed versus open-eruption techniques. J Oral Maxillofac Surg 2005;63:323–9.

24. Crescini A, Clauser C, Giorgetti R, Cortellini P, Pini Prato GP. Tunnel traction of intraosseous impacted maxillary canines: a three-year periodontal follow-up. Am J Orthod Dentofacial Orthop 1994;105:61–72.

25. Becker A, Caspi N, Chaushu S. Conventional wisdom and the surgical exposure of impacted teeth. Orthod Craniofac Res 2009; 12:82–93.

26. Becker A, Chaushu G, Chaushu A. An analysis of failure in the treatment of impacted maxillary canines. Am J Orthod Dentofacial Orthop 2010;137:743–54.

27. Becker A, Chaushu S. Success rate and duration of orthodontic treatment for adult patients with palatally impacted maxillary canines. Am J Orthod Dentofacial Orthop 2003;124:509–14.

28. Kornhauser S, Abed Y, Harari D, Becker A. The resolution of palatally-impacted canines using palatal-occlusal force from a buccal auxiliary. Am J Orthod Dentofacial Orthop 1996;110:528–34.

Anterior open bite malocclusion 22

INTRODUCTION

Anterior open bite (AOB) is present when there is no incisor contact and no vertical overlap of the lower incisors by the uppers.[1] The severity varies from almost an edge-to-edge relationship to a severe handicapping open bite (Figure 22.1a,b). It may occur with an underlying Class I, II or III skeletal pattern. The incidence in British children is 4% at age 9, falling to 2% by the early teens.[2]

AETIOLOGY

AOB can be broadly divided into two categories:

* *Dental open bite* – where the vertical skeletal pattern is not contributory
* *Skeletal open bite* – where the open bite is at least partly due to the vertical facial form.

The causes of AOB can be subdivided into a number of areas.

Digit Sucking Habits

Digit sucking is a common cause of AOB. The incidence of digit sucking is around 30% at 1 year of age, reducing to 12% at 9 years and 2% by 12 years. Most persist of suckers are female.[3] The severity of the malocclusion caused by the digit depends on the age of the patient and the intensity, frequency and duration of the habit.

The open bite caused by digit sucking is frequently asymmetrical, being greater on the side where the digit is inserted (Figure 22.2). The thumb or finger effectively acts as a barrier to the incisors erupting, while allowing excessive eruption of the posterior teeth. The upper incisors are invariably proclined whereas the effect on the lower incisors is more variable. Not infrequently there is a crossbite due to narrowing of the upper arch.

Teeth displacement correlates better with number of hours sucking per day than magnitude of pressure. Children who digit suck for 6 hours or more each day, particularly those who sleep with a digit between the teeth all night, can have a significant malocclusion.[4]

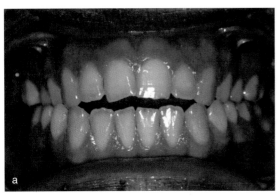
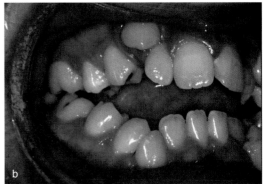

Figure 22.1 (a) Mild dental anterior open bite. (b) Severe skeletal anterior open bite.

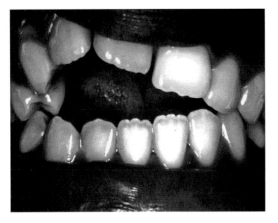

Figure 22.2 Severe anterior open bite due to avid thumb sucking. Note the asymmetrical appearance, the open bite being greater on the side the thumb is sucked.

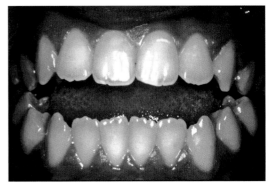

Figure 22.3 Anterior open bite due to aberrant tongue function and posture. Note the characteristic reverse curve of Spee in the lower arch.

Abnormal Tongue Function

A tongue thrust on swallowing is often noted in patients with an AOB. Two types of tongue thrust have been described:

- Primary (endogenous) tongue thrust
- Secondary (adaptive) tongue thrust.

Nearly all tongue thrust falls into the second category – the tongue is thrust forward on swallowing as an adaptive response to the presence of an AOB to prevent food/liquid/saliva escaping from the front of the mouth. The resting rather than dynamic position of the tongue has much greater influence on tooth position.[5] When the tongue is naturally kept in a forward position overlying the lower incisors, a reverse curve of Spee is present in the lower arch (Figure 22.3).

Endogenous tongue thrust is often associated with excessive circumoral contraction on swallowing. Treatment for AOB in a patient with an endogenous tongue thrust should not be attempted as relapse will almost certainly occur.

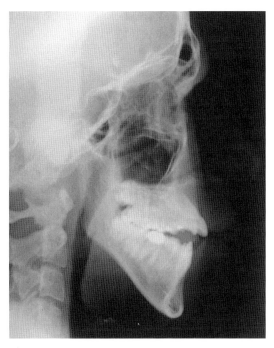

Figure 22.4 Lateral cephalogram of a patient with a skeletal open bite.

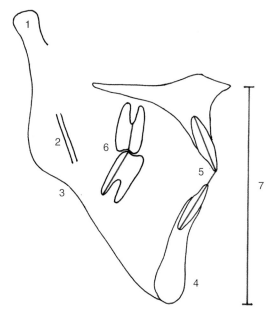

Figure 22.5 Bjork's features indicating a posterior mandibular growth rotation. 1: Backward inclination of condylar head; 2: straight mandibular canal; 3: antegonial notch; 4: receding chin; 5: reduced interincisal angle; 6: reduced intermolar angle; 7: increased lower anterior face height.

Skeletal Factors

Open bites may develop due to excessive vertical growth and are then termed 'skeletal open bites' (Figure 22.4). These are usually more severe in nature than dental open bites and only the terminal molars may be in contact. There is a significant increase in the lower anterior facial height (LAFH) and there may be vertical maxillary excess (VME). The Frankfort-mandibular planes angle (FMPA) is usually increased. Incisor eruption may be *increased* in relation to the underlying basal bone, although it still fails to compensate for the excessive vertical development of the jaws. Anterior facial heights are to a large extent under genetic control and hence taking a family history may be useful in growth prediction.[6]

In growing patients a skeletal open bite tendency is in large part synonymous with a backward (clockwise) rotation of mandibular growth, and hence study of the structural features as identified by Bjork[7] (Figure 22.5), may be more useful than conventional cephalometric analyses, in predicting how patients will grow and how they will respond to orthodontic treatment.

Other Environmental Factors

These include:

• Neuromuscular disorders such as muscular dystrophy
• Upper airway obstruction due to enlarged adenoids and/or tonsils,[8] deviated nasal septum and swollen turbinates
• Pathological open bite: acromegaly; trauma to the incisors (causing ankylosis) or facial

skeleton, such as condylar fractures or Le Fort fractures of the maxilla.

• Idiopathic condylar resorption is a rare cause of AOB developing in adults.

METHODS OF TREATMENT

Treatment is dependent on the age of the patient, his/her concerns and expectations, and the aetiology of the malocclusion.

Digit Habit Cessation

Management depends on the age of the patient at presentation (Box 22.1). If advice alone has not worked, then a deterrent appliance is effective in a compliant patient. This can be either removable or fixed in nature. It must be retained in place for a minimum of 6 months after sucking has apparently ceased, to ensure the habit has truly stopped (Figure 22.6; see also Chapter 20). These methods are likely to produce good spontaneous resolution of the

---

Box 22.1 Management protocol for digit-sucking habits

Primary dentition
• No treatment indicated
• If dummy-related, advise use of 'orthodontic dummy'
• Reassure parents that the AOB should resolve when habit stops

Early mixed dentition
• Advise patient to give up habit
• Use simple *aides memoire* or daily rewards

Late mixed dentition
• Consider deterrent appliance if advice has not worked
• May need orthodontic expansion of upper arch

Permanent dentition
• Spontaneous resolution of AOB unlikely
• Refer for specialist opinion

AOB in a pre-teen patient, but not in patients who have already passed the pubertal growth spurt.[9] In this case further orthodontic treatment may be indicated. However, it is essential that any digit habit is stopped first, otherwise not only will the treatment be unsuccessful, but there is also a risk of root resorption of the upper incisors due to the competing forces they will be subjected to.

Prevention of Habits

Use of an orthodontic dummy that flattens on use should be recommended to new parents as it is much easier to stop these than a digit.[10,11]

Myofunctional Therapy

Passive posterior bite-blocks are functional appliances that are used to open the bite 3–4 mm beyond the rest position. In growing patients, this inhibits the increase in height of the buccal dentoalveolar processes, thus preventing a downwards and backwards rotation of the mandible.[12] It also allows differential eruption to occur as the labial segments can erupt unhindered, hence closing the AOB. High-pull headgear to the bite-blocks increases their efficiency. Where the AOB is associated with a Class II skeletal pattern, a twin block appliance with high-pull headgear can be utilised to correct the

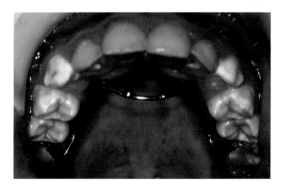

Figure 22.6 Fixed thumb dissuader.

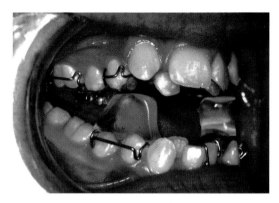

Figure 22.7 Twin block myofunctional appliance with extraoral traction tubes for high-pull headgear.

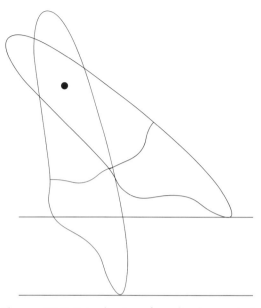

Figure 22.8 Retroclination of proclined upper incisors results in an extrusive movement as the crown is rotated around the centre of rotation of the tooth. The distance between the parallel lines indicates the increase in overbite.

anteroposterior discrepancy while controlling the vertical dimension (Figure 22.7).

The function regulator appliance (FRIV) is effective where the open bite is at least partly due to faulty postural activity of the orofacial musculature. It works by allowing vertical eruption of upper and lower incisors and retraction of the maxillary incisors, and may also encourage upward and forward mandibular rotation.[13]

Fixed Appliances

Anterior open bites can be closed using fixed appliances and vertical intermaxillary elastics to extrude the anterior teeth. This may be combined with a transpalatal arch (TPA) and high-pull headgear to limit vertical development of the maxillary molar teeth. The TPA functions to prevent buccal rolling of the first molars, which could cause the bite to be propped open on their palatal cusps. Use of anterior elastics may be successful in patients in whom a digit sucking habit has artificially inhibited eruption, but should not be used if the aetiology is primarily skeletal. Distal movement of teeth using headgear is contraindicated, as this will tend to worsen any AOB. Similarly class II or class III elastics should not be used as they cause molar extrusion.

Where anterior open bites are associated with proclined incisors, such as some bimaxillary proclination cases and Class II division 1 malocclusions, retroclination of the incisors results in an extrusive movement, as the crown is rotated around the centre of rotation of the tooth.[14] This reduces/eliminates the open bite (Figure 22.8). Stability depends on the tongue adapting to a new functional position after treatment.

Molar extractions have been utilised in an attempt to reduce the magnitude of the open bite by forward mandibular rotation and Mizrahi[15] has suggested limiting extractions to the posterior region of the arch where crowding is present. A multiloop edgewise archwire appliance used in conjunction with heavy anterior elastics has been shown to achieve molar intrusion and simultaneous incisor extrusion in the closure of anterior open bites.[16] The posterior teeth are distally uprighted using this technique, which may aid stability. Nanda has reported the successful use of extrusion arches to treat dental open bites.[17]

Extraoral Traction

Vertical pull chin-cup therapy has been used to limit excessive vertical growth and has been shown to close AOBs when combined with pre-molar extractions and fixed appliances.[18] However, chin-cup therapy generally has poor compliance rates and there is a concern that it may cause condylar damage.

High-pull headgear applied to the maxillary molar teeth and worn for 14 hours per day has been used to inhibit eruption of the posterior teeth and hence limit vertical growth. Headgear can be applied directly to the upper molar bands of a fixed appliance or used in conjunction with a functional appliance or maxillary intrusion splint. Headgear should not be used in Class III open bite cases as maxillary restraint may worsen the skeletal III discrepancy.

Molar Intrusion Using Skeletal Anchorage

Dental implants, mini-plates, mini-screws and ankylosed teeth have been used to provide absolute anchorage in orthodontic treatment. Mini-screws, also known as temporary anchorage devices (TADs), are rapidly gaining in popularity due to their ease of placement and their high success rate. A number of case reports have shown that TADs are effective in intruding molar teeth and closing anterior open bites.[19] This may become the most predictable way of closing anterior open bites of dental origin in the future, especially as it does not depend on patient compliance.

Orthognathic Surgery

A combination of fixed appliance orthodontics and orthognathic surgery may be required to treat skeletal open bites. This should not be commenced until growth has ceased, as further growth is very likely to be unfavourable. Presurgical orthodontics is aimed at individual arch alignment and arch coordination (see Chapter 25). Where there is an obvious step in the occlusal plane, this should not be levelled but maintained using segmental mechanics. Surgery may be segmental or involve the whole jaw. Surgery to the maxilla is mandatory and frequently bimaxillary surgery is required.[4]

STABILITY

AOBs tend to relapse in approximately 20% of treated cases.[20] As a rule, the greater the skeletal elements contribute to the aetiology of the malocclusion the poorer the prognosis for orthodontic treatment alone.[15] Relapse has been attributed to posterior mandibular growth rotation, unfavourable tongue posture; resumption of a digit habit; excessive incisor extrusion; and surgery which has increased the posterior face height.

References

1. Houston WJB, Stephens CD, Tulley WJ. A Textbook of Orthodontics, 2nd edn. Wright, Oxford, 1996:216.
2. O'Brien M. Children's Dental Health in the United Kingdom 1993. HMSO, Office of Population Censuses and Surveys, London.
3. Brenchley ML. Is digit sucking of significance? Br Dent J 1991;171:357–62.
4. Proffit WR, Fields HW, Sarver DM. Contemporary Orthodontics, 4th edn. Mosby, St Louis, 2007.
5. Proffit WR. Equilibrium theory revisited: Factors influencing the position of the teeth. Angle Orthod 1978;48:175–86.
6. Hartsfield JK. Development of the vertical dimension. Semin Orthod 2002;8:113–19.
7. Bjork A. Prediction of mandibular growth rotation. Am J Orthod 1969;55:585–99.

8. Behlfelt K, Linder-Aronson S, McWilliam J, Neander P, Laage-Hellman J. Cranio-facial morphology in children with and without enlarged tonsils. Eur J Orthod 1990;12(3): 233–43.

9. Larsson E. The effect of finger-sucking on the occlusion: a review. Eur J Orthod 1987;9:279–82.

10. Larsson E. Dummy and finger-sucking habits with special attention to their significance for facial growth and occlusion. 1. Incidence study. Sven Tandlak Tidskr 1971;64:667–72.

11. Development and Standards Committee. Dummy and Digit Sucking. British Orthodontic Society, London, 2006.

12. Iscan HN, Sarisoy L. Comparison of the effects of passive posterior bite-blocks with different construction bites on the craniofacial and dentoalveolar structures. Am J Orthod Dentofacial Orthop 1997;112: 171–8.

13. Erbay E, Ugur T, Ulgen M. The effects of Frankel's function regulatory therapy (FR-4) on the treatment of Angle Class I skeletal anterior open bite malocclusion.

Am J Orthod Dentofacial Orthop 1995;108: 9–21.

14. Sarver DM, Weissman SM. Nonsurgical treatment of open bite in nongrowing patients. Am J Orthod Dentofacial Orthop 1995;108:651–9.

15. Mizrahi E. A review of anterior open bite. Br J Orthod 1978;5:21–7.

16. Kim Y. Anterior openbite and its treatment with multiloop edgewise archwire. Angle Orthod 1987;57:291–21.

17. Nanda R. Biomechanics and Esthetic Strategies in Clinical Orthodontics. Elsevier/WB Saunders, St Louis, 2005: 164–5.

18. Pearson L. Vertical control in treatment of patients having backward-rotational growth tendencies. Angle Orthod 1978;48: 132–40.

19. Park YC, Lee HA, Choi NC, Kim DH. Open bite correction by intrusion of posterior teeth with miniscrews. Angle Orthod 2008; 78:699–710.

20. Huang GJ. Long term stability of anterior open-bite therapy: a review. Semin Orthod 2002;8:162–72.

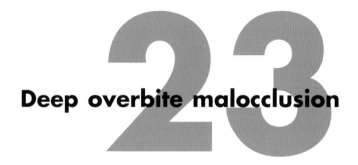

Deep overbite malocclusion

INTRODUCTION

Overbite may be defined as the degree of vertical overlap of the mandibular incisors by the maxillary incisors when the posterior teeth are in occlusion. Overbite depth is usually measured perpendicular to the occlusal plane, either in millimetres or as the amount/percentage of the total crown height of the mandibular incisors that is overlapped by the maxillary incisors. An average overbite occurs when the maxillary incisors overlap the incisal third of the mandibular incisor crowns. In a Class I incisor relationship where the mandibular incisor tips occlude with the cingulum plateau of the maxillary incisors, the overbite depth is 2–4 mm on average (Figure 23.1).

Overbite is described in terms of its **depth** and **incisor contact**. Therefore, overbite may be:

- Normal
- Reduced (decreased)
- Deep (increased)

and

- Complete to dentition or palatal mucosa
- Incomplete.

In addition, a deep overbite complete to the mucosa palatal to the maxillary incisors, known as an impinging overbite (Figure 23.2a), when combined with poor oral hygiene, may become traumatic, causing irritation and discomfort, and occasionally leading to significant soft tissue damage. In some Class II division 2 malocclusions with minimal overjet the retroclined maxillary incisors may impinge on the gingivae labial to the mandibular incisors (Figure 23.2b). Combined with poor oral hygiene this may lead to traumatic gingival recession.

Orthodontics: Principles and Practice, First Edition. Edited by Daljit S. Gill, Farhad B. Naini.
© 2011 Daljit S. Gill, Farhad B. Naini and Dental Update. Published 2011 by Blackwell Publishing Ltd.

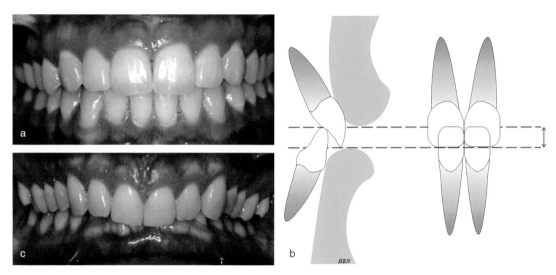

Figure 23.1 (a) A Class I incisor relationship with a normal overbite. (b) The maxillary incisors overlap the incisal third of the mandibular incisor crowns. (c) A deep anterior overbite with the maxillary incisors covering 100% of the mandibular incisor crowns.

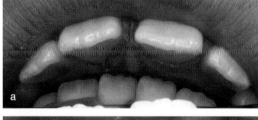

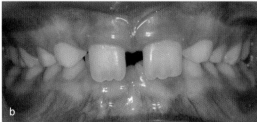

Figure 23.2 (a) Mandibular incisors impinging on the palatal mucosa. (b) Maxillary incisors impinging on the mandibular labial gingivae.

AETIOLOGY

Anterior deep overbite problems may result either from an upward and forward rotation of the mandible during growth, or from exces-sive eruption of the incisor teeth, notably the mandibular incisors. Anterior teeth generally erupt until they make contact, either with opposing anterior teeth, palatal mucosa or the resting tongue. The factors that contribute to an anterior deep overbite may be classified as follows:

* Skeletal
* Soft tissue
* Dental.

Skeletal

Forward rotation of the mandible, in the direction of mouth closing, is due to increased posterior vertical facial growth compared with anterior vertical facial growth (Figure 23.3a).[1] Bjork[2] described seven structural signs found on a lateral cephalometric radiograph, which may give an indication to the pattern of mandibular growth. The signs evident in forward growth rotators, which can give rise to an anterior deep overbite are shown in Figure 23.3b.

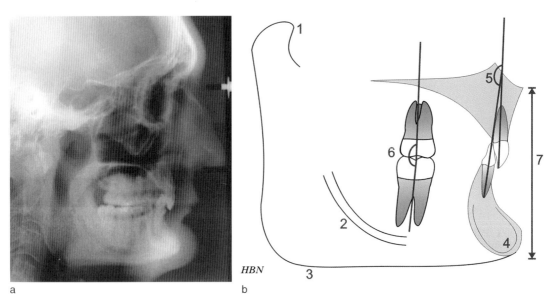

a   b

Figure 23.3 (a) Lateral cephalometric radiograph of a patient with a forward growth rotation of the mandible. (b) Bjork's seven structural signs indicating a forward mandibular growth rotation. 1: forward inclination of the condylar head; 2: an increased curvature of the inferior alveolar canal; 3: absence of an antegonial notch; 4: forward inclination of the mental symphysis; 5: increased interincisal angle; 6: increased intermolar (and interpremolar) angle; 7: a reduced lower anterior facial height.

Soft tissue

An important aetiological factor in Class II division 2 malocclusion is a high lower lip line, which is thought to guide the maxillary and mandibular incisors to erupt in a more retroclined position. Patients with a reduced lower anterior face height, often described as short face individuals, may have increased mentalis muscle activity. This is sometimes referred to as a strap-like lower lip. Depending on the vertical height of the lower lip, this may cause retroclination of the mandibular incisors, or if a high lower lip position is also present, bimaxillary retroclination of the maxillary and mandibular incisors.

If there is a forward resting tongue position and/or an adaptive tongue to lower lip swallow pattern occurs, the overbite may be deep, but just incomplete to the palatal mucosa.

Dental

Overeruption of the mandibular incisors often accompanies a Class II malocclusion. In Class II division 1 malocclusion with an increased overjet, the mandibular incisors erupt until they contact the palatal mucosa, unless there is a forward resting tongue position and/or an adaptive tongue to lower lip swallow pattern as discussed in the previous section.

In Class II division 2 malocclusion the deep overbite is often the result of retroclination of the incisor teeth. The maxillary incisor cingulum plateau is often poorly defined. The maxillary incisors may also have an increased crown/root angle.

It is important to note that a deep overbite may be partly due to over-erupted maxillary incisor teeth.

INDICATIONS FOR TREATMENT

Anterior deep bite may occur in the primary dentition. If so, it is often associated with a relatively short anterior lower face height, reduced mandibular plane angle and square gonial angles. That is, at this age it is primarily skeletal in nature. If the problem is treated in the primary dentition, it is likely to recur when the active treatment is discontinued. Therefore, at this stage of development, treatment is rarely indicated.

In the early permanent dentition, a deep overbite may need to be reduced if causing trauma to the soft tissues palatal to the maxillary incisors or labial to the mandibular incisors. It is important to note, however, that traumatic overbites are almost always associated with poor oral hygiene. The Index of Orthodontic Treatment Need (IOTN) is currently used in the UK hospital service to prioritise treatment by classifying malocclusions according to treatment need. Only patients with a deep overbite causing palatal or gingival trauma fall into the treatment need category (IOTN 4f).

Deep overbite is often associated with an increased overjet. During orthodontic treatment an increased overjet often cannot be orthodontically corrected until the overbite has been reduced.

METHODS OF OVERBITE REDUCTION

The method most suitable for each patient depends on the treatment objectives, which include the achievement of a stable end result. The dental movements required to reduce a deep anterior overbite may include one or more of the following:

• Relative intrusion of the incisors
• Absolute intrusion of the incisors
• Proclination of the labial segments.

Relative Intrusion of the Incisors

This may be achieved by eruption, extrusion or uprighting (distal tipping) of the premolar and molar teeth. Vertical facial growth is required if the overbite reduction achieved in this way is to remain stable. Molar and premolar extrusion may either be passive (e.g. using an anterior bite plane) or active (e.g. using vertical elastics on fixed appliances).

Absolute Intrusion of the Incisors

This can be difficult to achieve, and requires complex orthodontic mechanics. The mechanics tend to pit incisor intrusion against molar extrusion, thereby inevitably leading to some extrusion of the buccal segments as well as incisor intrusion. The only way to solely achieve true intrusion of incisors is with the use of implants or bone screws (absolute anchorage).

Proclination of the Labial Segments

Overbite depth reduces as the incisor teeth are proclined. A useful two-dimensional geometric model has been described, stating that there is approximately 0.2 mm change in overbite for every degree of incisal angular change e.g. 10° proclination leads to 2 mm reduction in overbite.[3] In clinical practice the actual change in overbite depth cannot be accurately predicted by this method alone due to other contributory factors, notably the intrusion or extrusion of the incisors and molars. It must be emphasised that in most cases the pretreatment labiolingual inclination of the incisors must be maintained for stability. Therefore, proclination of the incisors to reduce an overbite may only be used in select cases.

The other option is a combination of orthodontics and orthognathic surgery, in order to reduce a deep overbite surgically.

APPLIANCES AND TECHNIQUES FOR OVERBITE REDUCTION (TABLE 23.1)

Removable Appliances

Anterior Bite-plane

This may be used on a simple upper removable appliance as a preliminary stage of treatment, and is ideally fitted in a growing patient as the permanent dentition is establishing. Clip-over anterior bite-planes (Plint clip) may also be used with upper and lower fixed appliances, giving clearance for placement of lower anterior brackets in Class II division 2 deep bite cases. Overbite reduction occurs by preventing eruption of the mandibular incisor teeth, but allowing eruption of the posterior teeth (Figure 23.4). The lower anterior face height also increases. The addition of cold cure acrylic to the bite-plane allows further reduction of the overbite during treatment. A very useful appliance in a Class II deep bite case is the Ten Hoeve appliance, also known as a 'Nudger' (Figure 23.5).[4] This appliance, used in combination with headgear, combines the benefits of an anterior bite-plane with distal movement of the upper first molars to aid in Class II correction and bite opening.

Functional Appliances

These appliances are primarily indicated for correction of anteroposterior arch discrepancies in growing patients. However, capping of the mandibular incisors reduces mandibular incisor eruption while permitting buccal segment tooth eruption (the bite-plane effect), thereby flattening an increased curve of Spee and reducing a deep overbite. Furthermore, the use of functional appliances causes an increase in the lower anterior face height.[5]

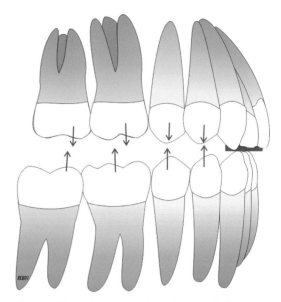

Figure 23.4 The anterior bite-plane works by allowing eruption of the posterior teeth.

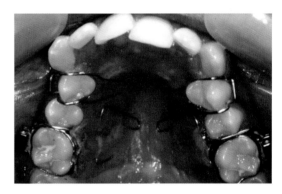

Figure 23.5 The 'Nudger' appliance. Finger springs, in addition to headgear, aid in distalisation of the maxillary first molars.

Fixed Appliances (Continuous Arch Mechanics)

Pre-adjusted Edgewise (Straight Wire) appliance

- *Continuous archwires.* Heavy flat stainless steel archwires may be used to level the occlusal plane, by a combination of mainly

Table 23.1 Appliances and techniques for overbite reduction

Removable appliances	Anterior bite-plane (or clip over bite-plane with fixed appliances)	
	Dahl appliance (removable)	
Functional appliances	Bite-plane effect, e.g. with activator-type appliances, such as the Medium Opening Activator	
Fixed appliances (continuous arch mechanics)	Pre-adjusted edgewise (straight wire) appliance	Continuous heavy flat archwires, e.g. 0.019 × 0.025 inch stainless steel
		Treating on a non-extraction basis, if possible
		Banding second molars early in treatment
		Placing an increased curve in the upper archwire, and a reverse curve of Spee in the lower archwire
		0.019 × 0.025 inch preformed counterforce nickel titanium archwires
	Tip Edge appliance	Anchor bends
	Lingual appliances	
	Dahl appliance (fixed)	
Fixed appliances (segmented arch mechanics)	Rickett's utility arch	
	Burstone's intrusion arch	
Auxiliaries	Class II intermaxillary elastics	
	Fixed bite-planes	Turbo props
		Composite bite-planes (direct or indirect)
Headgears	Wedge effect with distal movement	
	Cervical pull headgear to maxillary first molars	
	J-hook headgear to the upper labial segment	
Absolute anchorage	Implant anchorage	
	Micro-screw anchorage	
Orthognathic surgery	Mandibular advancement to three-point landing	
Segmental surgery	Lower labial segment set-down	
	Mandibulotomy	
	Upper labial segment impaction	

extrusion of posterior teeth and to a lesser extent intrusion of anterior teeth. The incorporation of the second molar teeth early in treatment will aid in arch levelling, but care must be taken to keep the tubes relatively occlusally positioned on the molar teeth for the maximum mechanical advantage (Figure 23.6). This allows for extrusion of the first molars and premolars as well as aiding incisor intrusion. Some patience on the part of the operator is required in allowing adequate time for levelling to occur. When using pre-adjusted edgewise bracket systems, it is also important to remember that the angulation (tip) built into the canine brackets, particularly distally angulated maxillary canines, will cause the initial archwires to extrude the incisors (Figure 23.7a). As the angulation or tip is expressed, the incisors will re-intrude and the arch will level (Figure 23.7b). This is known as vertical 'round tripping'. To counter this phenomenon, it is possible to use reduced tip maxillary canine brackets, or to initially by-pass the incisors in patients with very distally angulated canine teeth.

- *Placing curves in archwire.* It is possible to sweep a reverse curve of Spee into a lower

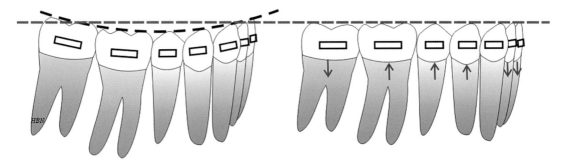

Figure 23.6 Banding the mandibular second molars to aid in arch levelling.

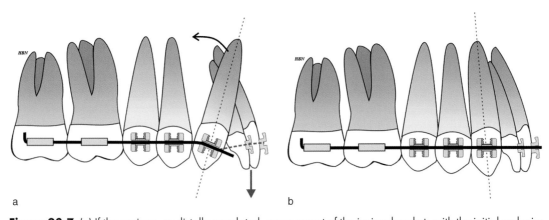

Figure 23.7 (a) If the canines are distally angulated, engagement of the incisor brackets with the initial archwire (red dotted line) will extrude the incisors. (b) The arch will level as the canine angulation is corrected.

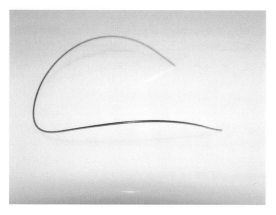

Figure 23.8 Counterforce nickel titanium archwires.

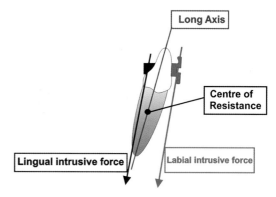

Figure 23.9 Diagram to illustrate the relationship between an intrusive force to the centre of resistance and long axis of a tooth (blue = lingual force; green = labial force).

stainless steel archwire and an exaggerated curve in an upper archwire. This allows extrusion of the buccal segments, especially the premolars, and some intrusion of the labial segments. However, as the area of force application in the brackets is anterior to the centre of resistance of the mandibular incisors, there will be an often-unwanted tendency for proclination of these teeth.

• *Counterforce NiTi archwires.* These rectangular nickel titanium archwires have built in pronounced curves of Spee (Figure 23.8). The disadvantage with these so-called 'rocking-chair' archwires is that they can cause distortion of the arch form if used for extended periods. Therefore their use requires close supervision.

Tip-Edge Appliance

So-called 'anchor' or 'anchorage' bends used in the first stage of the Tip-Edge appliance system are extremely useful in overbite reduction. An intrusive force is applied to the labial segments, and an extrusive force to the molars. The premolar teeth are not incorporated at this stage of treatment. Therefore, the archwire acts as a lever arm, allowing light forces to be used over

a relatively long range. The archwire of choice is a 0.016 inch round, high-tensile stainless steel archwire. The use of Class II elastics in the Tip-Edge system greatly facilitates the bite opening effect of the anchor bends.

Lingual Appliances

The brackets in these appliance systems are bonded to the lingual aspect of the teeth making the appliance more aesthetic than conventional fixed appliances. The anterior brackets may have a flat surface that occludes with the mandibular incisors, acting as an anterior bite-plane in deep bite cases. The point of force application is also different to conventional appliances. An intrusive force directed through a lingual bracket in a normally inclined tooth will pass closer to both the centre of resistance and the long axis of the tooth, thereby theoretically producing intrusion with less proclination than labially positioned brackets (Figure 23.9).[6]

Dahl Appliance

This appliance works along the same principle as the anterior bite-plane and is often used to

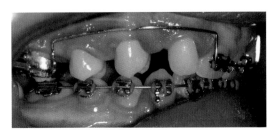

Figure 23.10 Rickett's utility arch.

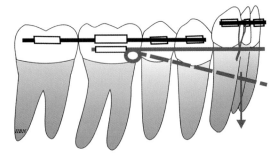

Figure 23.11 Burstone's intrusion arch.

give occlusal clearance for anterior restorations in prosthodontics.[7]

Fixed Appliances (Segmented Arch Mechanics)

A systematic review and meta-analysis of true incisor intrusion attained during orthodontic treatment concluded that in non-growing patients, 1.5 mm of true maxillary incisor intrusion and 1.9 mm of true mandibular incisor intrusion was attainable with the segmented arch technique.[8]

Rickett's Utility Arch

This technique is very valuable in allowing true intrusion of the incisor segment. The 'utility' archwire only engages the molars and incisors (Figure 23.10).[9] It is stepped away from the buccal segment teeth, allowing better load-deflection properties and reduced risk of archwire distortion during mastication. To reduce any extrusion of the molars, double buccal tubes are used on the first molar bands, in order to allow use of a sectional archwire linking the buccal segments as well as the utility arch. In order to limit proclination of the mandibular incisors, lingual crown torque must be built into the rectangular archwires used. Once the overbite has been reduced the canines are progressively ligated to the archwire and thereby intruded.

Burstone's Intrusion Arch

This appliance has been said to produce four times more incisor intrusion than molar extrusion – prior to the introduction of micro-screw anchorage, it was claimed to be the appliance of choice in adult patients where an increase in face height was not desired (Figure 23.11).[10] The anterior canine-to-canine region is aligned segmentally. The posterior molar and premolar teeth are also aligned as a segment and rectangular archwires as well as rigid palatal and lingual arches are placed, providing stable posterior vertical anchor units. The accessory archwire is vertically activated for labial segment intrusion by placing tip-back bends mesial to the molar tubes. It is placed in the additional buccal tubes on the first molars and ligated to the canine region of the anterior segment archwire.

Auxiliaries

Class II Intermaxillary Elastics

These are used bilaterally from the anterior maxillary dental arch to the mandibular first molar teeth. They are used in the correction of Class II malocclusion and the reduction of overjet. An often-unwanted effect is the resultant vertical forces on the mandibular molars. However, in low-angle, deep bite malocclusion the extrusion of the mandibular molars is beneficial in helping to reduce the anterior deep bite. An increased curve may be placed in the upper archwire to help reduce the unwanted maxillary incisor extrusion from the elastic force. However, the net effect of Class II elastics will be overbite reduction as the mandibular molars are closer to the condylar hinge axis than the maxillary incisors.

Turbo-props and Composite Bite-planes

Turbo props, also known as bite turbos, are bonded to the palatal aspect of the maxillary incisors. They have a bite-plane incorporated (Figure 23.12). These, as well as composite bite-planes, may be used with conventional fixed appliances, giving the advantage of allowing the placement of upper and lower fixed appliances from the start of treatment. Composite bite-planes may be made indirectly.[11]

Headgear

The direction of pull of the headgear largely depends on the patient's facial growth pattern. A combination-pull headgear or an Interlandi-type headgear may be used to provide straight-forward distal movement of the maxillary molars, causing the anterior bite to open. This is called the 'wedge' effect as the molar is

moved distally and therefore closer to the condylar hinge axis. Cervical pull headgear has an additional extrusive force on the maxillary molars, and is therefore ideal for use in low angle, deep bite Class II malocclusion. In cases where the maxillary incisors have overerupted, a J-hook headgear may be attached to the anterior aspect of the maxillary archwire to provide an intrusive force. This has the benefit of helping to reduce excessive gingival exposure; however, there are no safety features with this type of headgear and it may also place undesirably high intrusive forces on the maxillary incisors.

Absolute Anchorage

Absolute vertical anchorage may be used to produce true intrusion of incisor teeth. If rigid endosseous dental implants have been placed for future restoration of missing teeth, they can be incorporated into a fixed appliance to allow intrusive forces to be placed on surrounding teeth. However, these implants cannot be placed until the end of active facial growth. They also need to be placed in exactly the correct position for the placement of future prostheses. Therefore their use is restricted to skeletally mature adult patients and requires very precise joint planning between the orthodontist and prosthodontist.

Micro-screw anchorage on the other hand has a number of advantages over dental implants in that they are easier to place, cause minimal patient trauma and may be loaded immediately.[12] Due to their small size, they may be inserted into a number of locations allowing forces to be used in the required directions. Segments of teeth may therefore be intruded.

Orthognathic Surgery

Patients with a Class II division 1 malocclusion often have an excessive curve of Spee. In

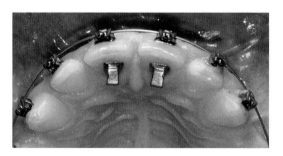

Figure 23.12 Turbo props (bite turbos) are bonded to the palatal aspect of the maxillary incisors.

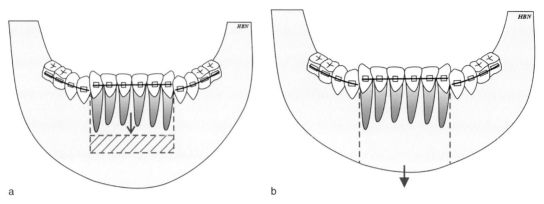

Figure 23.13 (a) Lower labial segment subapical set-down osteotomy. (b) Mandibulotomy.

patients with short faces, where an increase in the lower anterior face height is desired, the curve of Spee must be maintained prior to surgery by placing an increased curve of Spee in the mandibular archwires. When the mandible is advanced at surgery, there will be a three-point contact with the maxillary arch, in the incisor region and bilaterally in the terminal molar region. This is known as a three-point landing. The lower arch is then levelled after surgery by extrusion of the premolars. It is important to note that additional arch length is required for postsurgical levelling. This may be obtained by either maintaining some space in the lower arch before surgery, or allowing for some proclination of the lower incisors after surgery.

Segmental Surgery

This may be considered for adult patients where levelling the curve of Spee by orthodontic mechanics is not achievable. In cases where a natural step exists in the mandibular arch, the arch may be aligned and levelled in segments, usually with an anterior segment from canine to canine and two posterior segments. The arch may then be levelled surgically.[13] This has the advantage that no increase in arch length is required. However, care must be taken to diverge the roots of the teeth where the surgical cuts are to be made. If the lower anterior face height is to be maintained, a subapical osteotomy is undertaken to set down the lower labial segment (Figure 23.13a). If the face height is to be increased, a segmental osteotomy including the lower border is undertaken, sometimes referred to as a mandibulotomy (Figure 23.13b).

An anterior subapical maxillary segmental osteotomy may be undertaken to superiorly reposition the upper labial segment, particularly in cases of anterior vertical maxillary excess.

Conservative Management

Some patients with heavily restored and/or compromised dentitions presenting with deep overbites and recurrent palatal trauma may not be good candidates for orthodontics or orthognathic surgery. These patients may be managed conservatively by improvement of their oral hygiene, particularly palatal to the maxillary incisors, and possibly the provision of a baseplate, which they can wear as needed, usually at night.

CONSIDERATIONS IN TREATMENT PLANNING

Age

A patient with a deep traumatic overbite is best treated while still growing, when correction may be relatively straightforward and before any long-term periodontal damage occurs. Growth modification using various functional appliances with capping of the mandibular incisors or a simple upper removable appliance with an anterior bite-plane may be used.

In non-growing patients any extrusion of the buccal segments tends to be unstable due to stretching of the pterygo-masseteric sling. Therefore true intrusion of the incisor teeth is required, and possibly surgical correction using a combined orthodontic and orthognathic approach.

Upper Lip to Maxillary Incisor Relationship

The amount of maxillary incisor exposure in relation to the upper lip at rest should be about 2–4 mm. In patients with reduced incisor exposure at rest it may be prudent to intrude the mandibular incisors rather than the maxillary in order to prevent an aged appearance to the smile. Conversely, in patients with increased gingival exposure ('gummy smile') it is better to intrude the maxillary incisors.

Incisor Relationship

- *Class II division 1 malocclusion.* A significant Class II skeletal pattern, depending on age, requires growth modification or mandibular advancement surgery. However, if the Class II division 1 incisor relationship is on a Class I or mild Class II skeletal pattern, then treatment will involve orthodontic mechanics to correct the inclinations and vertical position of the incisor teeth.

- *Class II division 2 malocclusion.* If the skeletal pattern is Class I or mild Class II, as is often the case, treatment will centre on levelling the lower arch and intrusion and palatal root torque of the maxillary incisors. If the skeletal pattern is a moderate to severe Class II, the incisor relationship may be converted to a Class II division 1 malocclusion by proclining the upper labial segment, and then depending on age, will require growth modification or surgery.

- *Class III malocclusion.* Sufficient overbite is required at the end of treatment to maintain a stable incisor relationship. Examples include compensating for an underlying mild Class III malocclusion by retroclining the mandibular incisors and proclining the maxillary incisors, and also in cases where a maxillary incisor is to be moved labially to correct an anterior crossbite. It is the presence of a positive overbite that will prevent relapse at the end of treatment.

Vertical Skeletal Discrepancy

- *Short face, low-angle cases.* In growing patients, attempt to encourage extrusion of the buccal segments, using anterior bite-planes, functional appliances, cervical-pull headgear or the Tip-Edge appliance. In this way the increase in lower anterior face height will improve the facial profile as well as helping to reduce the overbite.

- *Increased face height, high-angle cases with deep bite.* It is important to avoid extrusive mechanics to the posterior teeth, in order to avoid any further increase in face height.

STABILITY OF OVERBITE CORRECTION

The stability of overbite reduction depends on a number of factors that must be taken into account from the treatment planning stage:

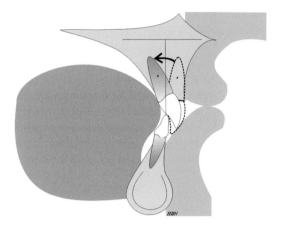

Figure 23.14 Incisor edge-centroid relationship. The dot in the maxillary incisor root is the centroid (centre of resistance).

- *Good interincisal angle.* The interincisal angle must be corrected (average 135°) in addition to the overbite being reduced in order to prevent re-eruption of the incisors after treatment.[14]
- *Correct mandibular incisor edge-centroid relationship.* Possibly the most important factor in overbite stability in all treated cases is correction of the relationship between the mandibular incisor edge and the maxillary incisor root centroid (Figure 23.14).[15] This is measured as the distance between the perpendicular projections of these two points on the maxillary plane (0–2 mm). This may be achieved by either retraction of the maxillary incisor root centroid using fixed appliances with palatal root torque, or proclination of the mandibular incisors to advance their edges. The decision depends on a number of factors including the facial profile and growth potential. If a patient has a retrognathic mandible, it is possible to procline the maxillary incisors and to either surgically advance the mandible or in a growing patient to use a functional appliance to help advance the mandibular incisors. In a patient with good facial profile aesthetics, the treatment may be carried out with fixed appliances alone, so long as the palatal alveolar process is thick enough to allow retraction of the maxillary incisor root centroid. The crowns of the incisor teeth should also be maintained within the zone of soft tissue equilibrium between the musculature of the tongue and the lips.[16] An interesting proposition is that in Class II division 2 malocclusions it may be possible to intrude and torque the maxillary incisor roots palatally, allowing the mandibular incisor crowns to be proclined and hence occupy the position previously occupied by the maxillary incisor crowns, thus maintaining the incisor complex within the zone of soft tissue equilibrium.[17]
- *Avoid change in intermaxillary height in non-growing patients.* The extrusion of molars in non-growing patients is unstable, as the muscular forces from the pterygo-masseteric sling will re-intrude the molars if the posterior vertical face height has not accommodated their extrusion.
- *Proclination of the lower labial segment in Class II cases.* This may still be unstable in the long term due to pressure from the lower lip.[18] Therefore, long-term retention may be required in such cases and must be discussed with the patient prior to treatment.
- *Vertical facial growth continues well into the late teenage years.* As the pattern of facial growth does not tend to change following treatment it is prudent to place a bite-plane on the maxillary removable retainer after the completion of orthodontic treatment. This may be worn on a part-time basis in order to maintain the corrected overbite until vertical facial growth has subsided.[19]

CONCLUSION

When faced with the correction of an anterior deep overbite, the clinician must follow a thorough diagnostic process, which must be worked through in order to reach the correct treatment goal. The patient's age, pattern of facial growth, type of malocclusion and the respective clinician's skill are all factors that must be taken into account. Knowledge of the skills of the orthodontist's prosthodontic and surgical colleagues is also vital if patients are to receive optimum treatment.

References

1. Bjork A. Facial growth in man, studied with the aid of metallic implants. Acta Odontol Scand 1955;13(1):9–34.
2. Bjork A. Prediction of mandibular growth rotation. Am J Orthod 1969;55(6):585–99.
3. Eberhart BB, Kuftinec MM, Baker IM. The relationship between bite depth and incisor angular change. Angle Orthod 1990;60(1): 55–8.
4. Cetlin NM, Ten Hoeve A. Nonextraction treatment. J Clin Orthod 1983;17(6): 396–413.
5. Naini FB, Gill DS, Payne E, Keel W. Medium opening activator: design applications for the management of Class II deep bite malocclusion. World J Orthod 2007;8(4):e1–e9.
6. Scuzzo G, Takemoto K. Biomechanics and comparative biomechanics. In: Invisible Orthodontics. Quintessence Books, Germany, 2003:55–60.
7. Dahl BL, Krogstad O, Karlsen K. An alternative treatment in cases with advanced localized attrition. J Oral Rehabil 1975;2(3): 209–14.
8. Ng J, Major PW, Flores-Mir C. True incisor intrusion attained during orthodontic treatment: A systematic review and meta- analysis. Am J Orthod Dentofacial Orthop 2005;128:212–19.
9. Ricketts RW. Bioprogressive Therapy. Rocky Mountain Orthodontics, Denver, 1979.
10. Burstone CJ. Deep overbite correction by intrusion. Am J Orthod 1977;72:1–22.
11. Philippe J. Treatment of deep bite with bonded biteplanes. J Clin Orthod 1996;30(7): 396–400.
12. Bae SM, Park HS, Kyung HM, Kwon OW, Sung JH. Clinical application of micro-implant anchorage. J Clin Orthod 2002;36(5): 298–302.
13. Kole H. Surgical operations on the alveolar ridge to correct occlusal abnormalities. Oral Surg 1959;12:277–88.
14. Schudy FF. The control of vertical overbite in clinical orthodontics. Angle Orthod 1968;38(1):19–39.
15. Houston WJB. Incisor edge-centroid relationships and overbite depth. Eur J Orthod 1989;11:139–13.
16. Proffit WR. Equilibrium theory revisited. Angle Orthod 1978;48:175–86.
17. Selwyn-Barnett BJ. Class II division 2 malocclusion: a method of planning and treatment. Br J Orthod 1996;23:29–36.
18. Mills JRE. The stability of the lower labial segment. Trans Br Soc Study Orthod 1968;54:11–24.
19. Nanda RS, Nanda SK. Considerations of dentofacial growth in long-term retention and stability: is active retention needed. Am J Orthod Dentofacial Orthop 1992;101: 297–302.

24
Hypodontia

INTRODUCTION

Hypodontia is the term used to describe the developmental absence of one or more primary or secondary teeth, excluding the third molars. The third molars are excluded as they are commonly missing to varying degrees in 20–25% of people.[1] The term anodontia is used to describe the total absence of teeth.

Hypodontia may be classified according to its severity, as mild (1–2 missing teeth), moderate (3–5 missing teeth) or severe (≥6 missing teeth). More than 80% of patients with hypodontia have mild, ≤10% moderate and ≤1% severe hypodontia. The prevalence of hypodontia in the primary dentition is 0.3–0.9% with the maxillary and mandibular lateral incisors being most commonly missing[2]. The prevalence of hypodontia in the permanent dentition is 4.5–6.5%.[3] Ethnic variation exists, with the common missing tooth types in Caucasians being lower second premolars > upper lateral incisors > upper second premolars > lower central incisors.[3] In some Asian populations, lower central incisors are reported to be commonly missing.[4] Overall, females are more commonly (×1.37) affected by hypodontia than males.[3]

AETIOLOGY OF HYPODONTIA

The aetiology of hypodontia is multifactorial with both genetic and environmental influences. Genetics is important as there is often a family history of hypodontia.[5] Several genes have been identified where mutations may be associated with hypodontia in humans, including *MSX1*, *PAX9* and *AXIN2*.[6] An example of an environmental factor is the absence of a maxillary lateral incisor associated with a cleft palate where the cleft causes a localised disruption of the dental

Orthodontics: Principles and Practice, First Edition. Edited by Daljit S. Gill, Farhad B. Naini.

lamina and a failure in formation of the lateral incisor tooth bud. Hypodontia may also be associated with childhood chemotherapy and radiotherapy.[7]

ORAL ANOMALIES ASSOCIATED WITH HYPODONTIA

Hypodontia can be associated with a number of dental anomalies and some medical conditions. Some dental anomalies include the following.

*   *Delayed dental development.* The second premolars are particularly prone to delays (Figure 24.1) in dental development and may not be visible radiographically until the age of 9 years. Hence, a diagnosis of their absence should be made with caution before this age.
*   *Microdontia.* This may be localised or generalised and its severity is often correlated with the severity of hypodontia. A common clinical example of microdontia is the presence of diminutive or peg-shaped lateral incisors (Figure 24.2).
*   *Maxillary canine impaction.* Impaction is associated with the absence, or the presence of a diminutive, maxillary lateral incisor. The

root of the lateral incisor may be important in guiding the canine into position (guidance theory). Up to 5% of those with absent lateral incisors may be affected by maxillary canine impaction.[8]

*   *Abnormal tooth position.* It is common for permanent teeth to migrate into any spacing present, for overeruption of teeth opposing edentulous spaces, and for teeth, particularly premolars, to be severely rotated.
*   *Infraocclusion of the retained primary molar when the successor is absent.* This can result in significant occlusal disruption when the infraocclusion is severe.
*   *Transposition between the maxillary canine and first premolars.*
*   *Taurodontism.* This is a developmental anomaly where the roots of the molars are shortened at the expense of an elongated pulp chamber. The roots of taurodont teeth may be more prone to orthodontically related root resorption and they offer less anchorage because of their reduced surface area. Additionally, endodontic treatment and extractions may be complicated by the abnormal root morphology.[9]
*   *Alveolar atrophy.* When a permanent tooth is absent and the deciduous tooth is lost, there will be localised alveolar atrophy which can complicate orthodontic space closure or later implant therapy.

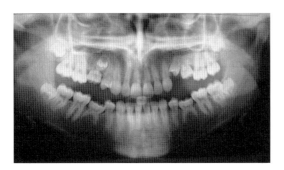

Figure 24.1 A late-forming upper right second premolar.

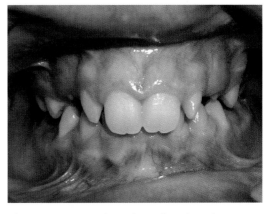

Figure 24.2 Peg-shaped maxillary lateral incisors.

MEDICAL CONDITIONS ASSOCIATED WITH HYPODONTIA

The ectodermal dysplasias are commonly associated with varying degrees of hypodontia or anodontia. These are a group of genetically transmitted conditions in which there is a defect within ectodermal tissues. Apart from hypodontia or anodontia, clinical features include hypohidrosis (failure to sweat leading to heat intolerance and dry erythematous skin, Figure 24.3a), hypotrichosis (sparse hair, Figure 24.3b), nail defects and xerostomia. Other medical conditions associated with hypodontia include Down syndrome, cleft lip and palate and hemifacial microsomia.

MANAGEMENT OF HYPODONTIA

The management of hypodontia involves a multidisciplinary team approach including the general dental practitioner, orthodontist, paediatric dentist, restorative dentist and oral surgeon. A clinical nurse coordinator can also play a valuable role in facilitating the transition of patient care within the hospital environment. The skills of a geneticist are often required when ectodermal dysplasia, or any other genetic disturbance, is suspected.

Treatment is dependent on the stage of development (Table 24.1), the severity of hypodontia and the patient's motivation for treatment. In the majority of patients treatment is undertaken because of aesthetic concerns

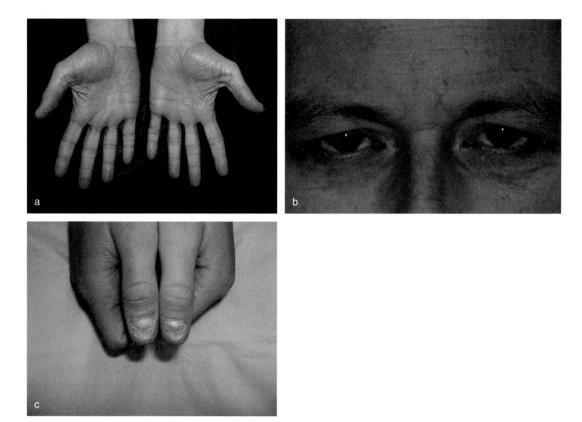

Figure 24.3 Signs of ectodermal dysplasia: (a) dry skin, (b) absence of eye lashes and (c) nail defects.

Table 24.1 Possible management strategies for hypodontia according to the age of the patient

Age	Treatment	Comments
<6 years (preschool) (deciduous dentition)	Removable dentures for psychological and functional reasons	Will require regular adjustments during growth. Retention and stability may be problematic in those with poorly developed alveolar ridges
7–12 years (mixed dentition)	Composite build-ups to improve aesthetics of microdont permanent teeth or worn deciduous teeth	
	Removable dentures	
	Consider interceptive extractions to guide eruption	Problems may include palatal maxillary canines and infraocclusion
	Simple orthodontic treatment for space redistribution	For example, a diastema that cannot be closed restoratively. Long-term retention will be required
>12 years (permanent dentition)	Orthodontic treatment	Pontics can be placed on the fixed appliances and the retainer following orthodontics as a temporary measure
	Resin-bonded bridges following orthodontics for tooth replacement	Other methods of tooth replacement include maintaining the deciduous predecessor, dentures, fixed bridges and transplantation
	Composite build-ups of microdont or hypoplastic teeth.	Disguising intense hypoplastic patches can be difficult
	Overdentures (severe hypodontia)	Abutments help maintain alveolar bone, improve retention and stability and provide proprioception
16–20 years	Single tooth implants or implant fixed bridges or implant-retained overdentures	Placed when the majority of growth is complete. Tends to be earlier in females than males. Bone augmentation procedures may be required before implant placement
	Orthodontics in combination with orthognathic surgery	For patients with severe skeletal discrepancies

relating to spacing,[10] as function is only affected in more severe cases. The main treatment options are:

- To maintain or idealise spacing present for tooth replacement or restorative build-up
- To orthodontically close spacing.

Deciduous Dentition

In severe hypodontia or anodontia early treatment may involve the placement of dentures to help improve aesthetics and function. If a few teeth are present serious consideration should be given to the placement of overdentures, as tooth abutments considerably improve support and retention. Dentures can be placed at a very young age but are especially important psychologically just before the start of schooling years.

Mixed Dentition

Dental development should be closely monitored and a high index of suspicion should be maintained for maxillary canine impaction when the lateral incisors are misshapen or absent. The psychological impact of hypodontia may not be apparent until eruption of the permanent incisors, when the child may notice spacing and be teased at school. If this is significant, it may be appropriate to build up microdont teeth with composite resin to help close space or provide dentures to replace missing anterior teeth. Simple orthodontic treatment can also be considered (e.g. diastema closure) but this does then commit the patient to retention for a number of years until definitive orthodontics is commenced. Some patients with marked Class II malocclusions may benefit from functional appliance therapy during the late mixed dentition stage as this can simplify overjet and overbite correction. Lessening anchorage requirements in the upper arch with functional appliances is particularly useful if space opening for missing dental units is the long-term plan.

Permanent Dentition

Once in the permanent dentition, patients will require a joint orthodontic-restorative assessment. It is essential that the orthodontist obtain a precise prescriptive plan from their restorative colleague about the exact planned space redistribution. Generally speaking, cases with severe hypodontia require more restorative than orthodontic input while milder cases can sometimes be treated with the use of orthodontics alone.

Fixed appliance treatment is often undertaken to correct any superimposed malocclusion, close or open missing tooth spaces and to make roots parallel for later implant therapy. Because of the general delay in dental development in patients with hypodontia, orthodontic treatment may commence at a later age compared to family and school friends not affected by the condition. Patients and parents can be warned that this may be the case at an early stage to reduce later frustration. For planning purposes, a trial diagnostic (Kesling) set-up, using duplicated study models, can be used to predict the final aesthetic and occlusal outcome for different treatment options.

In some cases, it may be feasible to keep retained deciduous teeth, especially the second deciduous molars, if these have a good long-term prognosis. Factors influencing the long-term prognosis of retained deciduous teeth include caries, toothwear, root resorption and submergence. An advantage of keeping these teeth include their ability to maintain alveolar bone height and width. A disadvantage is that retaining a primary molar, which is wider than a premolar, introduces a tooth size discrepancy that may make it difficult to achieve an ideal occlusal relationship. The mesiodistal width of the primary molar can be reduced by enamel reduction to minimise this complication.

Composite build-ups of microdont teeth can be undertaken before, during or after orthodontic treatment. Table 24.2 summarises the advantages and disadvantages of each approach.

It is recommended that a restorative opinion is obtained *before* orthodontic appliances are removed to ensure that teeth have been positioned ideally for restorative treatment. Long cone periapical radiographs should be obtained at potential sites of implant placement to ensure that roots have been separated adequately. Typically, at least 7 mm of space is required along the length between adjacent roots in order to facilitate implant placement. Following orthodontics, retention is important for space maintenance. Patients are often ready to consider wearing their retainers on a part-time basis following the first year of retention. This

Table 24.2 The relative advantages and disadvantages of timing the build-up of microdont lateral incisors before, during or after orthodontic treatment

Timing	Advantages	Disadvantages
Before orthodontics	Restoration acts as a space maintainer during treatment.	Space may not be available before treatment for a build-up. Altering the crown morphology may result in incorrect bracket placement. The restoration is at risk of damage during bracket removal at completion of the orthodontic treatment
During orthodontics	Excess space can be created temporarily to aid mesial and distal restorative finishing	Gingival inflammation can jeopardize bonding and ideal finishing.
	Restoration acts as a space maintainer.	If composite is added to the labial surface of the tooth it may be necessary to drop down archwires to correct the in-out tooth position
After orthodontics	Allows gingival inflammation to subside after appliance removal	A new retainer may need to be constructed after completion of restorative treatment. More difficult to finish interproximally correctly

is often a good time to have resin-bonded bridges placed so that the retainers can be worn part-time. It is important for the restorative dentist to liaise with the orthodontist closely so that the retainer can be adjusted with the bridgework in place, to avoid a period where the patient is left without a retention appliance.

In patients with severe hypodontia, removable dentures or overdentures may be the most effective treatment option until implant-retained prostheses can be offered following cessation of facial growth. Implants can only generally be placed once vertical facial growth had declined; as the implant has no eruptive mechanism, and will submerge as the surrounding teeth erupt to compensate for vertical skeletal growth. The precise timing of the completion of vertical growth is subject to considerable individual variation and requires serial standing height measurements and cephalometric superimposition to define accurately.

Orthodontics in combination with orthognathic surgery is used for the correction of severe skeletal discrepancies. This form of treatment must also be timed at the completion of facial growth. A team approach also involving an oral and maxillofacial surgeon is important for the success of this form of treatment.

References

1. Rozkovcová E, Marková M, Lánik J, Zvárová J. Agenesis of third molars in young Czech population. Prague Med Rep 2004;105(1):35–52.
2. Polder BJ, Van't Hof MA, Van der Linden FP, Kuijpers-Jagtman AM. A meta-analysis of the prevalence of dental agenesis of permanent teeth. Community Dent Oral Epidemiol 2004;32(3):217–26.
3. Daugaard-Jensen J, Nodal M, Skovgaard LT, Kjaer I. Comparison of the pattern of agenesis in the primary and permanent dentitions in a population characterized by agenesis in the primary dentition. Int J Paediatr Dent 1997;7(3):143–8.

4. Endo T, Ozoe R, Kubota M, Akiyama M, Shimooka S. A survey of hypodontia in Japanese orthodontic patients. Am J Orthod Dentofacial Orthop 2006;129(1):29–35.

5. Parkin N, Elcock C, Smith RN, Griffin RC, Brook AH. The aetiology of hypodontia: The prevalence, severity and location of hypodontia within families. Arch Oral Biol 2009;54(Suppl 1):52–6.

6. Cobourne MT. Familial human hypodontia – is it all in the genes? Br Dent J 2007;203(4): 203–8.

7. Kaste SC, Hopkins KP, Jenkins JJ 3rd. Abnormal odontogenesis in children treated with radiation and chemotherapy: imaging findings. AJR Am J Roentgenol 1994;162(6):1407–11.

8. Brin I, Becker A, Shalhav M. Position of the maxillary permanent canine in relation to anomalous or missing lateral incisors: a population study. Eur J Orthod 1986;8(1): 12–16.

9. Haskova JE, Gill DS, Figueiredo JA, Tredwin CJ, Naini FB. Taurodontism – a review. Dent Update 2009;36(4):235–6, 239–40, 243.

10. Hobkirk JA, Goodman JR, Jones SP. Presenting complaints and findings in a group of patients attending a hypodontia clinic. Br Dent J 1994;177(9):337–9.

Orthognathic management 25

INTRODUCTION

Orthodontics in combination with orthognathic surgery is undertaken for the comprehensive management of malocclusion associated with severe skeletal discrepancies in the anteroposterior (AP), vertical and transverse dimensions. This form of treatment is usually undertaken at the completion of facial growth to improve the prospect of stability of the corrected occlusion. Earlier treatment can be undertaken in certain circumstances, however, this is beyond the scope of this chapter.

A key to the successful management of the orthognathic patient is the multidisciplinary team approach involving an orthodontist, oral and maxillofacial surgeon, liaison psychiatrist, general dental practitioner, clinic nurse coordinator, dental technician and sometimes a restorative dentist. The skills of a plastic and reconstructive surgeon and an ear, nose and throat surgeon may also be called on in some situations. Without such a team approach the quality of treatment is likely to be compromised and there will not be a seamless transition of

care between specialists, which will almost certainly lead to patient dissatisfaction.

Figure 25.1 outlines the patient journey during a typical course of treatment involving orthodontics and orthognathic surgery. The duration of presurgical orthodontics varies but is typically 12–24 months and the duration of postsurgical orthodontics can vary between approximately 6 and 12 months.[1,2]

JOINT ORTHODONTIC-ORTHOGNATHIC CLINIC

The purpose of the first joint orthodontic-orthognathic consultation is to introduce the patient to the multidisciplinary team, identify the patient's main concerns, discuss the feasibility of treatment and the likely treatment plan and to obtain informed consent. It is essential to take considerable time to explore the patient's concerns in depth. This is because it is important that a treatment plan addresses these if patient satisfaction is to be achieved at the end of treatment. If all the patient's concerns can not

Orthodontics: Principles and Practice, First Edition. Edited by Daljit S. Gill, Farhad B. Naini.
© 2011 Daljit S. Gill, Farhad B. Naini and Dental Update. Published 2011 by Blackwell Publishing Ltd.

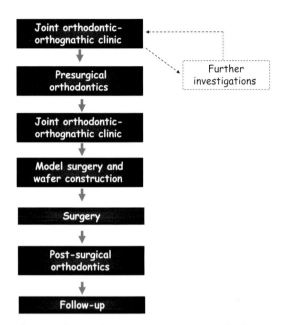

Figure 25.1 The stages in joint orthodontic-orthognathic care.

Table 25.1 The prevalence of altered sensation of the lip/chin (2 years postoperatively) following bilateral sagittal split osteotomy according to age at the time of surgery[7]

Age	Prevalence of altered sensation
<18 years	15%
18–31 years	17%
>31 years	29%

be addressed, it is essential that the patient understands this during the informed consent process. Patients who are specific about their concerns are more likely to make better patients than those who are vague.[3] Computerised prediction software (e.g. Dolphin) is now available to allow the visualisation of proposed treatment plans which can be useful, but should not be totally relied on, for patient consent.

It is important that the full risks of surgery are explained to the patient at this stage. It is worthwhile remembering that research suggests that patients will only be able to recall 40% of the information given to them about the risks of orthognathic surgery[4] and therefore it is important that time is spent providing this information both verbally and in written form. The possible complications will depend on the precise surgical procedure to be undertaken but commonly include the following:

- *Pain and swelling associated with any surgery.* Research suggests that it can take at least 6 months for facial swelling to fully resolve.[5]
- *Paraesthesia of the lower lip and chin in cases where a bilateral sagittal split procedure or a genioplasty have been performed.* The reported prevalence of altered sensation varies between 9% and 85% of the operated side. The prevalence of paraesthesia does appear to be affected by age at the time of surgery (Table 25.1). The combination of genioplasty and bilateral sagittal split procedure appears to be more detrimental to lip sensation than either of these procedures alone.[6]
- *Plate infection.* One study reported the prevalence of plate removal following bilateral sagittal split osteotomy as approximately 16% over 2 years.[8] The infection rate in the maxilla is likely to be lower.[9]
- *General complications such as bleeding and anaesthetic risk as associated with any surgical procedure.*

At the end of this joint consultation, there should be a clear idea of the orthodontic and surgical treatment plan unless further investigations are required. These may involve assessment by the liaison psychiatrist, investigations to assess the long-term prognosis of individual teeth, serial records to confirm the stabilisation of abnormal growth patterns (e.g. asymmetries; Class III malocclusion) and/or advanced imaging studies (e.g. computed tomography [CT] scans in those with complex asymmetries).

An assessment by a liaison psychiatrist is useful to investigate whether the patient is likely to be satisfied at the completion of treatment and can also be useful to detect patients with body dysmorphic disorder.

PRESURGICAL ORTHODONTICS

Presurgical orthodontics has the following aims:

- Alignment
- Decompensation of incisor and premolar/ molar inclinations
- Arch coordination
- Creation of space for interdental osteotomy cuts
- Facilitation of the placement of temporary intermaxillary fixation during surgery.

It is necessary to decompensate the incisors so that the true extent of the AP skeletal discrepancy is unmasked within the dentition to allow maximum repositioning of the maxilla and mandible. In Class II cases this will often involve retroclination of the lower incisors, and in Class III cases retroclination of the upper and proclination of the lower incisors. It is important to undertake a space analysis (Chapter 11) as extractions may be required, especially in those cases requiring significant incisor retraction. It is also important to ensure that adequate periodontal attachment is available to allow the dental movements required.

Anchorage may be reinforced with intermaxillary traction. Class II elastics are usually used in skeletal III cases and class III elastics in skeletal II cases. Decompensation unmasks the original malocclusion and makes the patient look worse before surgery is undertaken, and it is important that the patient is warned as part of informed consent about this before commencing treatment (Figure 25.2).

Arch coordination refers to coordinating the widths of the dental arches so that there is a normal transverse relationship following AP jaw movements. Treatment will often involve upper arch expansion in Class II and III cases using archwires or a quadhelix appliance. The degree of arch expansion required can be assessed by articulating the study models with the hands, such that the canines meet in a Class I relationship and reveals the transverse discrepancy. In those cases with significant transverse deficiency, surgical expansion may be the only alternative and this could involve surgically assisted rapid maxillary expansion or segmental surgery. In other severe cases it may be satisfactory to accept a bilateral crossbite at the completion of treatment provided there is no associated mandibular displacement.

In cases that require segmental jaw surgery, it is necessary to create space between the roots of teeth to enable surgical cuts to be made without causing damage (Figure 25.3). Extraction space is often necessary for this and one can also consider local bracket variations (e.g. transposing the canine brackets for cuts distal to the canines) to facilitate these cuts. A segmental surgical approach may be required in patients with transverse maxillary deficiency in whom upper arch expansion is required, and in those with an anterior open bite where there is a step in the maxillary occlusal plane. In rare cases a lower labial segment set-up or set-down may be the desired approach. In patients requiring segmental surgery it is prudent to place bands on the first molars with double tubes at the time of commencing orthodontics as a *continuous* auxiliary archwire can then be placed at the time of surgery to help stabilise the segments. Alternatively the surgical wafer can be left *in situ* following surgery for segment stabilisation.

At the end of presurgical orthodontics it is important to tie in passive 0.019 × 0.025 inch stainless steel archwires securely, using steel ligatures, and fix hooks onto the archwire that enable placement of temporary intermaxillary fixation during surgery. Full records including radiographs, standardised photographs and

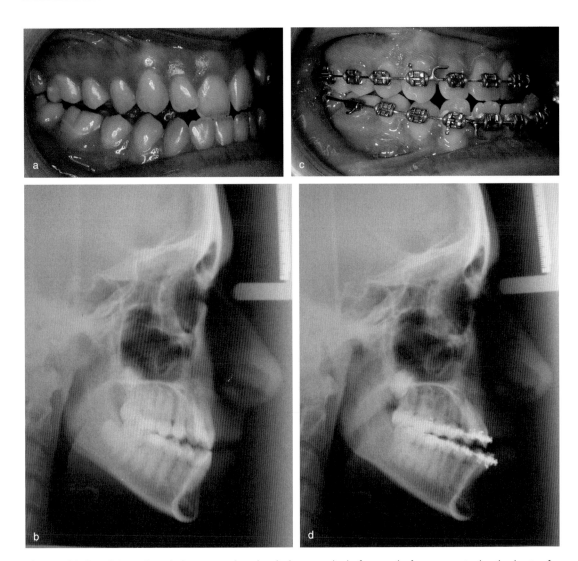

Figure 25.2a–d Lateral cephalogram and occlusal photographs before and after presurgical orthodontics for the management of Class III malocclusion. Note the increase in reverse overjet during decompensation.

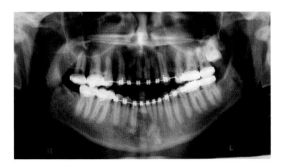

Figure 25.3 Preparation for segmental surgery in the maxilla. Note the space created for the interdental cuts distal to the maxillary canines. Also note the reverse tip of the canines produced intentionally to move the canine root away from the osteotomy site.

study models should be taken at the end of presurgical orthodontics and be available at the presurgical joint clinic appointment.

PRESURGICAL JOINT ORTHODONTIC-ORTHOGNATHIC CLINIC

At the end of presurgical orthodontics, the patients should be reassessed on the joint clinic in order to finalise the surgical movements. The original surgical plan may require slight alteration, based on the changes that have occurred during presurgical orthodontics. It is important to base the decision regarding the final surgical movements on a clinical assessment of the patient in three dimensions (Figure 25.4). The final plan is often based around establishing the correct upper incisor to lip relationship, at rest, in all three dimensions of space. The posterior vertical maxillary position is dependent on the lower anterior facial height and the need to establish the correct overbite. The details of orthognathic planning are beyond the scope of this chapter and the reader should consult text-

books dedicated to orthognathic surgery to gain further information.

MODEL SURGERY AND WAFER CONSTRUCTION

Model surgery, using study models mounted on a semi-adjustable articulator, is undertaken in those cases requiring maxillary surgery. This procedure allows an assessment of the effects of maxillary surgery on mandibular position (i.e. autorotation) and facilitates construction of surgical wafers. In cases requiring bimaxillary surgery, two surgical wafers have to be constructed. The first, or intermediary, wafer guides positioning of the maxilla in relation to the presurgical mandibular position. The second, or final, wafer positions the mandible in relation to the new maxillary position. In cases involving mandibular surgery alone, only one surgical wafer is required to guide positioning of the mandible in relation to the maxilla. In mandible only surgical cases, model articulation is not necessary.

SURGERY

Box 25.1 lists some of the more commonly performed surgical procedures. By far the most common procedures are the Le Fort 1 osteotomy (Figure 25.5a) and the bilateral sagittal split osteotomy (BSSO) (Figure 25.5b). Following introduction of rigid internal fixation, it has been common practice to use titanium plates and screws to stabilise osteotomy sites. This has a number of advantages compared with intermaxillary fixation, where the teeth are effectively wired together during the postoperative period, until bony healing has been achieved. Some of these advantages include increased safety of the airway in the immediate postoperative period, greater patient comfort, facilitation of oral hygiene and greater stability of surgical movements.

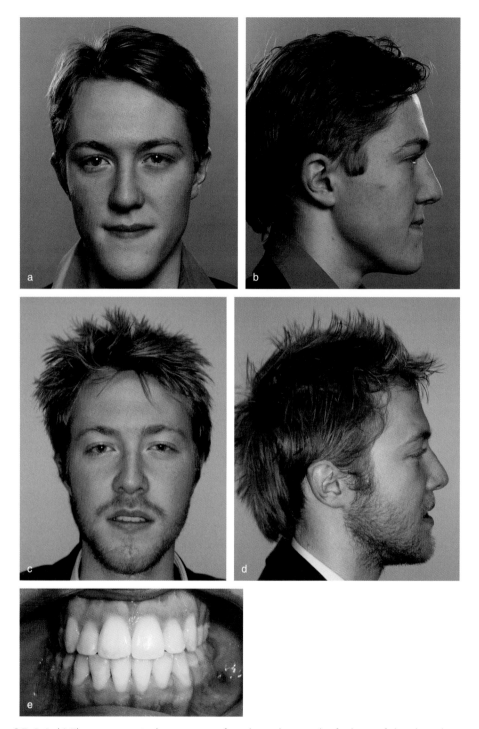

Figure 25.4 (a,b) The exact surgical moves are often dependent on the findings of the clinical examination following presurgical orthodontics. In this patient there is an anteroposterior deficiency of the maxilla and prognathism of the mandible. Therefore the patient would benefit from a maxillary advancement and a mandibular set-back. Vertically, the lower facial height, upper incisor display at rest and overbite are normal so there is no need for vertical repositioning of the maxilla. (c,d) Facial photographs following bimaxillary surgery show good facial balance. (e) The final occlusal result.

Box 25.1

Maxillary
- Le Fort 1
- Wassmund's

Mandibular
- Bilateral sagittal split osteotomy (BSSO)
- Genioplasty
- Total subapical osteotomy

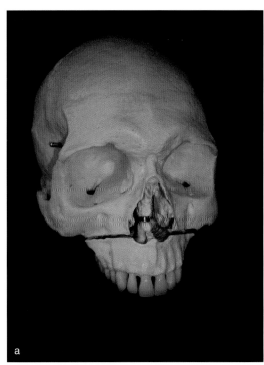

a

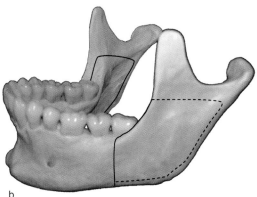

b

Figure 25.5 (a) The Le Fort 1 osteotomy. (b) Bilateral sagittal split osteotomy.

Maxillary surgery is undertaken utilising an incision around the full length of the sulcus to gain access to the underlying bone. The Le Fort 1 osteotomy is done to advance and/or vertically reposition the maxilla. The maxilla may be impacted posteriorly to reduce the lower anterior facial height and increase the overbite. The anterior vertical maxillary position is determined by the need to have 2–4 mm of incisor show at rest.

The BSSO can be undertaken using a posteriorly based intraoral incision. It can be used to advance, set back or asymmetrically reposition the mandible. The third molars are commonly removed at least 6 months before the procedure to facilitate the osteotomy.

POSTSURGICAL ORTHODONTICS

Some surgeons prefer to leave the second (final) wafer *in situ* following surgery to provide occlusal contacts which direct the mandible into its correct position. This may be unnecessary in those cases where there is a good postsurgical occlusion as the mandible is automatically guided into position. Intermaxillary elastics can be used in the immediate postsurgical period to help guide mandibular position as proprioception is often reduced due to altered nerve function.

The aims of postsurgical orthodontics are to produce a well-intercuspated occlusion that will help to improve the stability of surgery. This may involve the use of intermaxillary elastics and the fine tuning of arch coordination. Postsurgical orthodontics should take no longer than 6 months in the average case. Following debonding, patients should be provided with upper and lower orthodontic retainers.

RECALL

Patients should be reviewed on an annual basis following surgery for up to 5 years. This provides an opportunity to identify complications

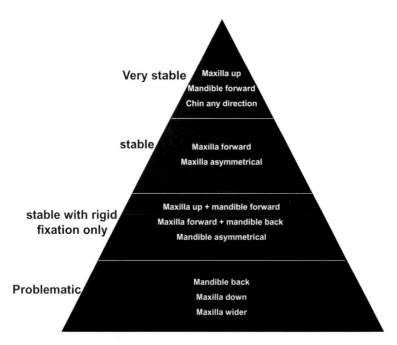

Figure 25.6 The hierarchy of surgical stability, with the most stable movements at the top.

and audit treatment outcomes. Complications following surgery include patient dissatisfaction with treatment, paraesthesia in the distribution of the inferior dental nerve, infection of bone plates and relapse. Some surgical procedures are more prone to relapse than others. One basic underlying principle that should be adhered to during surgical treatment is that the pterygo-masseteric sling should not be stretched as this will almost certainly lead to relapse. Figure 25.6 outlines the hierarchy of surgical stability, which can be used as a guide to predict the surgical moves that are more prone to relapse. Post-orthognathic condylar resorption is another factor that can contribute to relapse and is most likely in female patients with a high mandibular plane angle requiring mandibular advancement surgery.[10]

CONCLUSION

Joint orthodontic-orthognathic treatment is an extremely powerful treatment modality that can be used to correct large occlusal discrepancies and improve facial aesthetics. A multidisciplinary team approach is essential for the ideal management of patients. Orthodontic treatment plays an essential role in decompensating the dentition, to allow surgical movements, and a good final occlusal outcome may be important for surgical stability. A number of the important principles of delivering care have been outlined in this chapter. The reader is referred to more specialist texts for further details.

References

1. Luther F, Morris DO, Karnezi K. Orthodontic treatment following orthognathic surgery: how long does it take and why? A retrospective study. J Oral Maxillofac Surg 2007; 65(10):1969–76.
2. Luther F, Morris DO, Hart C. Orthodontic preparation for orthognathic surgery: how long does it take and why? A retrospective

study. Br J Oral Maxillofac Surg 2003;41(6):401–6.

3. Cunningham SJ, Feinmann C. Psychological assessment of patients requesting orthognathic surgery and the relevance of body dysmorphic disorder. Br J Orthod 1998;25(4): 293–8.

4. Brons S, Becking AG, Tuinzing DB. Value of informed consent in surgical orthodontics. J Oral Maxillofac Surg 2009;67(5):1021–5.

5. Day CJ, Robert T. Three-dimensional assessment of the facial soft tissue changes that occur postoperatively in orthognathic patients. World J Orthod 2006;7(1):15–26.

6. Gianni AB, D'Orto O, Biglioli F, Bozzetti A, Brusati R. Neurosensory alterations of the inferior alveolar and mental nerve after genioplasty alone or associated with sagittal osteotomy of the mandibular ramus. J Craniomaxillofac Surg 2002;30(5):295–303.

7. Westermark A, Bystedt H, von Konow L. Inferior alveolar nerve function after sagittal split osteotomy of the mandible: correlation with degree of intraoperative nerve encounter and other variables in 496 operations. Br J Oral Maxillofac Surg 1998;36(6):429–33.

8. Theodossy T, Jackson O, Petrie A, Lloyd T. Risk factors contributing to symptomatic plate removal following sagittal split osteotomy. Int J Oral Maxillofac Surg 2006;35(7): 598–601.

9. Schmidt BL, Perrott DH, Mahan D, Kearns G. The removal of plates and screws after Le Fort I osteotomy. J Oral Maxillofac Surg 1998;56(2):184–8.

10. Gill DS, El Maaytah M, Naini FB. Risk factors for post-orthognathic condylar resorption: a review. World J Orthod 2008;9(1):21–5.

Further Reading

Harris M, Hunt NP. Fundamentals of Orthognathic Surgery, 2nd edn. Imperial College Press, London.

26

The multidisciplinary management of cleft lip and palate deformity

INTRODUCTION

Clefts of the lip and palate are the most common congenital craniofacial deformity in the UK. The disrupted embryological development of the maxilla presents potentially as clefts of the nose and upper lip and may extend through the alveolus to involve the hard and soft palate. This has potential impact on infant feeding, facial appearance, tooth development, jaw growth, speech, hearing and psychological well-being. The majority of clefts are surgically repaired in the first year of life, restoring anatomical form and function. However, problems of a multifactorial nature may still present, which calls for a coordinated multidisciplinary approach to their management This is provided primarily by the members of a hospital cleft team, which include cleft surgeons, orthodontists, speech and language therapists, restorative dentists, psychologists, ENT surgeons and audiological physicians, but, also extends to healthcare workers in the primary and secondary care environments as part of a managed clinical network.

INCIDENCE

As mentioned above, clefts of the lip with or without cleft palate (CL/P) or cleft palate alone (CPO) are the most common congenital craniofacial anomaly in the UK (more than 1:1000 live births). There is also ethnic variation in the incidence being more common in oriental populations (1:500) and least common in African Caribbeans (1:2000).

PRESENTATION

CL/P is more common in boys, and the left side is affected twice as frequently as the right. Cleft lip may present unilaterally or bilaterally and may be associated with a cleft of the alveolus, primary or secondary palate (Figure 26.1). The cleft may be complete or incomplete and is caused by a failure of fusion between the frontonasal and maxillary processes of the embryo, at 6–7 weeks' gestation. CL/P make up approximately 60% of the clefts in newborn children and CPO the remaining 40%. CPO is more common in girls and has a greater association

Orthodontics: Principles and Practice, First Edition. Edited by Daljit S. Gill, Farhad B. Naini.
© 2011 Daljit S. Gill, Farhad B. Naini and Dental Update. Published 2011 by Blackwell Publishing Ltd.

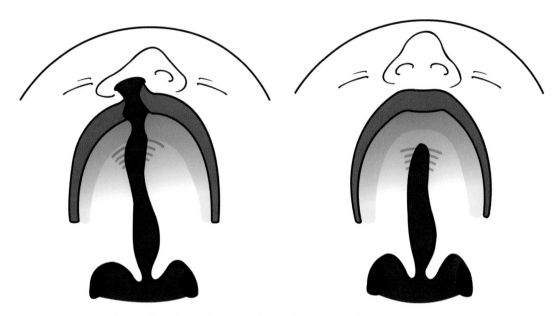

Figure 26.1 Complete unilateral cleft lip and palate and isolated cleft palate.

with syndromes (50%), for example, velocardiofacial syndrome. Failure of the palatal shelves to elevate or to fuse at 8 weeks' gestation results in a cleft of the secondary palate.

The cause of clefting remains unclear, but it is considered to be inherited as a complex condition, with both genetic and environmental factors contributing.

PROBLEMS ASSOCIATED WITH CLEFT LIP AND PALATE

As discussed, orofacial clefting creates a number of potential problems including infant feeding and breathing, speech, hearing, dental anomalies, facial growth and psychological wellbeing. For the purposes of this chapter we will concentrate on the dental and skeletal issues.

Dental Anomalies

Tooth development is delayed by between 0.3 and 0.7 years[1] and this delay increases with the increasing severity of the CL/P.[1] Tooth eruption may also be delayed locally in the area of the cleft alveolus.

Teeth are congenitally missing in both the primary and permanent dentitions, the most commonly affected tooth being the permanent maxillary lateral incisor on the cleft side. Hypodontia is not confined to the cleft site and its incidence increases with the increasing severity of the cleft (Figure 26.2). Supernumerary teeth are more common and occur most frequently, in the deciduous lateral incisor region of patients with cleft lip only.[2] The permanent lateral incisor in a complete cleft, if present, is almost always of abnormal morphology (Figure 26.3) and the central incisor may be similarly affected. The enamel of these teeth is often hypoplastic and hypomineralised (Figure 26.4).

Caries Risk

Cleft populations tend to have a higher caries incidence and this caries is often cleft site related.[3,4] Localised irregularity of the teeth in

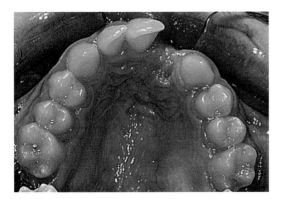

Figure 26.2 Missing permanent central and lateral incisor.

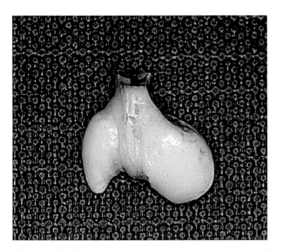

Figure 26.3 An upper lateral permanent Incisor of abnormal morphology.

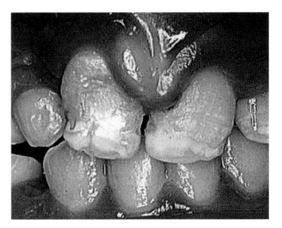

Figure 26.4 Enamel hypoplasia and hypomineralisation presenting on both permanent central incisors.

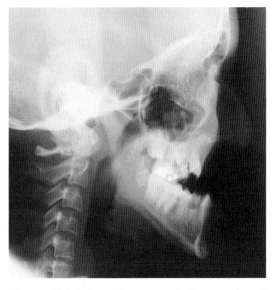

Figure 26.5 Severely restricted downward and forward growth of the maxilla.

the area of the cleft combined with reduced extensibility of the lip makes local hygiene in this area more difficult. Moreover, the teeth in this area have roughened hypoplastic enamel, which increases the risk of demineralisation and decay.

Growth

With any surgical intervention scarring of the lip and palate is inevitable and this may adversely affect downward and forward growth

of the maxilla.[5–7] This, coupled with the intrinsic skeletal hypoplasia due to the cleft, will inevitably cause progressive maxillary retrusion, resulting in a more skeletal III relationship (Figure 26.5). Intraorally this manifests as a narrowing of the transverse and anteroposterior dimensions of the upper arch, which leads to anterior and buccal crossbites (Figure 26.6).

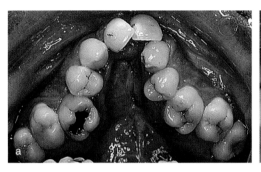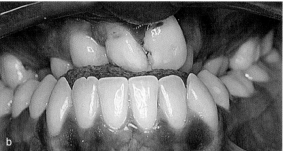

Figure 26.6a,b Severely restricted transverse growth of the maxilla.

MANAGEMENT

The aim of early surgical repair is to restore normal facial architecture, to separate the oral from the nasal cavity, and to reconstruct the velum (soft palate) so forming a valve in between the oro- and naso-pharynx that is both watertight and airtight.

Antenatal

Advances in ultrasonography have *in utero* enabled diagnosis of certain clefts. Parents are then able to meet key team members and discuss future care and to prepare psychologically for what lies ahead. Handled sensitively, this must be seen as an advantage.

Neonatal Care (0–12 Months)

The clinical nurse specialist and paediatrician will give advice on breathing and feeding and monitor progress during infancy. Dental advice at this stage will include brief mention of potential dental anomalies, oral hygiene advice and future interventions. Presurgical orthopaedics may be undertaken in neonates. This process involves fitting an active plate to reposition displaced alveolar segments, reducing the cleft lip separation, so facilitating surgical repair. The evidence for the long-term benefit from this intervention is equivocal and debate continues on its use.

3–12 Months

Surgical repair of the lip and nose and possibly the anterior hard palate is usually carried out between 3 and 6 months followed by repair of the soft palate before the start of speech development at 6–9 months of age. Opinion varies among cleft teams worldwide as to the ideal type and timing of the initial surgery. Most clinicians agree, however, that the extent of the surgery must be carefully managed to reduce scarring as much as possible.

1–7 Years

Patients will be regularly reviewed by the cleft team to assess all aspects of development. The general dental development must be assessed and it is vital that children are registered with a family dental practitioner. The premature loss of teeth may potentially result in loss of space, poor functional occlusion, poor dental aesthetics and may compromise future orthodontic and surgical management. The family dentist therefore has an essential role to play not only in delivering the message to parents on achieving and maintaining good oral health early on in infancy, but also identifying and rectifying problems early.

Simple orthodontic appliances may be used during this phase to correct crossbites and eliminate mandibular displacement.

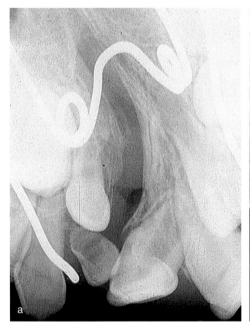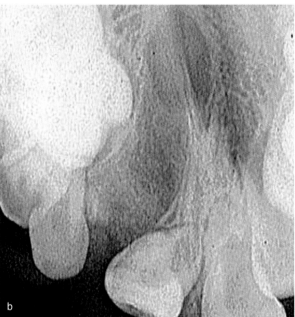

Figure 26.7a,b Pre- and postsurgical radiographs of secondary alveolar bone grafting.

7–12 Years

Secondary alveolar bone grafting needs to be considered for clefts of the alveolus and involves transplanting autogenous cancellous bone from a donor site, usually the pelvic bone, into the alveolar cleft region. The grafted area is closed by advancing a buccal mucoperiosteal flap. This new bone becomes fully integrated with the maxillary bone[8–10] (see Figure 26.7). This procedure is ideally carried out prior to the eruption of the upper canine. The substantial amount of sagittal and transverse maxillary growth is complete by 8–9 years of age, thereby limiting the adverse effects of alveolar surgery on future growth.[11]

Bone grafting facilitates:

- Closure of the osseous cleft of the alveolus and anterior palate while consolidating the maxilla
- Functioning bone into which teeth may erupt

- The closure of problematic oro-nasal fistulae
- Improved gingival and periodontal health of the teeth adjacent to the cleft site
- Orthodontic treatment
- Prosthodontic rehabilitation of the cleft area and possible osseointegrated implants.

Children are reviewed at 7–8 years and if indicated, a panoramic radiograph is taken. This allows the clinician to determine the stage of dental development (ideally the root of the upper canine should be one- to two-thirds formed) and the space available for surgical access, to place the bone graft. An upper anterior occlusal radiograph is taken to assess the quantity of missing bone and the morphology of the teeth in the cleft area. Often the upper arch width is contracted across the cleft site and using a simple removable or fixed appliance the orthodontist is able to open up the required space over a period of a few months. Any unwanted teeth need to be extracted, ideally, at least 1 month in advance of the surgery. A high standard of oral hygiene must be achieved both prior to and following surgery for successful grafting. The success is assessed radiographically 6 months postoperatively.

Over the next 2–3 years the orthodontist and family dentist will monitor the development of the permanent dentition and the craniofacial growth pattern.

12–16 Years

With establishment of the permanent dentition the orthodontist needs to consider how to achieve an ideal occlusion, without compromising dental and facial aesthetics. The most important determinant of success is the skeletal growth pattern and as already discussed the growth of the maxilla may be adversely affected. *For the patient who has a skeletal III pattern at the age of 10–12 years,, the prospect for successful orthodontic correction are reduced because of the potential for further unfavourable growth*

A full orthodontic assessment is required involving, a detailed clinical and radiographic examination, orthodontic study models and clinical photographs. The lateral cephalogram is used to assess skeletal growth and also the relative inclination of the upper and the lower incisor teeth. During growth the upper and lower incisors in general will tend to compensate for the position of the jaws. For example, in a skeletal III growth pattern the lower incisors tend to lean backwards and the upper incisors tend to lean forwards, normalising the incisor relationship. This then limits the scope to achieve solely orthodontic correction.

Orthodontic considerations for patients with cleft palate only are essentially the same as for routine management but, for clefts involving the alveolus, the effects on the associated dental, skeletal and soft tissue elements makes their management more complicated. Often the lateral incisor is missing, causing a shift of the upper dental centreline towards the cleft side.

Space therefore must either be re-created to make provision for prosthetic replacement or closed, which then necessitates camouflaging of the canine to appear as a lateral incisor. The shape, colour and position of the canine tooth will determine whether this approach is viable and needs to be planned jointly with the restorative dentist. Prosthetic replacement offers the potential advantage of improved dental symmetry along with a canine-guided occlusion but then requires long-term prosthetic maintenance.

The upper lip is often flatter in profile and one option is to increase the protrusion of the upper lip by advancing the upper incisors, at the expense of increasing the overjet. Despite requiring long-term retention this may be preferable for the patient.

Features to Assess, Particular to the Cleft Patient

- Upper incisor position with the lips at rest and with smiling
- Upper dental centreline
- Missing/additional teeth
- Prognosis of existing teeth (hypoplastic teeth)
- Upper lip morphology and position
- Lateral and anterior crossbites (may be indicative of unfavourable transverse and anteroposterior growth of the maxilla)
- Position, colour and shape of the canines
- Shape of the alveolar ridge (quality and quantity of alveolar bone)
- The potential to compensate the position of the teeth within the existing skeletal growth pattern to achieve an acceptable static and functional occlusion.

Assimilating this information the orthodontist must then decide if full correction is possible at 12–13 years of age. If it is not, one option is to carry out a short course of fixed appliance treatment in the upper arch to improve the dental aesthetics, deferring the decision on definitive orthodontic treatment until the growth pattern is more complete at 15–16 years of age. Joint discussion with relevant dental specialists is a vital part of the multidisciplinary treatment planning approach, so that the patient may be fully informed of all the potential options before they consent for treatment.

17–21 Years

For those patients with more severe skeletal discrepancies whose malocclusion is not amenable to treatment by orthodontics alone, a potential treatment option is surgical correction of the jaw position, orthognathic surgery. During routine orthodontic treatment the orthodontist will often *compensate* the position of the teeth within the existing jaw structure, to achieve a good occlusion. In the case of orthognathic management however, the orthodontist must first *decompensate* what has been produced by nature, to place the upper and lower teeth into a more normal physiological position prior to surgery. This usually has the effect of worsening the malocclusion and facial appearance, but places the teeth in the best possible position for achieving a good outcome following surgery. It is important that patients realise this beforehand to avoid short-term disappointment. The proposed treatment must be considered with the orthognathic surgeon and the restorative dentist so that a coordinated plan is formulated. In addition, advancing the maxilla will affect facial appearance and may affect speech, so the speech and language therapist and the cleft surgeon must also be involved. This allows the patient to be fully informed before consenting to treatment. The clinical psychologist is able to act both as an advocate, highlighting and addressing issues on behalf of the patient, and also as counsellor, managing psychological problems which may be encountered by the patient at this challenging time. Clinically, preparation is carried out with fixed orthodontic appliances over a period

of about 2 years. Once surgery is completed the occlusion must be detailed for a further 3–6 months with the fixed appliances in position.

It is generally the maxilla that is incorrectly positioned and surgery usually involves advancing the maxilla and altering its vertical position to optimise both facial aesthetics and the occlusion. If the discrepancy between the maxilla and mandible is severe, consideration needs to be given to lower jaw surgery also. The patient must be prepared for dramatic changes in their facial appearance (Figure 26.8). Advanced restorative dentistry is usually carried out at the completion of the orthodontic phase of treatment.

More recently a method of progressive advancement of the maxilla known as osseous distraction has been described. The maxilla is mobilised in the normal way but is gradually advanced forward by a force system. In this way the soft tissues are gradually stretched and new bone is able to fill in the defect that develops as the bone ends move apart, effectively growing new bone at the surgical site.

RECENT DEVELOPMENTS

Given the potential for missing incisors, osseo-integrated implants provide an alternative for prosthetic rehabilitation, with the advantage that they maintain alveolar bone in the cleft region so improving the gingival contour (see Figure 26.9).

Mini screw temporary anchorage devices when implanted into the bone provide a source of absolute anchorage against which forces may be applied to move teeth. The clinician now has greater control over the correction of cleft dental asymmetries without resorting to extractions to balance anchorage.

Following the recommendations of the CSAG report (1998),[12] cleft care has now been consolidated into regional centres in the U.K. which provide multidisciplinary teams with

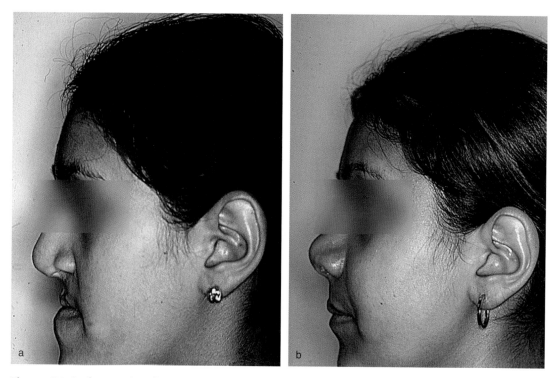

Figure 26.8a,b Lateral profile photographs showing pre- and post-surgical appearance following bimaxillary orthognathic surgery and rhinoplasty.

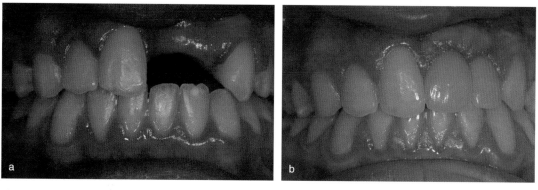

Figure 26.9a,b Pre- and post-treatment images of osseointegrated implant replacement of the missing central and lateral permanent incisors. Figure 26.9b was taken 2 years after placement.

expertise in the management of cleft patients. This provides patients with a coordinated multidisciplinary care pathway. Crucially this also increases the number of patients under the care of one team and with rigorous clinical research and audit, statistically meaningful comparisons may be made on treatment outcome over a shorter time frame, so that improvements to care pathways may be implemented more rapidly.

References

1. Ranta R. Comparison of tooth formation in non cleft and cleft-affected children with and without hypodontia. J Dent Child 1982;49:197–9.
2. Ranta R. A review of tooth formation in children with cleft lip/palate. Am J Dentofacial Orthop 1986;90(1):11–18.
3. Bokhout B, Hofman FXWM, van Limbeek J, Kramer GJC, Prahl-Anderson B. Incidence of dental caries in the primary dentition in children with cleft lip and/or deformity. Caries Res 1997;31:8–12.
4. Ahluwalia M, Brailsford SR, Tarelli E, et al. Dental caries, oral hygiene, and oral clearance in children with craniofacial disorders. J Dent Res 2004;83:175–9.
5. Ross RB. Treatment variables affecting facial growth in complete unilateral cleft lip and palate. Part 7: An overview of treatment and facial growth. Cleft Palate J 1987;28(2):71–7.
6. Mølstead K, Asher-McDade C, Brattström V, et al. A six-center international study of treatment outcome in patients with clefts of the lip and palate: Part 2. Craniofacial form and soft tissue profile. Cleft Palate Craniofac J 1992;29:398–404.
7. Brattström V, Mølsted K, Prahl-Andersen B, Semb G, Shaw WC. The Eurocleft Study: intercenter study of treatment outcome in patients with complete cleft lip and palate. Part 2: craniofacial form and nasolabial appearance. Cleft Palate Craniofac J 2005; 4(2/1):69–77.
8. Boyne PJ, Sands NR. Secondary bone grafting of residual alveolar and palatal clefts. J Oral Surg 1972;30:87–91.
9. Boyne PJ, Sands NR. Combined orthodontic/surgical management of residual palato-alveolar cleft defects. Am J Orthod 1976;70: 20–37.
10. Abyholm P, Bergland O, Semb G. Secondary bone grafting of alveolar clefts. Scan J Plast Reconstr Surg 1981;15:127–40.
11. Bergland O, Semb G, Abyholm F. Elimination of the residual alveolar cleft by secondary bone grafting and subsequent orthodontic treatment. Cleft Palate J 1986;23:175–205.
12. Clinical Standards Advisory Group. Cleft Lip and/or Palate Report of a CSAG Committee. The Stationery Office, London, 1998.

The multidisciplinary management of obstructive sleep apnoea

INTRODUCTION

Obstructive sleep apnoea (OSA) is a sleep-related breathing disorder, characterised by the repeated collapse of the upper airway during sleep, with cessation of breathing. Patients are at risk of severe cardiovascular and respiratory complications, secondary to the recurrent hypoxia and hypercapnia, and the overall quality of life for sufferers and their families may be reduced.

OSA is defined as the occurrence of five or more abnormal respiratory events per hour of sleep. These abnormal events include both apnoeas (cessation of breathing, lasting 10 or more seconds) and hypopnoeas (reduction in tidal volume, accompanied by a 4% or greater fall in oxygen saturation, lasting 10 or more seconds). It is estimated that 4 per cent of middle-aged men and 2 per cent of middle-aged women are affected by OSA.[1] This chapter describes the multidisciplinary management of OSA and highlights the important role dentistry can play.

AETIOLOGY OF OSA

The aetiology behind the collapse of the upper airway, during sleep, is complex and incompletely understood. OSA is thought to arise from a combination of anatomical and pathophysiological factors. A number of cephalometric studies have demonstrated the combination of a retropositioned facial skeleton and reduced oro-pharyngeal dimensions at one or more sites, between the soft palate, tongue and pharyngeal wall, which partly explains the underlying aetiology of this condition.[2–5] Functional impairment of the upper airway dilatory muscles, with patients demonstrating lower tonic and phasic muscle contraction during sleep, is also thought to be an important contributor to the development of OSA.[6]

CLINICAL SYMPTOMS

The symptoms of OSA can be readily classified into nocturnal and daytime. Nocturnal symptoms are:

Orthodontics: Principles and Practice, First Edition. Edited by Daljit S. Gill, Farhad B. Naini.
© 2011 Daljit S. Gill, Farhad B. Naini and Dental Update. Published 2011 by Blackwell Publishing Ltd.

- Snoring
- Witnessed apnoeas
- Choking/gasping
- Nocturia
- Restlessness.

Daytime symptoms are:

- Excessive daytime sleepiness
- Depression
- Impaired quality of life.

The severity of OSA can be worsened by a number of aggravating factors:

- Supine sleeping position
- Alcohol consumption
- Drug therapy which acts to suppress the central nervous system
- Obesity.

DIAGNOSIS

History and Examination

A comprehensive medical and sleep history should be obtained, ideally with the patient's sleeping partner present, to describe the degree of nocturnal disturbance experienced. Validated questionnaires, such as the Epworth Sleepiness Scale (ESS) have been designed to subjectively assess the severity of daytime sleepiness.[7]

Patients can also undergo an ear, nose and throat examination, in order to identify any obvious physical obstructions to breathing. Height and weight are also recorded and used to calculate the body mass index (weight in kilograms divided by the height in metres squared). Neck circumference can also provide a useful measure of upper airway compliance.

Investigations

A comprehensive medical and sleep history used in conjunction with the ESS questionnaire and clinical measures described can provide useful screening for OSA. However, the diag-

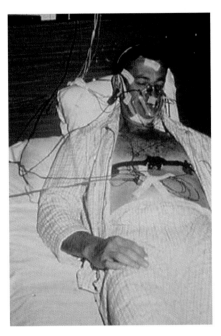

Figure 27.1 Overnight polysomnography.

nosis of OSA is established from an overnight sleep study. Overnight polysomnography (Figure 27.1) is regarded as the definitive investigation for the diagnosis of OSA, giving an objective measure of its severity in the form of an apnoea–hypopnoea index (AHI), in addition to oxygen saturation, brain, heart, muscle, eye activity, sleep sounds and patterns of respiration (Figure 27.2). The investigation is undertaken in a specially equipped sleep laboratory, attended by a sleep technician. OSA is typically classified as follows:

- Mild OSA – AHI 5–15 episodes per hour of sleep
- Moderate OSA – AHI 16–30 episodes per hour of sleep
- Severe OSA – AHI >30 episodes per hour of sleep.

More recently, a number of multichannel monitoring systems have been developed to permit domiciliary sleep studies to be per-

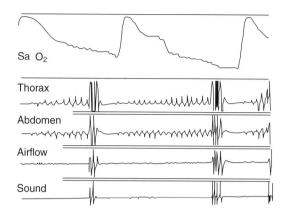

Figure 27.2 Printout from an overnight polysomnographic study of an OSA patient, illustrating repetitive episodes of apnoea and their resolution.

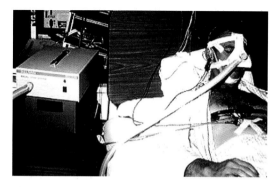

Figure 27.3 Continuous positive airway pressure application.

formed. Such limited sleep studies have been shown not only to accurately and reproducibly diagnose OSA in the home environment but also to provide reliable follow-up data during therapeutic trials in OSA subjects.[8] Studies performed in this way can save on the costs of accommodation in the sleep centre and the attendant staff costs.

TREATMENT

In view of the multifactorial nature of OSA, current management strategies focus around a multidisciplinary approach. Clinicians typically involved include:

- Thoracic physician (lead clinician)
- Orthodontist
- ENT surgeon.

In addition, a variety of other specialities may be called on, including oral and maxillofacial surgeons. Treatment for OSA is based on the following approach.

Conservative Treatment

Regardless of the severity of OSA, first-line treatment aims to eliminate co-existent condi-

tions that predispose to, precipitate or worsen upper airway dysfunction during sleep. Thus patients are advised to abstain from alcohol during the evening, avoid the use of other central nervous system depressants, ensure adequate control of any co-existing chronic obstructive airways disease, lose weight and avoid sleeping in the supine position.

Non-surgical Treatment

A variety of non-surgical approaches have been postulated but to date the only recognised treatments of proven value are overnight continuous positive airway pressure (CPAP) and mandibular advancement splints.

Continuous Positive Airway Pressure

CPAP is regarded as the major non-surgical, long-term treatment, the so-called 'gold standard' for moderate to severe OSA.[9] CPAP provides dramatic relief of symptoms and ensures airway patency during sleep by elevating the pressure in the pharynx. A continuous stream of filtered air, under pressure, is delivered to the pharynx by a nasal mask (Figure 27.3). The appropriate level of air pressure is determined by a process of CPAP titration undertaken in conjunction with overnight polysomnography. To be reliably effective, CPAP must be used for 4–6 hours per night, seven nights a week. However, the use of CPAP is not without adverse effects: problems are often encountered with the nasal mask (allergy, nasal congestion, air leaks, nasal abrasions) and the anti-social nature of the mask and headgear. Long-term compliance can be as low as 60%.[10]

Mandibular Advancement Splints

Mandibular advancement splints are now increasingly being recognised by sleep specialists as playing a valuable role in the management of OSA. Mandibular advancement splints are customised devices, designed to posture the mandible forwards during sleep. The principal mechanism of action of these appliances is anatomical. They act to increase the size of the pharyngeal airway by drawing the tongue forward through its muscular attachments, and by stretching the palatoglossal and palatopharyngeal arches they reduce airway collapsibility.[11,12] The American Academy of Sleep Medicine has issued the following recommendations for the use of mandibular advancement splints in OSA:[13]

- Mild to moderate OSA – in which patients express preference for a mandibular advancement splint, and are intolerant of *or* refuse nasal CPAP
- Severe OSA – these patients must always undergo a nasal CPAP trial and only if they are found to be intolerant of *or* refuse it, should they be offered a mandibular advancement splint. Furthermore, mandibular advancement splints should be offered to patients who are not suitable candidates for surgery.

Thus, it would appear that the mandibular advancement splints plays a very central role in the management of OSA, either as a primary or secondary treatment choice.

There is considerable variation in the design of mandibular advancement splints, but all posture the mandible forwards, to a varying extent, with a degree of vertical opening. They may be prefabricated or custom-made using a soft or hard plastic and as a one- or two-piece design. Despite the wide variety of appliances described in the literature, there are limited guidelines available in relation to the optimal design features important to their success.[14] The currently available appliances could be broadly classified into three types, based on a succession of design modifications, which importantly permit incremental advancement of the mandible:

- *First generation.* These were primarily one-piece in design, with no ability to incrementally advance the mandible, without a new appliance being fabricated (Figure 27.4).
- *Second generation.* This type of appliance was principally two-piece in design and offered the potential for incremental advancement (Figure 27.5). However, this would often necessitate laboratory support and potentially were more time-consuming at the chairside.
- *Third generation.* These appliances may be regarded as the 'gold standard' in design.

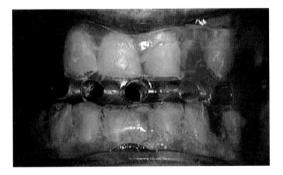

Figure 27.4 First generation vacuum-formed mandibular advancement splint.

They not only permit incremental advancement, which is self-adjustable, but also lateral movement of the mandible, and ensure the mandible is retained in its postured state during sleep (Figure 27.6).

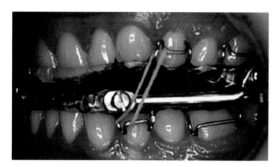

Figure 27.5 Second generation Herbst removable mandibular advancement splint.

A recent Cochrane review evaluated randomised trials comparing oral appliances with control appliances or other treatments in adults with OSA.[15] A total of 13 trials involving 553 subjects were included. The review found that while there was some evidence that these appliances improved subjective sleepiness and sleep-disordered breathing compared with a placebo, they were less effective than nasal CPAP. The authors concluded that based on the lack of definite evidence on their effectiveness, the use of oral appliances should be restricted to OSA subjects unwilling or unable to cope with nasal CPAP. However, the review found shortcomings in all the studies evaluated, such as small sample size, a lack of blinding and under-reporting of methods and data. In a subsequent randomised crossover trial involving

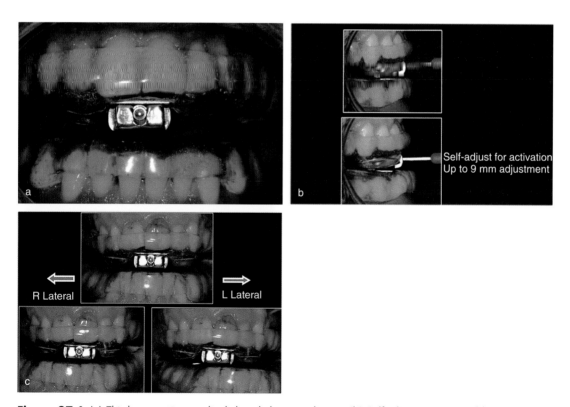

Figure 27.6 (a) Third generation medical dental sleep appliance. (b) Self-adjustment is possible anteroposteriorly in an incremental manner. (c) Right and left lateral movements.

80 patients with mild to moderate OSA, undertaken by Barnes et al.,[16] MAS were found to be subjectively as effective as CPAP. However, objectively CPAP performed superiorly.

It is important to note that mandibular advancement splints, like CPAP, do not provide a cure for OSA and as such will need to be used long term, requiring periodic adjustment, repair or replacement. Little is known about long-term compliance but short-term compliance is reported to range from 50% to 100%.[17] Short-term side effects are common, and include discomfort in the muscles of mastication, excessive salivation, dry mouth and abnormalities of the bite on awakening. These effects appear to be transient and tend to resolve with regular wear. Later complications which may preclude the use of a mandibular advancement splint is the risk of dentoalveolar changes.[18–20] In view of the long-term nature of this form of treatment and the potential for undesirable tooth movements to take place, patients should be followed up long term.

Surgical Treatment

A variety of surgical approaches have been developed and can be classified as follows:

- *Nasal surgery.* This form of surgery is designed to eliminate any obvious physical obstructions which can exacerbate the symptoms of OSA and inhibit the use of CPAP.
- *Pharyngeal surgery.* A number of surgical techniques have been developed in an attempt to increase the size of the pharyngeal airway in OSA patients. These have ranged in morbidity from uvulopalatopharyngoplasty (excision of the uvula, tonsils and a variable portion of the soft palate) to outpatient laser therapy. Unfortunately, their long-term value appears questionable and despite the reported short-term benefits these do not appear to last beyond 6–12 months. Tracheostomy has proven value, due to the fact the incision bypasses the pharyngeal airway. Naturally, the procedure is reserved for very severe obstructions which fail to respond to other treatment modalities, in view of its psychosocial morbidity.
- *Maxillofacial surgery.* A variety of surgical procedures have been described to treat OSA. While there appears to be short-term success, this appears to be highly variable and as such is not a recognised first-line approach in the management of OSA.

References

1. Young T, Palta M, Dempsey J, Skatrud J, Weber S, Badr S. The occurrence of sleep disordered breathing among middle-aged adults. N Engl J Med 1993;328:1230–5.
2. Lowe AA, Santamaria JD, Fleetham JA, Price C. Facial morphology and obstructive sleep apnoea. Am J Orthod Dentofacial Orthop 1986;90:484–91.
3. De Berry-Borowiecki B, Kukwa A, Blanks RHI, Irvine CA. Cephalometric analysis for diagnosis and treatment of obstructive sleep apnea. Laryngoscope 1988;98:226–34.
4. Johal A, Battagel JM, Kotecha B. A cephalometric comparison of subjects with snoring and obstructive sleep apnoea. Eur J Orthod 2000;22:353–65.
5. Johal A, Patel S, Battagel JM. The relationship between craniofacial anatomy and obstructive sleep apnoea: a case-controlled study. J Sleep Res 2007;16:319–26.
6. Deegan PC, McNicholas WT. Pathophysiology of obstructive sleep apnoea. Eur Respir J 1995;8:1161–78.
7. Johns MW. A new method for measuring daytime sleepiness: The Epworth Sleepiness Scale. Sleep 1991;14:540–5.
8. Redline S, Torteson T, Boucher M, Millman RP. Measurement of sleep-related breathing disturbances in epidemiologic studies. assessment of the validity and reproducibility of a portable monitoring device. Chest 1991;100:1281–7.

9. Sullivan CE, Berthon-Jones M, Issa FG, Eves L. Reversal of obstructive sleep apnoea by continuous positive airway pressure applied through the nares. Lancet 1981;1: 862–5.

10. Engleman HM, Martin SE, Douglas NJ. Compliance with CPAP therapy in patients with the sleep apnoea/hypopnoea syndrome. Thorax 1994;49:263–6.

11. Johal A, Battagel JM. An investigation into the changes in airway dimension and the efficacy of mandibular advancement appliances in subjects with obstructive sleep apnoea. Brit J Orthod 1999;26:205–10.

12. Ryan CF, Love LL, Peat D, Fleetham JA, Lowe AA. Mandibular advancement oral appliance therapy for obstructive sleep apnoea: effect on awake calibre of the velopharynx. Thorax 1999;54:972–7.

13. Kushida CA, Morgenthaler TI, Littner MR, et al. Practice parameters for the treatment of snoring and obstructive sleep apnea with oral appliances: An update for 2005. Sleep 2006;29;240–3.

14. Johal A, Battagel JM. Current principles in the management of obstructive sleep apnoea with mandibular advancement appliances. Brit Dent J 2001;190:532–6.

15. Lim J, Lasserson TJ, Fleetham J, Wright J. Oral appliances for obstructive sleep apnoea. Cochrane Database Syst Rev 2004; 4:CD004435.

16. Barnes M, Douglas R, Banks S, et al. Efficacy of positive airway pressure and oral appliance in mild to moderate obstructive sleep apnea. Am J Respir Crit Care Med 2004;170:656–64.

17. Schmidt-Nowara W, Lowe A, Wiegand L, Cartwright R, Perez-Guerra F, Menn S. Oral appliances for the treatment of snoring and obstructive sleep apnea: a review. Sleep 1995;18:501–10.

18. de Almeida FR, Lowe AA, Sung JO, Tsuiki S, Otsuka R. Long-term sequelle of oral appliance therapy in obstructive sleep apnea patients: Part 1. Cephalometric analysis. Am J Orthod Dentofacial Orthop 2006;129:195–204.

19. de Almeida FR, Lowe AA, Tsuiki S, et al. Long-term sequelle of oral appliance therapy in obstructive sleep apnea patients: Part 2. Study-model analysis. Am J Orthod Dentofacial Orthop 2006;129:205–13.

20. Marklund M. Predictors of long term orthodontic side effects from mandibular advancement devices in patients with snoring and obstructive sleep apnoea. Am J Orthod Dentofacial Orthop 2006;129: 214–21.

Appliance Techniques 4

28

Biological responses during orthodontic tooth movement

UPDATE ON BONE PHYSIOLOGY

Bone remodelling associated with orthodontic tooth movement has become clearer with an increased knowledge of osteoblast and osteoclast interactions. Bone comprises a matrix of mineral (70%) based on a type 1 collagen scaffold (27%). The remaining 3% of the matrix comprises minor collagens and other proteins including osteocalcin, osteonectin, osteopontin, phosphoproteins, sialoproteins, glycoproteins, lipids and glycosaminoglycans. The matrix also contains a wide variety of polypeptide growth factors. Many of these are bound to proteins (binding proteins) that render them inactive. These growth factors are liberated from the matrix as well as the binding proteins by osteoclast acid hydroxylases. Within the matrix are blood vessels and these features are important in cellular actions and bone function. The main bone cell types are osteoblasts, osteocytes and osteoclasts.

Osteoblasts

Osteoblasts arise from undifferentiated mesenchymal cells which differentiate through an immediate pre-osteoblast state to the mature and functional osteoblast state. In this mature state, the osteoblast synthesises both collagenous and non-collagenous bone proteins which constitute the organic matrix or osteoid. Within this osteoid, type I collagen accounts for 90% of the protein in bone. In addition to this bone-forming activity, the osteoblast is responsible for osteoclast recruitment and activation in response to hormonal and mechanical challenges. It is the osteoblast that has receptors for most of the bone-resorbing hormones such as parathyroid hormone (PTH) and the cytokines. This is important when osteoblast and osteoclast interactions are considered further (see below).

Osteocytes represent terminally differentiated osteoblasts, and are cells that have produced sufficient matrix to encase themselves

Orthodontics: Principles and Practice, First Edition. Edited by Daljit S. Gill, Farhad B. Naini.
© 2011 Daljit S. Gill, Farhad B. Naini and Dental Update. Published 2011 by Blackwell Publishing Ltd.

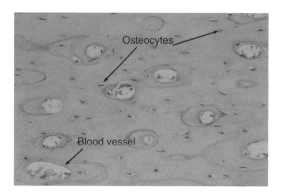

Figure 28.1 Haematoxylin and eosin section of bone illustrating the position of osteocytes within a calcified matrix. The large lacunae are blood vessels and both the osteocyte and the blood vessel are clearly marked.

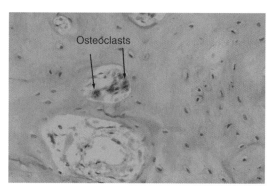

Figure 28.2 The lineage of osteoclasts is important. This haematoxylin and eosin section demonstrates a blood vessel in bone and within the blood vessel three osteoclasts, two of which are clearly marked.

within bone. They remain connected to other osteocytes and the surface-lining osteoblasts through canaliculi. Entombed within a fairly rigid matrix, they are ideally positioned to detect any mechanical forces that might be placed on bone such as in orthodontic tooth movement. The osteocytes can then send signals to the osteoblasts, which may recruit and activate osteoclasts to cause bone resorption. Figure 28.1 shows the position of osteocytes within the bone, each lying within its own lacunae.

Osteoclasts

Osteoclasts are the main bone resorption cells. Their appearance in culture is striking, and each has a large number of nuclei and a highly active peripheral cytoplasm. The latter is a crucial morphological feature since it allows the osteoclasts to 'seal' off a portion of bone matrix and then create an acid environment for the dissolution of bone as well as the cleavage of growth factors from their binding proteins. These growth factors are usually cleaved in a latent (inactive) form but the acidity will release the growth factors from this latency, enabling them as active growth factors.

Osteoclasts are formed by fusion of circulating monocytes in response to specific signals from the osteoblasts. Figure 28.2 shows very clearly the importance of this vascular origin. Within the blood vessel are several osteoclasts and these can be recruited to specific regions of resorptive activity. These osteoblast–osteoclast interactions have been an area of exciting discovery in the past few years. The osteoclast by contrast to the osteoblast has very few receptors for hormones, e.g. calcitonin and retinoic acid. Most of the hormones that the osteoclast has receptors for have inhibitory actions (e.g. prostaglandin E_2) and these result in a decrease of osteoclast activity. A number of hormones elevate intracellular cyclic AMP levels and this second messenger seems to be a major pathway for inhibition of osteoclast activity.

Osteoblast–osteoclast Interactions

Osteoclasts in isolated culture have relatively little activity and are not stimulated with bone-seeking hormones such as PTH or cytokines. It is only when co-cultured with osteoblasts and bone-seeking hormones that osteoclasts start to demonstrate motility or to resorb calcified matrices such as bone or dentine. Thus osteo-clasts cannot resorb bone without prior activation by osteoblasts but for many years what these signals comprised was not known. Furthermore the control mechanisms and feed-back loops to control the bone remodelling could only be guessed at. Recently a number of important discoveries have helped clarify the situation.

The first significant step was the recognition that three members of the tumour necrosis factor (TNF) and TNF receptor superfamily are involved in the formation and activation of osteoclasts. A well-known step in the formation of osteoclasts is the action of the macrophage colony-stimulating factor (M-CSF) which stimulates differentiation and proliferation of hae-mopoietic progenitors or pre-osteoclasts. These pre-osteoclasts express a receptor called RANK (receptor activator of nuclear factor [NF]-κB) and the ligand for this receptor (RANKL) is produced by osteoblasts. RANKL is important for the differentiation of osteoclasts from mono-cytic precursors as well as maintaining osteo-clast function.

Unfortunately, a feedback loop makes this a bit more complicated. Osteoblasts also produce and secrete osteoprotegerin (OPG), which acts as a decoy receptor that can block RANKL/RANK interactions. Bone-resorbing hormones can increase RANKL expression in osteoblasts, and some can also decrease OPG expression.[1] Bone cells appear to express the membrane-bound form of RANKL, and, thus, osteoblasts must physically interact with osteoclast precur-sors in order to activate RANK. This complex picture can be seen clearly in studies where, in mice, the genes for OPG are manipulated so that OPG is overexpressed. Since OPG blocks RANKL/RANK interactions, osteoclast func-tion is diminished and excess bone is laid down. The mouse becomes osteopetrotic. This osteo-petrotic state can be reversed by injection of the RANKL protein. Similarly the gene for OPG can be deleted in mice with a resultant increase in osteoclast activity and the development of an

osteoporotic state, sufficiently severe to cause bone fractures.[2] Potentially all of these findings could provide information to develop a strat-egy to deal with the consequences of osteopo-rosis, osteopetrosis and other crippling diseases. No doubt other pathways which modulate osteoblast and osteoclast interactions will be found and modify our thinking on bone remod-elling. These complex interactions are sum-marised in Figure 28.3 and the osteoblast, osteoclast and osteocyte relationships in Figure 28.4.

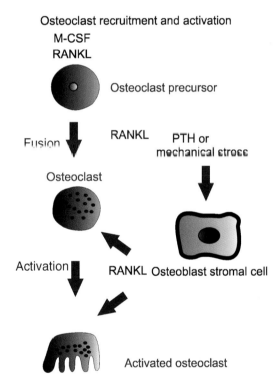

Figure 28.3 The 'missing link' between osteoblasts and osteoclast interactions can be explained in part through RANK ligand (RANKL). Osteoblasts produce RANKL in response to stimuli such as mechanical stress or hormones such as parathyroid hormone (PTH). RANKL is responsible for formation of osteoclasts from haemopoietic progenitor cells and also for increasing the activity of osteoclasts and thus increasing bone resorption. M-CSF, macrophage colony-stimulating factor.

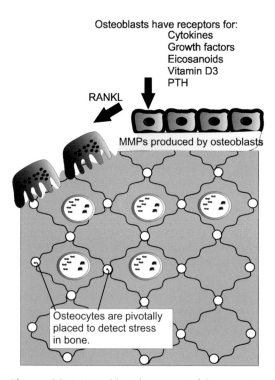

Osteoblasts have receptors for:
Cytokines
Growth factors
Eicosanoids
Vitamin D3
PTH

RANKL

MMPs produced by osteoblasts

Osteocytes are pivotally placed to detect stress in bone.

Figure 28.4 Osteoblasts have most of the receptors for bone-seeking hormones, some of which are shown within the schematic. In response to these hormones or indeed mechanical stress, RANK ligand (RANKL) is produced, which is responsible for recruitment and activation of osteoclasts. The osteoblast in response to bone-seeking hormones also produces matrix metalloproteinases (MMPs), which remove the thin collagenous osteoid layer. This is important for osteoclast dissolution of mineralised tissue. PTH, parathyroid hormone.

Matrix Regulation

The regulation of extracellular matrix is an integral and crucial part of bone remodelling. The extracellular matrix degrading metallo enzymes are known collectively as matrix metalloproteinases (MMPs). This family of enzymes are also regulated by endogenous inhibitors called tissue inhibitors of metalloproteinases (TIMPs). The family of MMPs is constantly increasing; they are called metallo because they depend on zinc and calcium ions for activity. They act at

neutral pH and are important because they digest the major macro molecules of connective tissues. It must be emphasised that tissue breakdown occurs where MMPs are in excess of TIMP. The significance in bone resorption is that the thin layer of osteoid covering bone must be removed before osteoclasts can remove calcified matrix. Osteoblasts, when stimulated, produce the MMPs (principally collagenase) responsible for removal of the osteoid layer.

In summary, a hormone or mechanical force stimulates osteoblasts to produce a soluble mediator for activation and recruitment of osteoclasts (RANKL/RANK). In addition, osteoblasts produce MMPs for breakdown of the non-mineralised osteoid layer. Once osteoid is removed, the mineralised matrix is exposed and the osteoclasts can then remove bone. The osteocytes are situated in a rigid matrix and are thus ideally positioned to detect changes in mechanical stresses. They are able to signal to surface-lining osteoblasts, and either bone formation or bone resorption results.

BIOLOGICAL RESPONSES DURING ORTHODONTIC TOOTH MOVEMENT

The various theories of tooth movement have by and large been discounted or at least placed in context by an improved understanding of biological responses seen during remodelling of tissues. How biological responses to mechanical stress result in bone resorption and bone formation is not fully understood but it is relevant to first consider how these forces are transmitted to cells. Teeth move in the direction of the force applied to them. Tooth movement is achieved by bone being resorbed in front of the direction of travel (pressure site) and bone being deposited behind the tooth in the so-called tension site. This simplistic view is not understood by orthopaedic surgeons who will interpret bone responses to pressure and tension sites very differently. If a long bone is

Bone bending

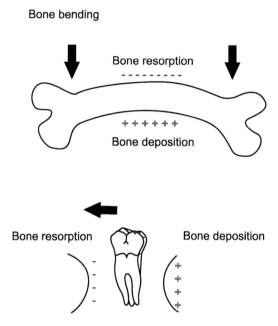

Figure 28.5 Teeth move in the direction of the force applied to them. It is achieved by bone being resorbed in front of the direction of travel (pressure site) and bone being deposited behind the tooth (the 'tension' site). When a long bone is bent, bone is resorbed at tension sites but bone formation is seen where bone is compressed. Bone bending is also seen during tooth movement. The shape of the alveolar bone housing a tooth is altered by the stretching of periodontal ligament fibres, which produces a concave configuration of the alveolar bon, identical to that seen in the concave long bone where compression of the molecules results in bone formation. By contrast, where the periodontal ligament is compressed, the adjacent alveolar bone surface becomes convex and bone is resorbed.

bent (see Figure 28.5), bone is resorbed in tension sites and compression results in bone formation. Essentially we may be looking at the same thing. The shape of the alveolar bone housing a tooth is altered by the stretching of periodontal ligament fibres, which produces a concave configuration of the alveolar bone, identical to that seen in the concave long bone where compression of the molecules results in bone formation. By contrast where the periodontal ligament is compressed, the adjacent

alveolar bone surface becomes convex and bone is resorbed.

It is important to also consider how the forces are transmitted to cells and there are several areas which appear to have received scant attention in the majority of texts. The immediate response after the application of an external force is strain in the matrix of the periodontal ligament and the alveolar bone, which results in fluid flow in both tissues.[3] The fluids flow from an area of compression to a zone of tension and this flow will cause a strain in cells and also stretch the intracellular cytoskeleton which is attached through the cell wall to the extracellular matrix. All these changes result in force on the cell membrane, the cytoskeleton and the surrounding matrix (Figure 28.6). In response to these forces, the cells in the periodontal ligament, osteoblasts and osteocytes are activated and a variety of biological responses follow. The periodontal ligament is remodelled and bone is either synthesised or resorbed to allow the tooth to move. What is not clear is how cells recognise when to produce molecules which destroy matrix or build matrix.

Immediate Cellular Responses

The immediate cellular responses are those associated with cell membranes and the triggering of intracellular second messenger pathways which invoke a nuclear response. Thereafter, further signalling molecules are generated which are responsible for osteoclast recruitment and activation, or secretion of bone-forming growth factors. An indirect pathway of activation exists whereby membrane enzymes (phospholipase A_2) make substrate (arachidonic acid) available for the generation of prostaglandins and leukotrienes. These compounds have both been implicated in tooth movement. These eicosanoids activate the intracellular second messengers cyclic AMP and inositol phosphates. These both raise intracellular calcium, which may also enter the cell via G-protein-controlled ion channels.[4]

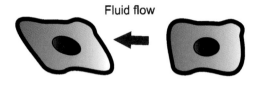

Fluid flow

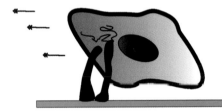

Cytoskeleton distortion

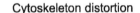

Extracellular matrix

Membrane distortion of phospholipid bilayer

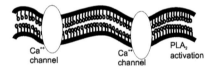

Ca^{++}
channel

Ca^{++}
channel

PLA_2
activation

Figure 28.6 The immediate response after the application of an external force is strain in the matrix of the periodontal ligament and the alveolar bone which results in fluid flow in both tissues. The fluid flow will cause a strain in cells and also stretch the intracellular cytoskeleton which is attached through the cell wall to the extracellular matrix. All these changes result in force on the cell membrane, the cytoskeleton and the surrounding matrix. The cytoskeleton distortion triggers activation of a number of signal pathways. The mechanical deformation of the bi-lipid cell membrane will result in activation of calcium channels and the enzyme phospholipase A_2 (PLA_2), which cleaves arachidonic acid from the membrane. The latter is a substrate for cyclo-oxygenases and the result is the formation of prostaglandins and leukotrienes, agents known to be involved in orthodontic tooth movement.

Cytokines, Cell-cell Signalling Molecules and Enzymes

Much of the improvement in understanding of events associated with tooth movement has arisen from advances in molecular biology. One

approach has been the use of cDNA microarrays, which allows a shotgun, non-hypothesis-driven strategy to simply look at which genes are up- or down-regulated in compressed tissue. This technology allows the screening of thousands of genes. Once identified, the proteins they code for can be examined for function *in vivo*. A good example is the work which identified up-regulation of the *MMP3* gene when osteoblast-like cells were compressed in a three-dimensional gel *in vitro*. This was followed up by identifying that the protein was also produced by these compressed cells with a western immunoblot analysis and finally corroborated *in vivo* using immunohistochemistry to look at orthodontically compressed tissues in 'volunteer' patients.[5] MMP3, a stromelysin, has broad catabolic activity on a variety of extracellular matrix molecules, including proteoglycans, fibronectin, gelatin, collagen types IV and IX, and laminin. This study also corroborated that the gene for cyclo-oxygenase enzymes (eventually producing prostaglandins) was also up-regulated, an observation reported previously in many studies of compressed tissue. Using a similar approach, others have shown a different response when cells derived from the periodontal ligament were stretched rather than compressed. Under these conditions the periodontal ligament cells show markers of osteoblast differentiation through up-regulation of genes associated with bone formation (bone morphogenetic proteins and alkaline phosphatase) including differentiation through the chondrogenic pathway (*Sox9*). This makes sense as, clearly, mechanically perturbed cells need at some point to make new matrix and lay down new bone.[6]

Having described the RANKL-RANK control of bone turnover, not surprisingly, this has been examined during tooth movement. Some initial work showed that gene transfer of RANKL to the periodontal ligament increased the rate of tooth movement and this was followed by a study in humans undergoing orthodontic tooth movement. Here the resorption site of tooth movement showed higher expression of TNF-α, RANKL and MMP-1, whereas the bone forming site showed higher expression of interleukin (IL)-10, TIMP-1, OPG and osteocalcin. The latter group of molecules are all associated with anabolic activities and thus bone formation.[7]

Chemokines are a superfamily of small chemotactic cytokines that regulate inflammatory processes and migration. They are known to be involved in cell precursor development for osteoblasts and osteoclasts. They are therefore potential modulators of bone remodelling associated with orthodontic tooth movement. Osteoclast precursors express chemokine receptors and the chemotactic signals provided by chemokines may invoke their migration to bone tissues as well as the differentiation, survival and activation of osteoclasts. The latter function also requires the involvement of RANK-RANKL. Osteoblasts are also found to express several chemokine receptors, and the binding of chemokines induces both proliferation and collagen type I mRNA expression in osteoblasts. They also promote cell survival. There is evidence of differential expression of chemokines in compressed and stretched periodontal ligament during orthodontic tooth movement suggesting that chemokines may contribute to the differential bone remodelling in response to orthodontic force as well as the establishment of distinct microenvironments in compression and tension sides.[8]

OPTIMAL FORCES FOR INDUCING TOOTH MOVEMENT

Classically, ideal forces in orthodontic tooth movement are those which just overcome capillary blood pressure. In this situation bone resorption is seen on the pressure side and bone deposition on the tension side (Figures 28.7, 28.8). Teeth rarely move in this ideal way. Usually force is not applied evenly and teeth move by a series of tipping and uprighting movements. In some areas excessive pressure

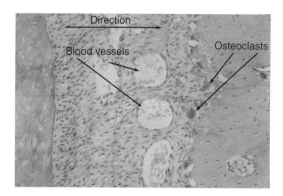

Figure 28.7 Haematoxylin and eosin section of a tooth being moved in the indicated direction. True frontal resorption is evident with numerous osteoclasts resorbing bone. The periodontal ligament is highly vascular, which is the likely conduit for recruitment of osteoclasts.

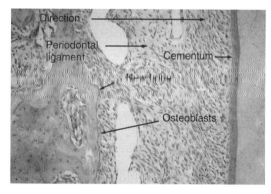

Figure 28.8 Haematoxylin and eosin section of a tooth being moved in the indicated direction. Bone deposition is evident as a pale pink eosinophilic area with no osteocytes. The large surface-lining osteoblasts are obvious and line the area of new bone formation.

results in hyalinisation where the cellular component of the periodontal ligament disappears. The hyalinised zone assumes a ground-glass appearance but this returns to normal once the pressure is reduced and the periodontal ligament repopulated with normal cells. In this situation a different type of resorption is seen whereby osteoclasts appear to 'undermine' bone rather than resorbing at the 'frontal' edge

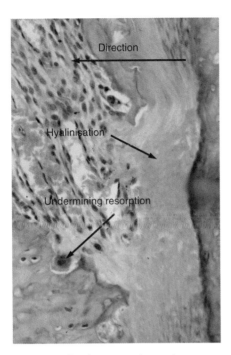

Figure 28.9 This haematoxylin and eosin section shows an area of periodontal ligament which has been subjected to excessive pressure resulting in a 'ground glass appearance' of the cells commonly referred to as hyalinisation. There is no vascularity and no cell architecture (compare with Figures 28.7 and 28.8). Undermining resorption is evident on one aspect of this section. This is a slow and inefficient way of moving teeth.

(Figure 28.9). The forces used should therefore be light and it is recognised that very low levels of force are capable of moving teeth.

Evidence on applying different forces to bone suggests that intermittent forces generate more bone turnover than continuous forces. In practice this is difficult to apply clinically but the 'intermittent' effect of occlusal contact during mastication may provide this effect in bone adjacent to teeth and account for the efficiency of orthodontic tooth movement. In a systematic review of crevicular changes during orthodontic tooth movement it has been suggested that associations exist between PGE_2

and IL-1β and pain, velocity of tooth movement, and treatment mechanics. IL-1β and PGE_2 show different patterns of up-regulation, with IL-1β being more responsive to mechanical stress and PGE_2 more responsive to synergistic regulation of IL-1β and mechanical force. The results support the concept of using light continuous forces for orthodontic treatment.[9] The current vogue for ascribing an ability of a single bracket type (self-ligating) to change these basic biological concepts seems unlikely. These commercially driven claims need to be supported with evidence. There is, moreover, a growing body of evidence that the clinical advantages of self-ligating brackets are completely unfounded and that they do not align teeth more quickly, cause less pain or grow more bone than other types of brackets.[10–12]

References

1. Suda T, Takahashi N, Udagawa N, Jimi E, Gillespie MT, Martin TJ. Modulation of osteoclast differentiation and function by the new members of the tumor necrosis factor receptor and ligand families. Endocrinol Rev 1999;20:345–57.
2. Bucay N, Sarosi I, Dunstan CR, et al. Osteoprotegerin-deficient mice develop early onset osteoporosis and arterial calcification. Genes Dev 1998;12:1260–8.
3. Henneman S, Von den Hoff JW, Maltha JC. Mechanobiology of tooth movement. Eur J Orthod 2008;30:299–306.
4. Krishnan V, Davidovitch Z. Cellular, molecular, and tissue-level reactions to orthodontic force. Am J Orthod Dentofacial Orthop 2006;129:469.e1–32.
5. Chang HH, Wu CB, Chen YJ, et al. MMP-3 response to compressive forces in vitro and in vivo. J Dent Res 2008;87:692–6.
6. Wescott DC, Pinkerton MN, Gaffey BJ, Beggs KT, Milne TJ, Meikle MC. Osteogenic gene expression by human periodontal ligament cells under cyclic tension. J Dent Res 2007;86:1212–16.

7. Garlet TP, Coelho U, Silva JS, Garlet GP. Cytokine expression pattern in compression and tension sides of the periodontal ligament during orthodontic tooth movement in humans. Eur J Oral Sci 2007;115: 355–62.

8. Garlet TP, Coelho U, Repeke CE, Silva JS, Cunha F, Garlet GP. Differential expression of osteoblast and osteoclast chemoattractants in compression and tension sides during orthodontic movement. Cytokine 2008;42:330–5.

9. Ren Y, Vissink A. Cytokines in crevicular fluid and orthodontic tooth movement. Eur J Oral Sci 2008;116:89–97.

10. Scott P, Sherriff M, Dibiase AT, Cobourne MT. Perception of discomfort during initial orthodontic tooth alignment using a self-ligating or conventional bracket system: a randomized clinical trial. Eur J Orthod 2008;30:227–32.

11. Scott P, DiBiase AT, Sherriff M, Cobourne MT. Alignment efficiency of Damon3 self-ligating and conventional orthodontic bracket systems: a randomized clinical trial. Am J Orthod Dentofacial Orthop 2008; 134:470.e1–8.

12. Pandis N, Polychronopoulou A, Eliades T. Self-ligating vs conventional brackets in the treatment of mandibular crowding: a prospective clinical trial of treatment duration and dental effects. Am J Orthod Dentofacial Orthop 2007;132:208–15.

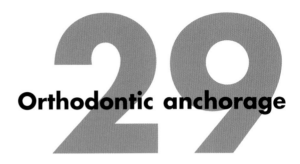

Orthodontic anchorage

INTRODUCTION

Orthodontics involves moving teeth from positions of malalignment into alignment. This requires the application of a force through an archwire, an elastic or a spring. Unless the orthodontist is using a screw or plate attached to the jaw bone (see Chapter 30), the force used to move the tooth is applied from other teeth within the same or opposite arch. These teeth may be in the correct position and therefore the orthodontist will not want them to move. Anchorage is the term used by orthodontists to describe the process of ensuring that desirable tooth movements occur and undesirable tooth movements, in all three dimensions, are prevented. In brief, it is the *control of unwanted tooth movement*.

No discussion of orthodontic anchorage is complete without mentioning Newton's third law of motion. It is also known as the law of reciprocal action or as summarised by Newton 'Every action has an equal and opposite reaction'. An example of Newton's third law of motion is that of a canoe being propelled

forward by the backward force of paddling (Figure 29.1).

When a force of sufficient size and duration is applied to a tooth it will generally move in the direction of the force, unless steps are taken to prevent it. Early studies suggested that the rate of tooth movement was associated with the size of the force applied and the surface area of the root of the tooth.[1–6] Partly as a result of these studies, clinicians have undertaken various steps in order to prevent the anchor teeth from moving, also known as **conserving** anchorage. These include:

- Involving as many teeth in the anchorage unit as possible to distribute the force over a larger root surface area
- Only moving one tooth at a time per quadrant
- Using a light force sufficient to move the tooth, but not large enough to move the anchor unit.

Recent work carried out under more controlled conditions has cast doubt on this approach to

Orthodontics: Principles and Practice, First Edition. Edited by Daljit S. Gill, Farhad B. Naini.
© 2011 Daljit S. Gill, Farhad B. Naini and Dental Update. Published 2011 by Blackwell Publishing Ltd.

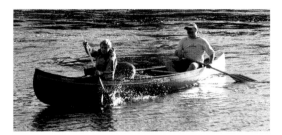

Figure 29.1 Newton's third law of motion in action. The canoe is being propelled forward by the backward force of the paddling.

anchorage conservation. Pilon et al.,[7] working with experimental dogs, found no difference in the mesial movement of the anchorage unit between three different clinically relevant forces. The authors suggest that the individual's biological response to the force was a more significant factor in determining the rate of tooth movement than was the size or duration of the force. Ren et al.[8] combined the data from several animal studies to produce a mathematical model to describe the relationship between force magnitude and the rate of tooth movement, which they then tested on data from clinical research. They concluded that there are insufficient data to determine whether there is a threshold of force below which tooth movement does not occur. They also identified a wide range of forces (104–454 cN) over which the maximum rate of movement could be achieved.

It would therefore appear that the traditional clinical approaches to anchorage conservation might not be as reliable as was once thought and the orthodontist should consider alternative means of **reinforcing** anchorage when required, in order to achieve the best treatment results.

ANCHORAGE IN CLASS I CASES

The anchorage requirements in a patient with a Class I malocclusion will depend on the exact

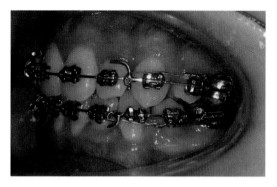

Figure 29.2 An example of reciprocal anchorage. Residual space following extraction of first premolars to create space for alignment of crowded incisors is being closed by equal movement of anterior and posterior teeth.

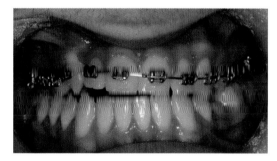

Figure 29.3 Loss of vertical anchorage during the alignment of the upper right ectopic canine.

cause of the malocclusion. If a patient with crowded arches has space created by the extraction of premolars, then after alignment of the teeth it is usually sufficient to close any residual extraction spaces by equal movement of both anterior and posterior teeth. This equal movement of teeth on either side of the force is sometimes known as **reciprocal** anchorage (Figure 29.2). In cases where vertical movements are required, for example with an ectopic canine, vertical reinforcement of anchorage may be required (Figure 29.3). This might involve the use of a transpalatal arch (TPA) attached to bands on the upper first molars (Figure 29.4). Some clinicians use an upper removable

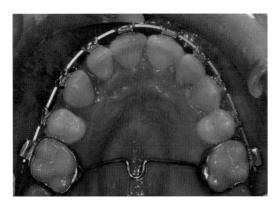

Figure 29.4 A transpalatal arch providing additional vertical anchorage during alignment of the ectopic upper right canine.

appliance, with acrylic palatal coverage for additional vertical anchorage support.

ANCHORAGE IN CLASS II CASES

In patients with a Class II malocclusion the orthodontist is generally aiming to reduce the overjet, but might also need additional space to align crowded teeth. Space requirements are therefore usually critical in the upper labial segment. The undesirable tooth movement in this situation is for the upper posterior teeth to move forward, using up the space required to align the labial segment and reduce the overjet. Many orthodontists use a functional appliance to reduce the overjet and correct a Class II molar relationship thereby improving the anchorage requirements. Another way to reinforce anchorage is to place headgear to the upper molars to prevent their forward movement (Figure 29.5), but this is unpopular with patients and there is the risk, albeit rare, of serious injury.[9]

The TPA is another traditional method of preventing excessive forward movement of the upper posterior teeth in patients in situations where the anchorage requirements are not too

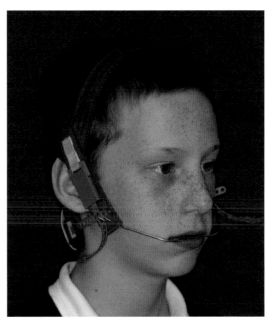

Figure 29.5 An extraoral or headgear appliance being used to provide additional anchorage support.

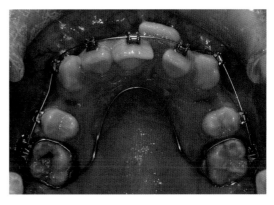

Figure 29.6 A transpalatal arch with an acrylic Nance button providing additional anchorage support from the palate.

critical. A Nance button, made of acrylic, can be placed in the palate to provide additional resistance (Figure 29.6), but care needs to be taken to remove this before active space closure, otherwise it can cause trauma and ulceration by becoming embedded in the tissues.

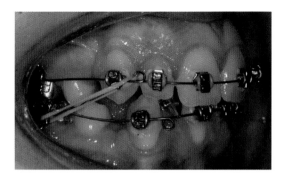

Figure 29.7 A Class II intermaxillary elastic being used with the Tip-Edge appliance.

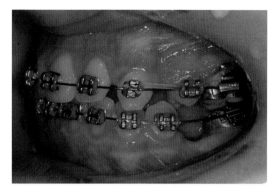

Figure 29.8 A Tip-Edge bracket being used on the upper left canine to tip it distally, creating space to correct the upper centreline, which was significantly displace to the right. Pre-adjusted edgewise brackets have been placed on the remaining teeth to prevent tipping and conserve anchorage.

The anchorage balance might be changed in a Class II patient by using intermaxillary elastics (Figure 29.7). A class II elastic, placed around the hook on the lower molar and taken to a loop or hook anteriorly in the upper arch will cause retroclination of the upper incisors. It will also encourage forward movement of the lower posterior teeth with minimal retroclination of the lower incisors and a consequent reduction in overjet.

In theory, lighter forces are required to tip teeth rather than move them bodily therefore anchorage can be conserved by allowing the tooth you want to move to tip, but preventing tipping in the anchor unit, so they have to move bodily. This is the basis of the Begg appliance and the more modern Tip-Edge appliance (see Chapter 33) (Figure 29.7), where the upper anterior teeth are allowed to tip distally using the force of the intermaxillary class II elastic, but the molar is prevented from moving forward by a 'tip-back bend'. The tip-back bend also helps to overcome the vertical extrusive effect of the elastic on the anterior teeth.

This principle can also be used to advantage in the pre-adjusted edgewise appliance. Figure 29.8 shows a Tip-Edge bracket being used on the upper left canine to allow this tooth to be tipped distally into a Class I relationship with the lower canine from the force of an intra-arch elastic. This is creating space to correct the upper centreline, which was significantly displaced to the right. The anchor unit of the second premolar and first molar are prevented from tipping by the edgewise bracket slot. They can only move forward by bodily movement, which requires a larger force.

Proponents of the newer self-ligating brackets suggest that because there is less friction in the system, lighter forces can be used and that this will be 'lighter' on anchorage. To date, there is little evidence to support this assertion.

ANCHORAGE IN CLASS III CASES

In patients with Class III malocclusions the undesirable tooth movements are retraction of the upper labial segment and/or proclination of the lower labial segment. Either of these movements might lead to loss of a positive overjet and appearance of a negative overjet. The risk of this happening can be reduced by maintaining torque (i.e. the inclination) in the upper incisor teeth with a full size rectangular stainless steel archwire and preventing torque expression in the lower incisors by using a

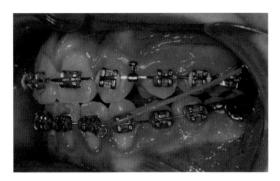

Figure 29.9 A class III intermaxillary elastic being used to bring the upper molar forward and help preserve a positive overjet for a patient with a missing upper lateral incisor undergoing orthodontic space closure.

round archwire. The anchorage balance can also be altered in favour of forward movement of the upper posterior teeth by using Class III intermaxillary elastics from the hook on the upper molar to a loop or hook anteriorly on the lower archwire (Figure 29.9). If extractions are required to relieve crowding then it is usually best to extract teeth further back in the upper arch, for example, by removing the second premolars rather than the first premolars.

SUMMARY

The careful planning of anchorage is crucial to the success of any orthodontic treatment plan. All patients should undergo a comprehensive space analysis (see Chapter 10) to estimate the anchorage requirements of the case. The concepts of anchorage conservation developed following early clinical experiments examining the relationship between force applied and movement of teeth might not be as successful as once thought. There are, however, various techniques that the orthodontist can use to ensure that desirable tooth movements are

achieved and undesirable tooth movements are kept to a minimum. The recently introduced orthodontic bone anchorage devices (see Chapter 30) have opened up greater possibilities for anchorage management.

References

1. Andreasen GF, Zwanziger D. A clinical evaluation of the differential force concept as applied to the edgewise bracket. Am J Orthod 1980;78:25–40.
2. Boester CH, Johnston LE. A clinical investigation of the concepts of differential and optimal force in canine retraction. Angle Orthod 1974;44:113–19.
3. Hixon EH, Aasen TO, Clark RA, Klosterman R, Miller SS, Odom WM. On force and tooth movement. Am J Orthod 1970;57:476–8.
4. Hixon EH, Atikian H, Callow GE, McDonald HW, Tacy RJ. Optimal force, differential force, and anchorage. Am J Orthod 1969;55:437–57.
5. Smith R, Storey E. The importance of force in orthodontics. Austr J Dent 1952;56:291–304.
6. Storey E, Smith R. Force in orthodontics and its relation to tooth movement. Austr J Dent 1952;56:11–18.
7. Pilon JJ, Kuijpers-Jagtman AM, Maltha JC. Magnitude of orthodontic forces and rate of bodily tooth movement. An experimental study. Am J Orthod Dentofacial Orthop 1996;110:16–23.
8. Ren Y, Maltha JC, Van 't Hof MA, Kuijpers-Jagtman AM. Optimum force magnitude for orthodontic tooth movement: a mathematic model. Am J Orthod Dentofacial Orthop 2004;125:71–7.
9. Samuels RH, Willner F, Knox J, Jones ML. A national survey of orthodontic facebow injuries in the UK and Eire. Br J Orthod 1996;23:11–20.

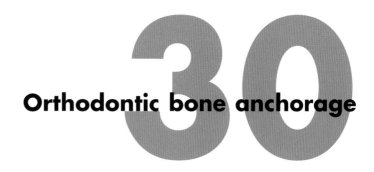

Orthodontic bone anchorage

INTRODUCTION

The subject of orthodontic anchorage has been revolutionised since the late 1990s through a combination of product innovations and both technique and research publications on skeletal anchorage. Indeed, within a few years the resultant paradigm shift has both rapidly and radically altered orthodontists' expectations of clinically absolute three-dimensional anchorage control. On one hand, many routine orthodontic movements may become more efficient and effective. Indeed, a recent prospective study of the retraction of incisors indicated that while headgear use results in anchorage loss, bone anchorage not only prevents anchorage loss, but can actually result in an anchorage gain (distalisation of molars).[1] On the other hand, the range of orthodontic treatment possibilities has been greatly expanded, e.g. it is now possible to correct anterior open bites by true orthodontic intrusion of the posterior teeth. This chapter describes the principles and types of bone anchorage, and provides an insight into its clinical potential.

BONE ANCHORAGE DEVICES

The first orthodontic bone anchorage devices were developed by several independent teams during the 1990s by utilising and adapting existing technology from two distinctly separate sources: restorative dental implants and maxillofacial bone plating kits (Figure 30.1). In turn, these developments have produced three categories of orthodontic devices: implants, mini-plates and mini-implants. Unfortunately, this has also resulted in a confusing array of names for these anchorage fixtures. In order to demystify the terminology it is probably best to use an umbrella term such as bone or temporary anchorage devices (BADs or TADs) to describe all types of osseous-based anchorage reinforcement. The acronym TAD is frequently used in the USA because it avoids any confusion with permanent restorative implants and the concept of bone surgery. However, it does not indicate the fundamental fact that these devices rely directly on osseous rather than tooth or superficial tissue stabilisation. As such many authors prefer to use specific terms which

Orthodontics: Principles and Practice, First Edition. Edited by Daljit S. Gill, Farhad B. Naini.
© 2011 Daljit S. Gill, Farhad B. Naini and Dental Update. Published 2011 by Blackwell Publishing Ltd.

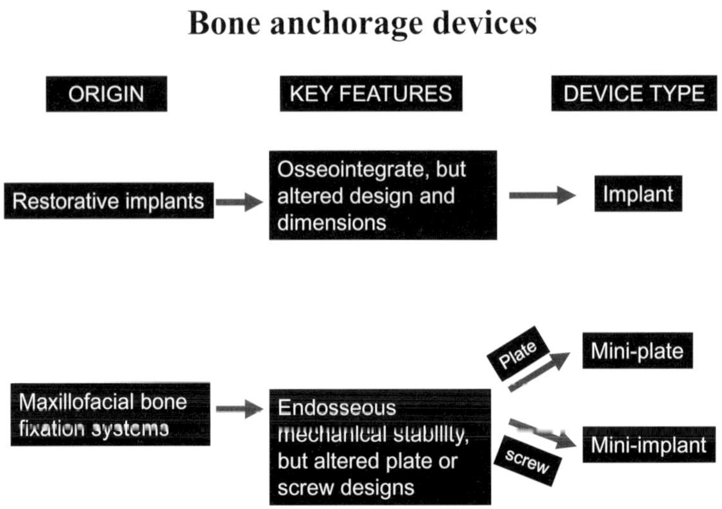

Bone anchorage devices

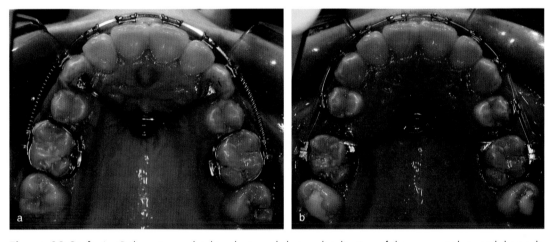

Figure 30.1 The origins and distinguishing features of the three principal types of orthodontic bone anchorage.

Figure 30.2a,b An Orthosystem palatal implant used during distalisation of the upper molars and then subsequent retraction of the anterior teeth. Indirect anchorage is achieved using a transpalatal arch between the implant head and the canines followed by the first molars.

signify the skeletal basis of this anchorage and the device's design, such as mini-implant or mini-screw. The term micro-implant is commonly misused, having erroneously arisen during translation into English, and should be avoided since none of these anchorage devices have microscopic dimensions.

In the first instance, adaptation of osseointegrating dental implant designs resulted in orthodontic-specific fixtures with shorter lengths (typically 4–6 mm) and wider diameters (typically 3–4 mm) than their restorative counterparts, e.g. the Orthosystem implant.[2] However, these dimensions limit their insertion into edentulous sites, typically the mid-palate (Figure 30.2) and retromolar areas. Other disadvantages is that these anchorage devices rely on osseointegration, which requires a 3 months' delay in orthodontic loading; their success rate is diminished by technique sensitivity, especially at the insertion stage; and they involve relatively complex indirect anchorage connections and associated laboratory work.[3] Consequently, while orthodontic implants may provide absolute anchorage they appear unlikely to be adopted into mainstream orthodontics, and essentially they have been superseded by mechanically retentive fixtures.

Mini-plates, e.g. the Bollard and Skeletal Anchorage (SAS) systems, arose from the adaptation of maxillofacial bone plates. In particular, the orthodontic versions have transmucosal necks and customised heads to facilitate their connection to fixed appliances (Figure 30.3). While mini-plates appear to be successful for a range of *en masse* tooth movements, and even intermaxillary skeletal traction (such as maxillary protraction in Class III cases), their insertion is limited to extra-alveolar sites such as the zygomatic process and inferior mandibular body.[4] In addition, they require much more invasive surgical placement and removal than other devices, and require an experienced surgical operator to insert them. Therefore, their potential for widespread clinical usage is likely to be limited.

Orthodontic mini-implants, like mini-plates, are derived from bone plating technology, but are much more user friendly to both the orthodontist and patient than the two aforementioned devices.[5,6] Consequently, and as indicated by the large number of recent publications on them, it is highly likely that mini-implants will be the form of bone anchorage adopted by most orthodontists. These fixtures are derived from the screw components of bone-plating systems e.g. Absoanchor, Infinitas, Vector. They typically consist of head, neck and body sections (Figure 30.4) with endosseous dimensions of 1.3–2.0 mm diameter and 5–10 mm length. In general, an approximate diameter of 1.5 mm is recommended for interproximal sites in order to maximise the surface area of bone engagement yet limit the proximity to dental roots and the (0.25 mm wide) periodontal ligament. To place these dimensions in context, the mean interproximal distance between the upper second premolar and first molar mesiobuccal root is 3.5 mm (Figure 30.5).

The latest mini-implant designs result from substantial modifications since the original bone screws were used in the 1990s, especially in terms of their head and neck configuration, and self-drilling insertion capabilities (Figure

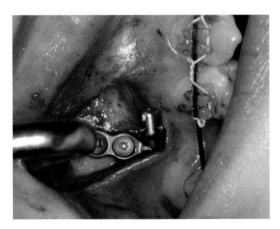

Figure 30.3 A Bollard mini-plate fixed to the inferior aspect of the zygomatic buttress by bone screws (after elevation of a mucoperiosteal flap). The cylindrical head will remain exposed in the buccal sulcus. Photograph courtesy of Dr Lars Christensen.

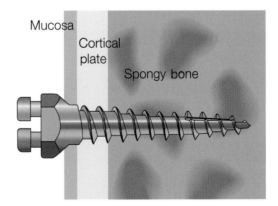

Mucosa
Cortical plate
Spongy bone

Figure 30.4 Diagram of a mini-implant showing its three principal parts: the intraoral bracket-like head, the transmucosal neck and the tapered threaded endosseous body (in both cortical and cancellous bone).

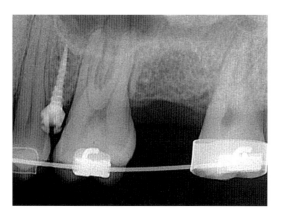

Figure 30.5 Radiograph showing a 1.5 mm diameter Infinitas mini-implant inserted buccally and interproximally between the maxillary second premolar and first molar teeth. This is being used for direct protraction of the third molar.

30.4). For clarity, it is worth explaining screw insertion behaviour: all bone screws are able to form a thread within the adjacent bone, i.e. they are self-tapping, but the addition of self-drilling properties entails more distinctive cutting (body) threads and a sharper body tip. These features frequently obviate the need for pre-drilling (except to perforate the dense mandibular cortex). Since mini-implants are by far the most commonly used bone anchorage devices the rest of this chapter will be restricted to them.

PARAMETERS AFFECTING BONE ANCHORAGE SUCCESS

Multiple publications, albeit mostly retrospective, reporting the results of large case series and published since the mid-2000s, indicate a consensus of approximately 80% and 90% mini-implant success rates for mandibular and maxillary alveolar insertions, respectively.[7–9] This is explained by relative differences between the jaws in terms of the density and thickness of the cortical plate, whereas the cancellous bone is much less influential. As such, it is apparent

that a mini-implant needs to engage a minimum of 1 mm thickness of cortical plate for primary (immediate) stability. However, if the insertion torque (the resistance encountered during insertion) is excessive then it is likely that secondary failure will occur because of ischaemic pressure effects on the adjacent alveolar bone.[10,11] At present, more research is needed to define the optimum range of clinical torque, especially for the latest range of self-drilling mini-implants.

Research also indicates that mini-implant success rates are better in sites with attached gingiva rather than mobile mucosa, probably because of less soft tissue inflammation and effects of tissue mobility.[12] Aside from patient anatomy, variations in success rates also occur in relation to different mini-implant design features (Figure 30.4), such that higher stability may be achieved with self-drilling (rather than pre-drilled) insertion, relatively larger body diameter (minimum 1.5 mm body diameter), conical (tapered) body shape and a relatively low head emergence profile (neck-to-body length ratio).[13]

MINI-IMPLANTS: CLINICAL STEPS

Mini-implant insertion techniques should aim for optimal use of the available interproximal bone volume, while avoiding adjacent anatomical structures such as adjacent dental roots, the naso-maxillary cavities and neurovascular tissues. In particular, close proximity to tooth roots is likely to contribute to reduced success rates, especially in the mandible.[14] However, several animal and clinical studies have provided clear reassurance that even when pilot drills or mini-implants have been used to directly traumatise the periodontal and root tissues, these heal without clinically detectable damage (in terms of loss of vitality, irreversible root resorption, ankylosis).[15] Therefore, the main reason to avoid root proximity is to maximise mini-implant success rates. This is achieved by careful planning, possibly the use of an insertion guidance stent, and oblique (rather than horizontal) insertion.[16]

Mini-implants are easily inserted under either local or topical anaesthesia. Crucially only the superficial soft tissues (gingiva/mucosa and periosteum) should be anaesthetised. This means that patient discomfort is minimised by the avoidance of a large anaesthetised area, yet after insertion pain levels are very low and analgesics seldom required after 24 hours.[5,6] Crucially, a profound 'deep' level of anaesthesia is actually counterproductive, since the patient's sensory feedback from the periodontal tissues can warn if the mini-implant begins to approximate the root of an adjacent tooth. Most mini-implants are inserted transmucosally, especially where the soft tissues are less than 1.5 mm thick, e.g. at the frequently used buccal site between the upper second premolar and first molar roots (Figures 30.5, 30.6). A manual insertion technique, using a customised screwdriver, is recommended for most insertions, although slow motor-driven insertion may be used, especially in palatal sites. Various forms of insertion guidance devices or stents have also been recommended to improve positional accuracy, especially where interproximal space is limited and/or surgical access is difficult.[13]

It is feasible to apply an orthodontic (unidirectional) force immediately after insertion, although it is commonly recommended that full force application be delayed for the first month, especially in adolescents (where there is a higher failure rate).[17] One of the great benefits of mini-implant anchorage is that forces may truly be applied in three dimensions, which particularly makes tooth intrusions much more achievable than with conventional treatment mechanics (Figure 30.7). In addition there is great flexibility in clinical application since it is possible to utilise both direct and indirect anchorage, where traction is applied to the mini-implant or anchor teeth are connected to form a stable unit, respectively. The orthodontist also has more control over both the timing and duration of force application, especially since there is frequently an option of 'resting' the mini-implant without loading.

Once the anchorage demand has abated, the mini-implant may be left *in situ* or removed. There have been no clinical case reports of mini-implant osseointegration, despite the experimental histological observation of areas of mini-implant and bone direct physical contact.[18] Consequently, explantation is frequently performed simply by unwinding the mini-implant, with the resultant defect healing uneventfully within days.

INTEGRATING BONE ANCHORAGE INTO ORTHODONTIC TREATMENT

Bone anchorage is easily integrated into fixed appliance treatments, but case selection and specific treatment planning considerations are important in order that the full benefits of both maximum and three-dimensional anchorage may be realised, yet biomechanical side effects

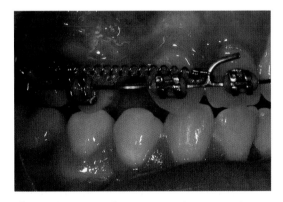

Figure 30.6 An Infinitas mini-implant inserted at an oblique angle (the body is more apical than the head) mesial to the upper right first molar. A coil spring has been attached to its head for direct retraction of the anterior teeth.

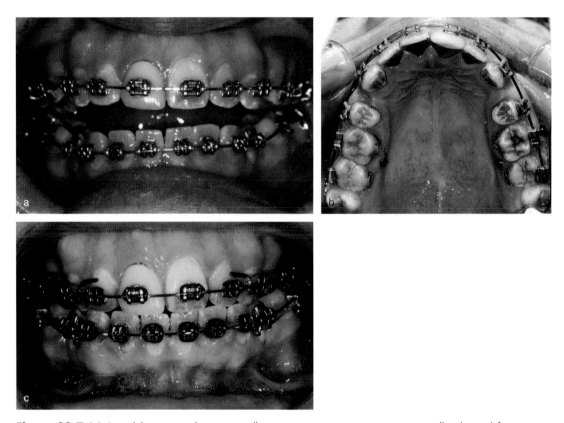

Figure 30.7 (a) An adult patient where a maxillary impaction osteotomy was originally planned for anterior open bite correction. (b) Instead, bilateral mini-implants were inserted on the palatal aspect of the maxillary alveolus and used to intrude the molars. The palatal view, after three months, shows movement of the molar crowns towards the mini-implant heads, and intrusion of the second molars relative to the third molars. (c) A positive overbite was achieved after 5 months of maxillary molar intrusion only.

minimised. Otherwise, unexpected movements may occur, e.g. the development of lateral open bites. While these can be resolved, it is preferable to avoid them in the first instance in normal or deep overbite cases. Conversely, molar intrusion is a key component of the treatment plan in anterior open bite cases. Therefore, on balance it is strongly advisable that treatment planning and the orthodontic treatment itself are both performed by an orthodontist. Who places the anchorage device is a different consideration. Mini-implants may be easily inserted by both dentists and orthodontists with a small amount of further training.

However, mini-plates should be placed by an oral surgeon with experience of maxillofacial plating.

References

1. Upadhyay M, Yadav S, Nagaraj K, Patil S. Treatment effects of mini-implants for en-masse retraction of anterior teeth in bialveolar dental protrusion patients: a randomized controlled trial. Am J Orthod Dentofacial Orthop 2008;134:18–29.
2. Wehrbein H, Feifel H, Diedrich P. Palatal implant anchorage reinforcement of poste-

rior teeth: a prospective study. Am J Orthod Dentofacial Orthop 1999;116:678–86.

3. Cousley R. Critical aspects in the use of orthodontic palatal implants. Am J Orthod Dentofacial Orthop 2005;127:723–9.

4. Cornelis MA, De Clerck HJ. Maxillary molar distalization with miniplates assessed on digital models: a prospective clinical trial. Am J Orthod Dentofacial Orthop 2007;132:373–7.

5. Kuroda S, Sugawara Y, Deguchi T, Kyung H, Takano-Yamamoto T. Clinical use of miniscrew implants as orthodontic anchorage: success rates and postoperative discomfort. Am J Orthod Dentofacial Orthop 2007;131:9–15.

6. Lee TCK, McGrath CPJ, Wong RWK, Rabie ABM. Patients' perceptions regarding microimplant as anchorage in orthodontics. Angle Orthod 2008;78;228–33.

7. Moon C, Lee D, Lee H, Im J, Baek S. Factors associated with the success rate of orthodontic miniscrews placed in the upper and lower posterior buccal region. Angle Orthod 2008;78:101–6.

8. Park H, Jeong S, Kwon O. Factors affecting the clinical success of screw implants used as orthodontic anchorage. Am J Orthod Dentofacial Orthop 2006;130:18–25.

9. Wiechmann D, Meyer U, Buchter A. Success rate of mini- and micro-implants used for orthodontic anchorage: a prospective clinical study. Clin Oral Implants Res 2007;18: 263–7.

10. Motoyoshi M, Hirabayashi M, Uemura M, Shimizu N. Recommended placement torque when tightening an orthodontic mini-implant. Clin Oral Implants Res 2006; 17:109–14.

11. Wilmes B, Rademacher C, Olthoff G, Drescher D. Parameters affecting primary stability of orthodontic mini-implants. J Orofac Orthop 2006;67:162–74.

12. Cheng SJ, Tseng IY, Lee JJ, Kok SH. A prospective study of the risk factors associated with failure of mini-implants used for orthodontic anchorage. Int J Oral Maxillofac Implants 2004;19:100–6.

13. Cousley RRJ. A stent-guided mini-implant system. J Clin Orthod 2009;43:403–7.

14. Kuroda S, Yamada K, Deguchi T, Hashimoto T, Kyung H, Takano-Yamamoto T. Root proximity is a major factor for screw failure in orthodontic anchorage. Am J Orthod Dentofacial Orthop 2007;131:S68–73.

15. Kadioglu O, Buyukyilmaz T, Zachrisson BU, Maino BG. Contact damage to root surfaces of premolars touching miniscrews during orthodontic treatment. Am J Orthod Dentofacial Orthop 2008;131:353–60.

16. Wilmes B, Su Y, Drescher D. Insertion angle impact on primary stability of orthodontic mini-implants. Angle Orthod 2008;78: 1065–70.

17. Motoyoshi M, Matsuoka M, Shimizu N. Application of orthodontic mini-implants in adolescents. Int J Oral Maxillofac Surg 2007;36:695–9.

18. Serra G, Morais LS, Elias CN, et al. Sequential bone healing of immediately loaded mini-implants. Am J Orthod Dentofacial Orthop 2008;134:44–52.

The straight wire appliance

INTRODUCTION

The straight wire appliance, also termed the pre-adjusted edgewise appliance, was originally described by Larry Andrews in 1976.[1] Over the following three decades this system revolutionised fixed orthodontic appliance treatment, due to the detail of design in the brackets and the associated reduction in archwire bending required by the orthodontist. The appliance is termed the **straight wire appliance** because of the minimal amount of archwire bending required. The angle at which the bracket slot is cut and the thickness of the bracket base determine the final tooth position.

The origins of fixed orthodontic appliance treatment date back to the turn of the 20th century with Edward Angle's appliance systems.[2] The original system went through several modifications culminating in the production of the edgewise appliance in 1928 (Table 31.1). Previous attempts at pre-adjusted systems have been described[3,4] and while these systems showed developments in bracket design with aspects of pre-programming, complexities

associated with their use prevented their widespread uptake. A classification of fixed appliance systems is outlined in Table 31.2.

The brackets used in fixed orthodontic appliances are usually composed of a base that fits onto the tooth surface, a slot on the outer surface into which the archwire fits, and some form of retaining item or tie-wing to allow the archwire to be held securely within the slot (Figure 31.1). The dimension of the bracket slot can vary depending on the appliance system used, however the majority of systems fall into either 0.018 inch or 0.022 inch slot sizes. These figures relate to the vertical height of the slot in thousandths of an inch, and the normal depth of these slots would be 0.025 inch or 0.028 inch, respectively. The 0.022 inch slot is the most commonly used worldwide and has the advantage that larger sized archwires can be used, which improves the control of tooth movement.

The forerunner to the straight wire appliance, the non-programmed standard edgewise fixed appliance system is designed to use identical or 'standard' brackets on each tooth. This

Orthodontics: Principles and Practice, First Edition. Edited by Daljit S. Gill, Farhad B. Naini.
© 2011 Daljit S. Gill, Farhad B. Naini and Dental Update. Published 2011 by Blackwell Publishing Ltd.

Table 31.1 Angle's developments in fixed appliance design

Appliance	Year of production
E-Arch	1887
Pin and tube	1910
Ribbon arch	1916
Edgewise	1928

Table 31.2 Classification of fixed appliance systems

Fully or part-programmed	Andrews' series (fully)
Non-programmed	Standard edgewise
Custom appliances	Incognito lingual appliance (individual tooth specific)
Semi-Custom appliances	Reversal of lower canine brackets to stop the canine tip in Class III incisor cases for camouflage orthodontics

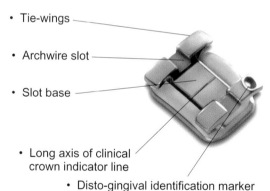

• Tie-wings

• Archwire slot

• Slot base

• Long axis of clinical crown indicator line

• Disto-gingival identification marker

Figure 31.1 Features of a pre-adjusted straight wire appliance bracket.

then requires bending of the archwire in three planes of space when orthodontically aligning teeth with the bends determining the final tooth position. Andrews' concerns in relation to this system centred around the time required to bend the respective archwires, as well as the difficulties faced in establishing an ideal occlusion at the end of appliance treatment. With the latter in mind, Andrews analysed study models of non-orthodontic ideal occlusions to ascertain any specific occlusal relationships present on these study models which should be accurately replicated at the completion of active orthodontic treatment. From the 120 non-orthodontic cases Andrews' analysed, he formulated the six keys to normal occlusion, which he published in 1972:[5]

• Class 1 molar relationship
• Correct crown angulation (tip)
• Correct crown inclination (torque)
• No rotations
• No spacing
• Flat occlusal plane.

To clarify how these untreated ideal occlusions differed from post-orthodontic treatment cases, Andrews analysed the models of 1150 post-orthodontic cases in the late 1960s. He concluded that if dental or skeletal relationships vary significantly from the norm or 'central tendency', one or more of these six keys may not be met even with the greatest clinical proficiency. Andrew's speculated that based on a normal distribution no more than 5% of patients would fall outside this population norm, however, this is quite a conservative estimate with the figure being nearer 20%. It should also be borne in mind that iatrogenic factors such as inaccurate bracket placement by the orthodontist, inappropriate treatment planning and mechanics, and poor patient compliance may prevent achievement of an ideal occlusion.

The advantages and disadvantages of this appliance system are listed in Table 31.3. There are three features that characterise the Andrew's straight wire appliance:

• Slot siting features
• Auxiliary features
• Convenience features.

Table 31.3 Advantages and disadvantages of the straight wire appliance

Advantages	Disadvantages
Reduced wire bending	Often requires minor wire adjustments
Sliding mechanics	Friction
Precision and finishing	Anchorage demands
Flexible biomechanics	Does not account for biological variation in tooth position
Multiple bracket designs	Multiple bracket designs

SLOT SITING FEATURES

The design features of a straight wire bracket are illustrated in Figure 31.1. To achieve a successful outcome with the use of a pre-adjusted appliance, one of the key factors is accuracy of bracket placement. The midpoint of the long axis of the clinical crown (LACC), which is known as the LA or FA point, is the central point on the surface of the crown of a tooth, onto which a straight wire appliance bracket should be located. For the straight wire appliance to function as initially designed, it is imperative that the centre of the bracket is placed on this point. In addition there must be a normal root and crown morphology to comply with the design of the appliance and achieve ideal objectives.

The compound contoured bracket base, as described by Andrews, allows ease of horizontal and vertical location of the straight wire brackets. It also minimises the need for additional bending of the archwire due to the torque values being built into this bracket base.

AUXILIARY FEATURES

With the straight wire appliance the prescription for the final angulation and inclination of each individual tooth is built into the respective bracket (as opposed to the entire bracket being angulated). This minimises any potential for rocking of the bracket when fitting the appliance. It also allows the tie-wings to be aligned parallel to each other and so again reduces the need for further archwire adjustment.

Andrews also incorporated a 10° molar offset in the upper molar attachments, which avoids the need for a molar offset to be placed in the archwire as in the standard edgewise appliance system. This integrated offset allows 'en masse' closure of spaces using a straight archwire, while ensuring the correct final occlusal relations of the first molar teeth.

The original bracket design described by Andrews uses power arms or hooks on the canine brackets to allow auxiliaries for space closure to be active closer to the centre of resistance of the teeth, i.e. approximately two-thirds along the height of the root length. This design feature is now less commonly used as the force application to the hooks often resulted in a degree of unwanted rotation and tipping of the canine itself, and hygiene around the hooks was compromised.

CONVENIENCE FEATURES

Each bracket also has an orientation marker, on the disto-gingival tie wing, and some of the current manufacturers etch number markings on this same tie-wing to clarify the tooth specificity for each bracket. The shape of individual brackets can facilitate the accuracy of their location on the tooth surface. With Andrews' design, as originally marketed through 'A company', the bracket shape has been contoured such that the sides of the brackets are parallel with the LACC for each tooth.

The factors of accuracy of bracket position and that of normal tooth-crown morphology may prove to be difficult to establish. Consistently exactly locating the LA point is not as accurate as Andrews initially presumed, and the latter point of root and crown morphology can vary, in particular for the upper lateral incisors. Therefore the concept of a true 'straight wire

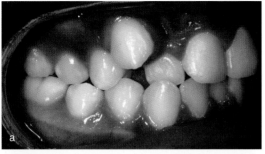
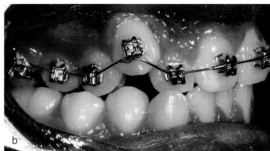
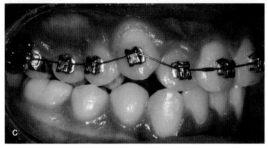

Figure 31.2a–c Stages of initial alignment.

appliance to produce an ideal occlusion may be unachievable in certain cases, and this is exemplified by the large number of variations in individual bracket prescription available today.[6]

Based on the difficulty of establishing an ideal occlusion at the completion of orthodontic treatment, Ronald Roth developed an appliance prescription[7] (the Roth prescription) with a degree of overcorrection to accommodate for the settling of teeth into non-orthodontic 'normal' positions after treatment. McLaughlin, Bennett and Trevisi also developed a prescription (MBT)[8] to improve clinical control and treatment efficiency.

STAGES OF TREATMENT IN THE USE OF THE STRAIGHT WIRE APPLIANCE

Level and Align the Dentition

In the initial phase of straight wire appliance treatment, the dentition is aligned commonly through the use of round 0.014 inch or 0.016 inch nickel-titanium archwires (Figure 31.2). Nickel-titanium has the advantage of superelasticity, which means that the wires deliver a constant force, and shape memory, which means that the wire will return to its pre-set shape. Anchorage (see Chapter 29) must be well controlled throughout treatment, but it is often particularly important during this alignment phase. This is in part due to the pre-programming of the brackets within the system, which tends to throw the teeth forwards. This aligning stage is routinely followed by levelling (i.e. lining up the bracket slots in the vertical dimension), if required, which is commenced using a 0.018 inch round stainless steel archwire. More recently, efficiency-based practice with the MBT philosophy has led to immediate progression from the aligning nickel titanium wire to a 0.018 inch × 0.025 inch rectangular nickel-titanium wire; thus omitting the round steel wire stage. Early progression to a rectangular wire helps to express torque, which determines the final inclination of teeth, and also facilitates progression onto a 0.019 × 0.025 inch stainless steel archwire.

Overbite and Overjet Reduction

The next phase in straight wire appliance treatment requires the use of rectangular stainless steel archwires (both 0.017 inch × 0.025 inch and 0.019 inch × 0.025 inch) to level the curve of Spee, which, based on Andrews' six keys, should be flat. Levelling of the curve of Spee helps to reduce the overbite, which permits full retraction of the upper incisors and space closure. Reduction of the overjet also takes place in the larger of these two rectangular wires and is often corrected as part of the space closure process.

Space Closure

In the main, spaces can be closed by one of two ways: either by using loop mechanics or most commonly with sliding mechanics. With the former the archwire has a closing loop bent into it, which is then activated once the wire is ligated. Loop mechanics was the mainstay of space closure in standard edgewise treatment. As the archwire is static when using closing loops, this process does not generate any significant frictional forces.

The most commonly used archwire for space closure is a 0.019 × 0.025 inch rectangular archwire within the 0.022 inch bracket. The fuller the dimension of the archwire, the greater the control of tooth movement during space closure. However, a degree of clearance between the archwire and bracket slot is required (0.022 − 0.019 = 0.03 thousandths of an inch) in order to reduce friction and permit the wire to slide through the bracket to allow space closure by sliding mechanics. This clearance, which is also termed 'slop', does reduce the control of tooth movement and particularly torque (inclination) control.

A number of different tools are available to the orthodontist to allow the closure of spaces using sliding mechanics. These can be employed within the same arch (intra-arch traction, Figure

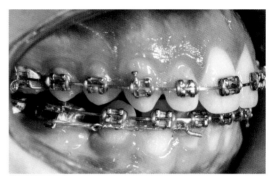

Figure 31.3 Space closure with intra-arch mechanics.

31.3) or from the maxillary to the mandibular arch (inter-arch traction). A drawback of sliding mechanics is that friction is generated between the archwire sliding through the bracket slots which necessitates higher space closing forces to overcome frictional resistance. Higher forces may make anchorage management more problematic as the anchor teeth are more likely to move. However, sliding mechanics do overcome the problem of bending complex loops into an archwire and the reduced flexibility of the archwire helps in better control of arch form. As always, anchorage control is a key element to achieving the final objectives of treatment (see Chapters 29 and 30). If anchorage is lost, it is not possible to correct the interincisal relationship fully.

Finishing

While the straight wire appliance was designed to avoid the need for wire bending, in reality some degree of finishing is frequently required, as indicated previously. This may be due to inaccurate bracket placement, a variation in tooth morphology or other desired variations in final tooth position. A light round stainless steel archwire, or a rectangular titanium-molybdenum alloy archwire, would be most frequently used in the finishing process. Alternatively, brackets can be repositioned on the incorrectly positioned teeth and a flexible nickel-titanium archwire can be used to achieve alignment.

MODIFICATIONS OF THE CLASSIC STRAIGHT WIRE APPLIANCE

The issue of frictional resistance and its impact on anchorage management is one of the drawbacks of the straight wire appliance system. The use of sliding mechanics, while allowing a straight wire to be maintained during space closure, also leads to the negative effect of friction developing between the archwire and the brackets, as the latter (which are most commonly held in by elastomeric ligatures) move along the archwire. The development of self-ligating brackets (see Chapter 32) has clearly assisted in reducing the impact of friction when sliding mechanics are employed.

The Tip-Edge appliance is also described in this textbook (see Chapter 33), and this particular low-force system (being the successor to the Begg appliance), has benefited from the incorporation of pre-programmed brackets. The stages of treatment and mechanics employed in Tip-Edge are, however, different from those followed with the conventional straight wire appliance.

This chapter has aimed to provide an oversight into the history and recent developments of the straight wire appliance, with a degree of insight into how the appliance works.

References

1. Andrews LF. The straight wire appliance. J Clin Orthod 1976;10:99–114, 170–95, 282–304, 360–79, 425–41, 507–29, 581–8.
2. Angle EH. Treatment of Malocclusion of the Teeth and Fractures of the Maxilla, Angle's System. SS White Dental Manufacturing Company, Philadelphia, 1900.
3. Steiner CC. Is there one best orthodontic appliance? Angle Orthod 1933;3:277–94.
4. Holdaway R. Bracket angulation as applied to the Edgewise appliance. Angle Orthod 1952;22:227–36.
5. Andrews LF. The 6 keys to normal occlusion. Am J Orthod 1972;63:296–309.
6. Metasa CG. Preadjusted appliance: one shoe fits all ? (Questioning the 'universality' of the prescriptions). Phoenix Without Arbor, April 1993.
7. Roth RH. Functional occlusion for the orthodontist, Parts 1–4. J Clin Orthod 1981;32–50, 100–23, 174–98, 246–66.
8. Bennett JC, McLaughlin KP. Orthodontic Management of the Dentition with the Preadjusted Appliance. Isis Medical Media, Oxford, 1997.

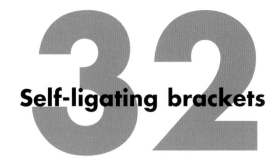

Self-ligating brackets

INTRODUCTION

Self-ligating brackets have an inbuilt labial face which can be opened and closed to retain and release engagement of the archwire. This labial face is usually metal but can be ceramic or plastic resin and is usually referred to as a clip or slide. Brackets incorporating their own ligation system have existed for a surprisingly long time in orthodontics but they have made a major impact in orthodontics only in the past decade. New designs continue to appear, with at least 20 new brackets since 2000. Several earlier designs had deficiencies, for example the clips or slides were too awkward to open and close or were prone to distortion or fracture or to inadvertent opening between visits. There are now some excellent self-ligating brackets available. Two popular and representative brackets are the Damon MX (Figure 32.1) and the In-Ovation (Figure 32.2). The author has a fairly wide range of experience of self-ligation, having used 15 types of such bracket since 1982 with exclusive use of self-ligating brackets since 1995. Claims for the advantages for such brackets have ranged from the straightforward

to the more surprising. A straightforward and easily tested claim is that these brackets are quicker to use than conventional ligation. A more thought-provoking and challenging claim is that self-ligation enables the low forces from the lips to influence the direction and extent of tooth movement during alignment. This chapter aims to briefly examine these claims and summarise the current and probable future place of self-ligation.

THE DEFICIENCIES OF CONVENTIONAL LIGATION

Conventional wire or elastomeric ligatures have significant failings. Wire ligatures are usually secure and robust but are very slow to place and remove. Studies[1,2] have shown that wire ligation is very slow compared to elastomerics with the use of wire ligatures adding almost 12 minutes to the time needed to remove and replace two archwires. This difference in speed of use is the largest and very understandable reason why so few wire ligatures are now used. Elastomeric ligatures, while being much

Orthodontics: Principles and Practice, First Edition. Edited by Daljit S. Gill, Farhad B. Naini.
© 2011 Daljit S. Gill, Farhad B. Naini and Dental Update. Published 2011 by Blackwell Publishing Ltd.

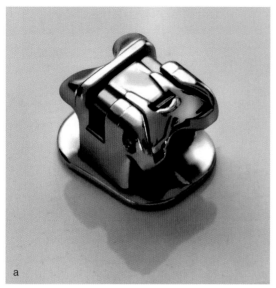

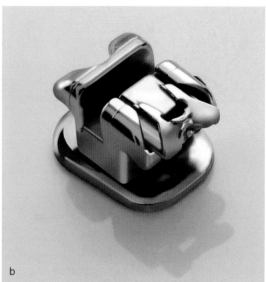

Figure 32.1a,b The Ormco Damon MX is a popular passive self-ligating bracket.

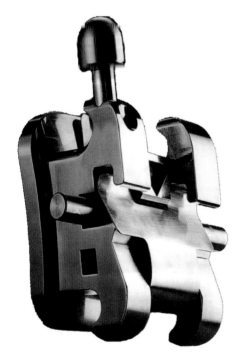

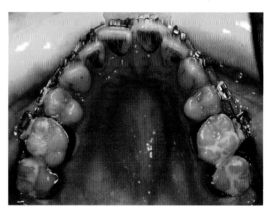

Figure 32.3 Failure of elastomeric ligatures to fully engage a 0.014 inch aligning wire on several brackets.

Figure 32.2 The GAC IN-Ovation bracket is a popular active self-ligating bracket. The flexible clip intrudes into the slot, decreasing its labiolingual dimension.

more rapid to place, have two inherent deficiencies, inadequate ligating performance and high friction. The force they provide decays with time and this can lead to loss of full archwire engagement and consequent loss of tooth alignment. The force decay of elastomerics has been well documented.[3,4] Figure 32.3 shows failure of elastomeric rings to achieve

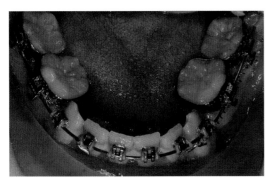

Figure 32.4 Failure of elastomerics ligatures to maintain full engagement on three of the six ligated teeth. This necessitated a backward step in treatment.

full archwire engagement and Figure 32.4 shows loss of control by elastomeric ligatures later in treatment. Elastomeric ligatures also have a high coefficient of friction, which inhibits the majority of desired tooth movements. Looking at other potential deficiencies, there is some reason to believe that elastomeric ligatures inhibit good oral hygiene, while the ends of wire ligatures can traumatise the oral mucosa.

CORE ADVANTAGES OF SELF-LIGATION

In the past two decades, a consensus has emerged on the potential core advantages of self-ligation. These address all the deficiencies of conventional ligation:

- More certain full archwire engagement
- Faster archwire removal and ligation
- Low friction between bracket and archwire
- Less chairside assistance required
- Better oral hygiene.

Self-ligating brackets vary in their capacity to reliably deliver these potential core advantages, but the best deliver on all of them. The first three advantages in the list can be considered proved beyond reasonable doubt, the fourth is

self-evident since no passing to and fro of ligatures is required and the last core advantage on the list is a tenable hypothesis but is not yet proven.

Secure, Full Archwire Engagement and Low Friction

A self-ligating clip or slide achieves and maintains full archwire engagement. The friction between bracket and archwire has been clearly demonstrated and quantified in many studies to be much lower with self ligation than with elastomerics.[2,5,6] This combination of very low friction and very secure full archwire engagement is currently only possible with self-ligating brackets and it uniquely enables teeth to slide along an archwire using much lower and more predictable forces and yet under complete control. This may be particularly beneficial in the alignment of very irregular teeth. It also reduces the need for extractions to create space for crowded teeth if that is the desired treatment goal (Figure 32.5).

Faster Ligation/Archwire Removal?

This is well supported by studies. Shivapuja and Berger[2] showed a large reduction in time required using SPEED brackets compared with wire ligation and a smaller but still significant reduction advantages (approximately 2 minutes per pair of archwires) compared with elastomeric ligation. Turnbull and Birnie[7] found very similar time savings with Damon2 brackets and it is very probable that more recent bracket types such as the Damon 3MX would show much greater savings in time for archwire changes because the mechanism is so easy and rapid even for a novice. An additional factor which should be remembered is that archwire changes using self-ligating brackets do not require a chairside assistant to speed the process, because self-ligating brackets require

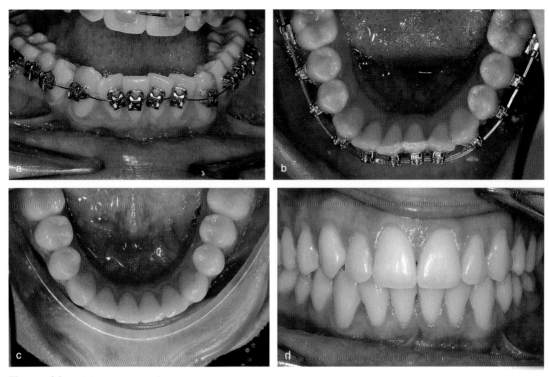

Figure 32.5 (a) A 0.012 inch wire fully engaged in spite of very small inter-bracket spans on crowded lower incisors. This wire were changed for a 0.018 inch archwire after 10 weeks. (b) 0.014 × 0.025 inch nickel-titanium wire fully engaged after a further 5 weeks at the third visit to complete the alignment. (c, d) Full resolution of the rotations and other irregularities.

no passing of elastomeric or wire ligatures to the operator.

Active or Passive Slide?

The part of a self-ligating bracket that retains the wire in the slot can be classified as active or passive. This is an issue which has attracted heated debate and some misunderstanding.[8,9] SPEED and In-Ovation, are examples of brackets which have a flexible spring clip that encroaches on the slot from the labial aspect, potentially placing an additional active force on the archwire. In contrast, Damon[10] and Vision LP are examples of passive brackets which have a slide that creates a rigid labial surface to the slot.

The principal intended benefit of an active clip is that a given wire will have its range of labiolingual action extended and produce more alignment than would a passive slide with the same wire. A consequence is that for a given archwire, the force applied to the tooth will be higher than with a passive bracket and with thicker wires, a lingually directed force will remain on the wire even when the wire is passive. An active clip therefore has higher friction. Hain et al.[11] and several other authors have demonstrated substantially lower friction with passive brackets and this may facilitate dissipation of binding forces and the ability of teeth to push each other aside as they align. A passive slide requires a slightly larger archwire to achieve full labiolingual and rotational control. The choice of an active clip or passive slide is also influenced by other related factors such as security of ligation or ease of use.

Does Self-ligation Deliver More Efficient Treatment?

The studies previously mentioned have demonstrated a definite and worthwhile saving in chairside time with self-ligation. It is also a firm clinical impression and a very tenable hypothesis that the combination of good tooth control and low friction will shorten treatment times and facilitate high-quality treatment. Several studies have investigated this suggestion. Three cohort studies with control groups[12-14] have found that self-ligation with earlier versions of Damon brackets was quicker, with fewer patient visits and good or better final alignment and occlusion than with conventional appliances used by the same operator/s. These were consecutive case series. However, more recent randomised controlled trials[15-17] have not confirmed these findings. It seems very probable that self-ligation does not confer a blanket advantage of more rapid treatment and that factors such as appointment interval, archwire sequence and case mix are also significant. Further studies are in progress with a variety of bracket types and this is a rapidly moving field of enquiry. It is certainly sensible to exploit the increased effectiveness of light forces and the better archwire control by starting mesiodistal tooth movement on lighter, more flexible wires and from the first visit in many instances. This may be expected to shorten treatment times (Figure 32.6).

Qualitative Differences in Tooth Movement with Self-Ligation?

A number of case reports, publications and lecture presentations have in recent years proposed additional clinical benefits deriving from the combination of the core advantages dis-cussed above.[18] Essentially, these reflect the belief that self-ligation – and particularly passive self-ligation – enables tooth-moving forces to be sufficiently light that forces from the soft tissues can compete with them and influence the resulting tooth movement. It has for example been proposed that the lips can restrain labial movement of the incisors and that the alignment of crowded teeth on a non-extraction basis will result in more lateral arch expansion and less labial incisor movement than would be the case with heavier forces and higher resistance to sliding. A large volume of research is in progress with this research technology. Figure 32.7 shows a case where very substantial alignment has occurred with light forces and without the significant labial movement of the incisors which might have been anticipated. This case underwent orthognathic treatment at a later stage and proclination of the upper incisors was contraindicated in that plan.

It has also been claimed that expansion brought about by such light forces is more likely to achieve an arch form which is in balance with the tongue and cheeks and can establish a wider arch that will be relatively stable because of altered tongue position. Such hypotheses have inconclusive research support or are yet to be formally investigated, but research is rapidly growing in these areas.

CONCLUSION

Self-ligating brackets have become reliable and several types are very easy to use. The core advantages of speed of use, security of archwire engagement and low friction are well documented in good research and in clinical use. These are reason enough to explain their very rapidly growing popularity. They undoubtedly expand the potential choice of treatment aims and treatment mechanics. The less intuitive claims concerning interaction with soft tissues are very interesting and starting to be thoroughly investigated, but are far from proven. The next few years will be of great interest in

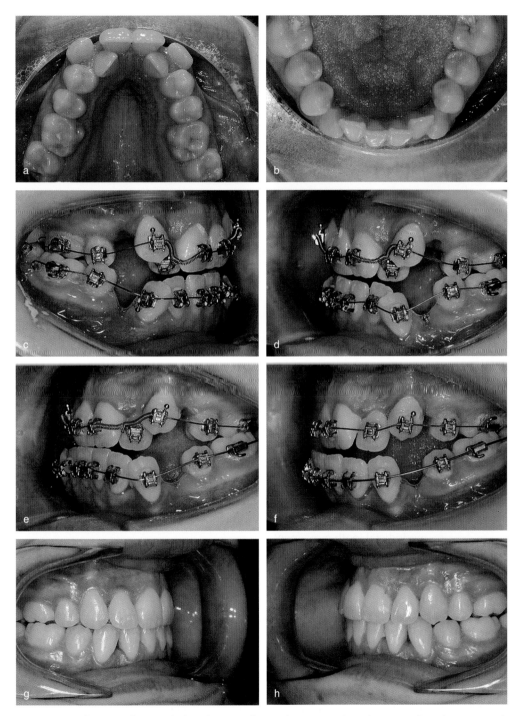

Figure 32.6 (a, b) Severely crowded arches. (c, d) Initial 0.014 inch archwires with coil springs to begin canine retraction from the first visit. (e, f) Second and third visits showing canine alignment with good rotational control. (g, h) End of active treatment. The anterior open bite was the principal reason for extractions.

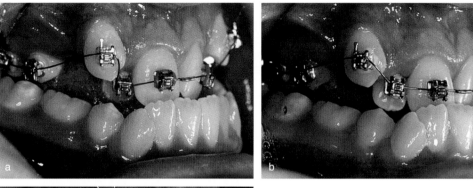

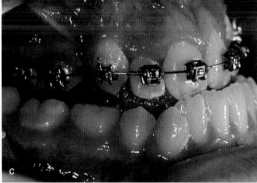

Figure 32.7 (a, b) Initial alignment with a 0.012 inch archwire causing little detectable incisor proclination. (c) Insertion of a 0.014 × 0.025 inch archwire after 16 weeks.

this area of orthodontics. It is very possible that self-ligation will soon become the conventional means of ligation.

References

1. Maijer R, Smith DC. Time saving with self-ligating brackets. J Clin Orthod 1990;24: 29–31.
2. Shivapuja PK, Berger J. A comparative study of conventional ligation and self-ligation bracket systems. Am J Orthod Dentofacial Orthop 1994;106:472–80.
3. Taloumis LJ, Smith TM, Hondrum SO, Lorton L. Force decay and deformation of orthodontic elastomeric ligatures. Am J Orthod Dentofacial Orthop 1997;111:1–11.
4. Eliades T, Bourauel C. Intraoral aging of orthodontic materials: the picture we miss and its clinical relevance. Am J Orthod Dentofacial Orthop 2005;127:403–12.
5. Thomas S, Birnie DJ, Sherriff M. A comparative in vitro study of the frictional characteristics of two types of self ligating brackets and two types of preadjusted edgewise brackets tied with elastomeric ligatures. Eur J Orthod 1998;20:589–96.
6. Thorstenson BS, Kusy RP. Resistance to sliding of self-ligating brackets versus conventional stainless steel twin brackets with second-order angulation in the dry and wet (saliva) states. Am J Orthod Dentofacial Orthop 2001;120:361–70.
7. Turnbull NR, Birnie DJ. Treatment efficiency of conventional versus self-ligating brackets: the effects of archwire size & material. Am J Orthod Dentofacial Orthop 2007;131:395–9.

8. Matasa CG. Self-engaging brackets: passive vs. active. Orthod Mater Insider 1996;9: 5–11.

9. Rinchuse DJ, Miles PG. Self-ligating brackets: Present and future. Am J Orthod Dentofacial Orthop 2007;132:216–22.

10. Damon DH. The rationale, evolution and clinical application of the self-ligating bracket. Clin Orthod Res 1998;1:52–61.

11. Hain M, Dhopatkar A, Rock P. A comparison of different ligation methods on friction. Am J Orthod Dentofacial Orthop 2006; 130:666–70.

12. Harradine NWT. Self-ligating brackets and treatment efficiency. Clin Orthod Res 2001;4:220–7.

13. Eberting JJ, Straja SR, Tuncay OC. Treatment time, outcome and patient satisfaction comparisons of Damon and conventional brackets. Clin Orthod Res 2001;4:228–34.

14. Tagawa D. The Damon system vs. conventional appliances: a comparative study. Clin Impressions 2006;15:1 9.

15. Miles PG. SmartClip versus conventional twin brackets for initial alignment: is there a difference? Austr Orthod J 2005;21: 123–7.

16. Miles PG, Weyant RJ, Rustveld L. A clinical trial of Damon 2 vs conventional twin brackets during initial alignment. Angle Orthod 2006;76:480–5.

17. Pandis N, Polychronopoulou A, Eliades T. Self-ligation vs. conventional brackets in the treatment of mandibular crowding: A prospective clinical trial of treatment duration and dental effects. Am J Orthod Dentofacial Orthop 2007;132:208–15.

18. Damon DH. Treatment of the face with biocompatible orthodontics. In: Graber TM, Vanarsdall RL, Vig KWL (eds) Orthodontics: Current Principles and Techniques. Elsevier/Mosby, St Louis, MO, 2005.

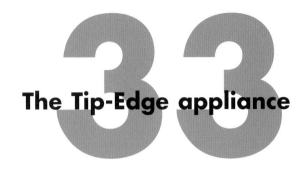

The Tip-Edge appliance

INTRODUCTION

A plethora of fixed appliances are available to orthodontists, many offering variations of specification and detail refinements, although the majority continue to be based on the edgewise or straight wire bracket. Tip-Edge Plus, however, exploits radical new thinking in many areas not seen before in orthodontics. A single chapter can be no more than introductory in nature and the reader is advised to obtain instruction in the technique before exploiting its many potential advantages over conventional bracket systems.

Tip-Edge is gaining worldwide recognition for its ability to handle difficult malocclusions beyond the expectation of established fixed appliances.

DERIVATION AND DESIGN

Tip-Edge is a relatively recent and highly innovative fixed appliance technique of great promise. It breaks much new ground in orthodontics, both in terms of speed of tooth movement and accuracy of finishing. However, the root of its thinking and the inspiration behind its development goes back to the former Begg appliance.[1] It was Dr Begg who first showed the extraordinary ease and rapidity with which teeth will respond to very light forces if allowed to tip during translation. Unfortunately, his primitive bracket and intricate means of uprighting the teeth to complete the case called for exceptional technique skills and was difficult to control. Nevertheless, Begg established the principle of 'differential tooth movement' – moving the crowns into corrected positions, by means of simple tipping, prior to uprighting the roots to the new crown positions. For reasons that we do not fully understand, teeth come with us much more willingly by this method than by bodily movement, which is imposed by the design of straight wire-derived bracket systems.

In fact, as a bracket, Tip-Edge is the son of edgewise rather than Begg, since it originated from a single straight wire bracket. Merely by

Orthodontics: Principles and Practice, First Edition. Edited by Daljit S. Gill, Farhad B. Naini.
© 2011 Daljit S. Gill, Farhad B. Naini and Dental Update. Published 2011 by Blackwell Publishing Ltd.

removing two opposite corners from a parallel archwire slot, Kesling[2,3] allowed free tipping in the desired direction. In Figure 33.1, the intact surfaces F are the finishing planes, while T are the tip limiting surfaces that prevent each tooth from tipping too far. CR are the central ridges against which torque will be developed later in treatment. An ingenious design feature is that these ridges are not directly opposed, but offset to the lateral of the midline. Because of this, the bracket has the unique property of increasing its vertical archwire space as the tooth tips during translation, from 0.022 inch up to a pos-

sible 0.028 inch, greatly speeding levelling and aligning, as well as reducing friction (Figure 33.2). The treatment sequence (upper right canine) is depicted in Figure 33.3. From the outset of treatment (A), the tooth tips distally, opening up the archwire slot (B). With the crown now in its corrected position, overall root uprighting commences (C), powered by a full arch nickel-titanium wire running through 'deep tunnels'. With a passive rectangular archwire in the main archwire slot, torque will be imparted as the tooth is untipped, so that when the finishing surfaces have closed into firm contact with the upper and lower flats of the rectangular archwire (D) both torque and tip will have been fully expressed. Impossible? Let us see how it goes in the mouth.

OUR PATIENT

The patient presented with a severely crowded Class II division 1 malocclusion with nearly 10 mm of overjet on the upper central incisors (Figure 33.4). Both lower lateral incisors are bodily displaced lingually with marked forward displacement of both lower canines and there is a supernumerary upper right lateral incisor. The overbite is increased and complete. With so much crowding, there are no prizes for guessing that four first premolars were the extractions of choice in this case (plus the supernumerary lateral incisor).

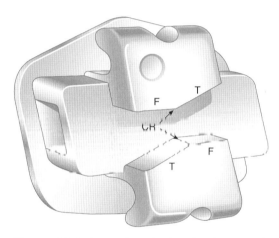

Figure 33.1 A Tip-Edge Plus bracket (upper right canine) showing the finishing surfaces (F), tip limiting surfaces (T) and central ridges (CR). Reproduced with permission from Elsevier.

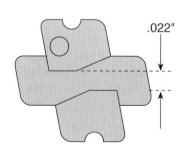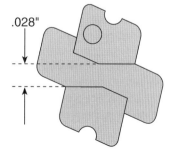

Figure 33.2 The archwire slot increases its vertical dimension from 0.020 inch (left) up to 0.028 inch (right) as the bracket tips during initial tooth translation. Reproduced with permission from Elsevier.

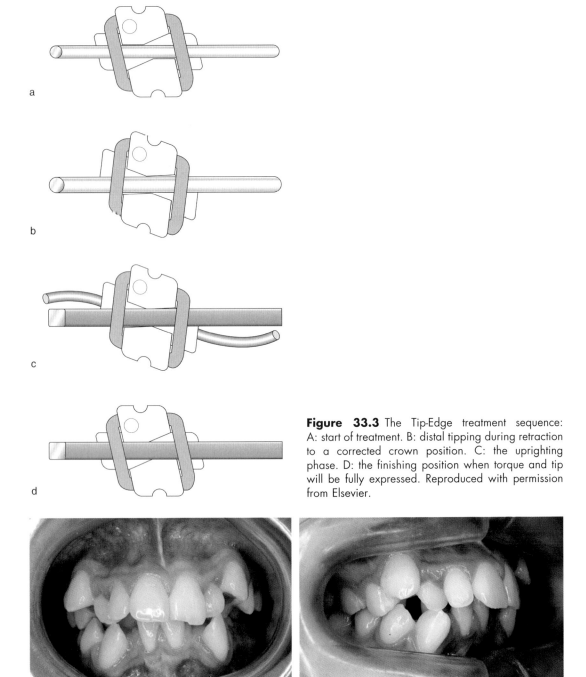

a

b

c

d

Figure 33.3 The Tip-Edge treatment sequence: A: start of treatment. B: distal tipping during retraction to a corrected crown position. C: the uprighting phase. D: the finishing position when torque and tip will be fully expressed. Reproduced with permission from Elsevier.

a

b

Figure 33.4a,b A severely crowded Class II division 1 malocclusion with nearly 10 mm of overjet. Reproduced with permission from Elsevier.

Stage I

Differential tooth movement requires three distinct stages of treatment, whatever the malocclusion. Stage I concerns the anterior segments: correction of crowding or spacing, overjet and overbite. One great advantage of Tip-Edge is that all three can be tackled simultaneously from the outset (Figure 33.5).

The main archwires are high-tensile stainless 0.016 inch round, with small vertical bends mesial to the molar tubes to prevent mesial migration of the first molars, concurrent with intrusion of the upper and lower anterior teeth. The premolars are by-passed so as not to interfere with the intrusive forces. The instanding incisors are ligated to an anterior sectional nickel-titanium 'underarch' running through the main archwire slots, while the overjet will be taken care of by very light (50 gm) Class II intermaxillary elastics. We are pitting bodily resistance of two lower molars against six upper anterior teeth, all of which are free to tip distally, therefore consuming very little anchorage. Freedom to tip is also the reason why canines do not need to be retracted first. Lower canines drift distally in natural response to the instanding incisors seeking space. This cannot happen with conventional brackets which, by their very design, impart bodily control from first engagement.

After only 3 months, the crowding, the overjet and the overbite, have all been corrected (Figure 33.6). The premolars are picked up in readiness for the next stage.

Stage II

This is generally the briefest stage, primarily concerned with closure of any residual spacing (Figure 33.7). High-tensile 0.020 inch stainless steel archwires are used, with horizontal elastomeric 'E-links' across the extraction spaces, from first molar hooks to the small circles (adjustable hooks) on the archwires mesial to the canines. Modest bite sweeps, as in the straight wire technique, prevent overbite recurrence.

Stage III – How Does it Work?

Stage III is the final phase, involving correction of torque and tip angles for each individual tooth to achieve the finishing prescription written into each bracket base. Recovery from such angles of tip would be extremely difficult with straight wire-type brackets, but with Tip-Edge has come an entirely revolutionary method of precision root movement,[4,5] which, particularly with the latest Plus version of the bracket, has become simple to use. Previously,

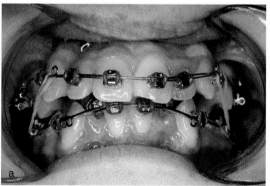

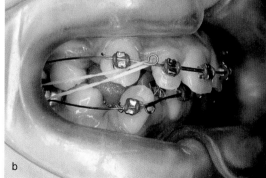

Figure 33.5a,b Stage 1 begins alignment of the anterior teeth, together with overjet and overbite reduction. Reproduced with permission from Elsevier.

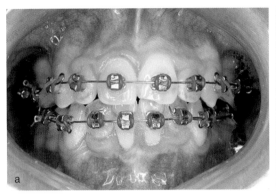
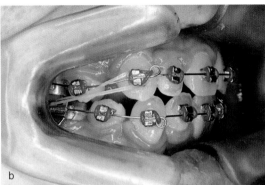

Figure 33.6a,b At 3 months, alignment, overjet and overbite reduction are already achieved. Reproduced with permission from Elsevier.

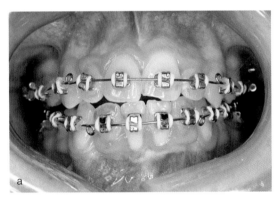
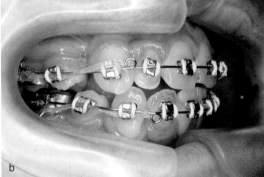

Figure 33.7a,b Stage II is required to close small residual extraction spaces. Reproduced with permission from Elsevier.

uprighting was performed by Side-Winder uprighting springs, one to each bracket, which was laborious. The Plus 'deep tunnel' system, which runs through the bracket bases, uses nickel-titanium uprighting instead of multiple springs. Because the tunnels have no labial access, they require to be threaded, which the flexibility of nickel-titanium readily allows. As can be seen from the left of the bracket illustrated in Figure 33.1, the entry and exit are funnel shaped to facilitate this. It can readily be visualised (Figure 33.8) that a 0.014 inch round nickel-titanium in the deep tunnels will exert an overall uprighting effect. But how can torque be delivered synchronously with tip by the action of this wire?

Refer back, if you will, to Figure 33.2. We are about to reverse the angle changes (right to left). By correcting tip to the new crown position, we are closing the vertical archwire space down again towards its 0.022 inch dimension. So it is that we fit a passive 0.0215×0.028 inch rectangular archwire (Figure 33.9) which goes in easily with the slots open at up to 0.028 inches. Now view the action down the long axis of the archwire (Figure 33.10). At A, the day of fitting, the oversize vertical slot dimension can accommodate up to approximately 14° of torque discrepancy in either direction without binding. However, as tip correction progresses, energised from the deep tunnels, two-point compression is achieved (B) denoted by the

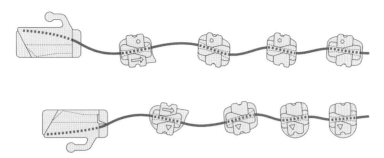

Figure 33.8 In Stage III, the levelling action of the underlying nickel-titanium archwire running through the deep tunnels can readily be visualised. It is essential that stainless steel main archwires be used simultaneously (see Figure 33.9). Reproduced with permission from Elsevier.

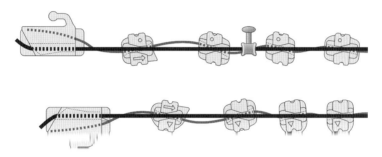

Figure 33.9 A Stage III passive 0.0215 × 0.028 inch stainless steel main archwire preserves arch stability and imparts full torque expression during tip correction. Reproduced with permission from Elsevier.

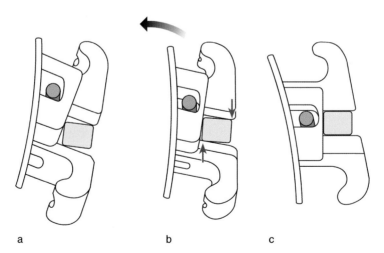

a   b   c

Figure 33.10 The interaction of the deep tunnel and main archwires viewed down the long axis of the archwires. A: initial placement of archwires. By B, the uprighting action of the deep tunnel wire is producing a torque reaction off the rectangular main archwire (see text) which is progressive until C, when torque and tip are fully expressed. Reproduced with permission from Elsevier.

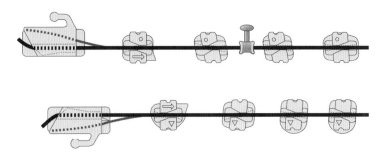

Figure 33.11 The action is self-limited with no residual 'torque slop' between bracket and main archwire. Reproduced with permission from Elsevier.

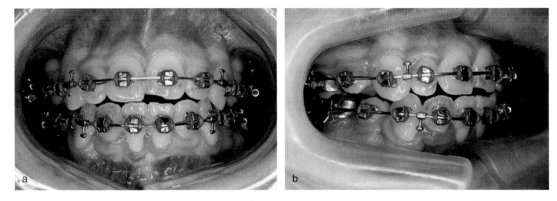

Figure 33.12a,b The start of Stage III, 7 months into treatment. Reproduced with permission from Elsevier.

small arrows, which induces a torque force as the vertical archwire space continues to reduce, until finally (C) the finishing surfaces of the slot are perfectly approximated to the archwire. The action is self-limited at this point (Figure 33.11). (The tunnels are slightly angled within the brackets to ensure adequate activation right up to the finish.) Unlike straight-wire, there is no remaining tolerance or torque slop between archwire and bracket. It should be noted that the heavy rectangular arch has a passive function. Each bracket becomes adapted to the archwire, instead of the archwire itself doing the work by being 'sprung' on insertion into a conventional bracket.

Stage III

Still only 7 months into treatment, the deep tunnels are threaded with full 0.014 inch

nickel-titanium archwires, before fitting the main 0.0215 × 0.028 inch archwires (Figure 33.12). Very little bite sweep is required in the latter, as the overbite appears slightly over corrected. Unusually, in order to preserve a full facial profile in this case, the passive rectangular wires incorporate some proclination at the front.

Frequently, visits during this final stage are no more than maintenance checks and 5 months of uprighting brings us to the finish (Figure 33.13). A small space distal to the upper lateral incisor has been maintained to allow augmentation of its rather small crown. Active treatment has taken only 13 months. A comparison of Figure 33.14a and 33.14b illustrates the improvement in aesthetics, and the treatment changes are shown in the superimposed profile tracings (Figure 33.15).

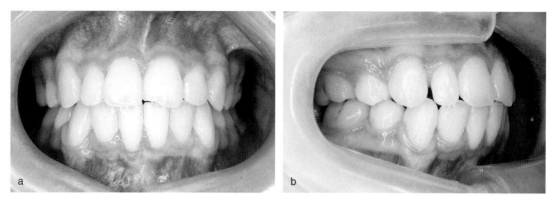

Figure 33.13a,b After 5 months in Stage III and 13 months of active treatment, the case is complete. Reproduced with permission from Elsevier.

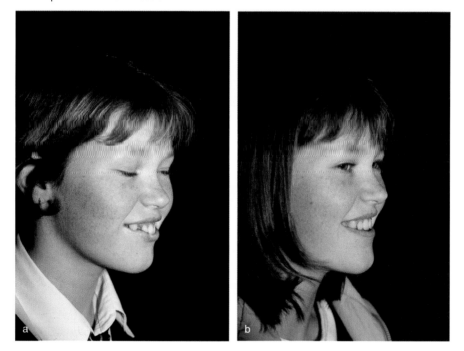

Figure 33.14 Facial views (a) before and (b) after treatment. Reproduced with permission from Elsevier.

Tip-Edge Versatility

A single chapter cannot illustrate the flexibility and the many treatment options that become possible with Tip-Edge. The appliance has proved itself effective in all categories of malocclusion, with or without extraction, although its benefits are perhaps seen to best advantage in the deep bite cases and big overjets, where arguably straight wire appliances are least convincing. For example, Figure 33.16 shows a 12 mm overjet treated with upper first and lower second premolar extractions in 1 year 5 months, without requiring headgear or implant anchorage. The Class II division 2 case in Figure 33.17, treated with four second premolar extractions, took 1 year 11 months, again powered only by very light Class 2 elastics. Class III cases, too, handle easily, even with complex reverse overjets. The case in Figure 33.18 took 1 year 8 months. Each of these three cases used only three main archwires in each arch – the usual number for Tip-Edge.

SUMMARY AND CONCLUSION

As with any appliance, expertise must be gained by experience before comparisons can be made. However, the treatment efficiency of Tip-Edge can be expected to compare favourably with conventional appliance systems.[6] In cases of simple non-extraction alignment, it may have few advantages over Siamese twin brackets beyond improved aesthetics. However, the more difficult the case – particularly in terms of tooth translation, big overjets and deep overbites – the more the advantages become apparent. Because the appliance is so light on anchorage,[7,8] it places less demand on both operator and patient, frequently resulting in better compliance and quicker treatment, particularly with the Plus bracket.

Because Tip-Edge Plus is radically different in its treatment progression from any conventional appliance, the reader is strongly advised to obtain instruction in its use before treating cases. The appliance is exclusive to TP Orthodontics, which will be pleased to advise on availability of courses. TP also produces the Tip-Edge Plus Guide,[9] while the author's textbook *Tip-Edge Orthodontics*,[10] published by Mosby, is now in its second edition, with the addition of the Plus bracket.

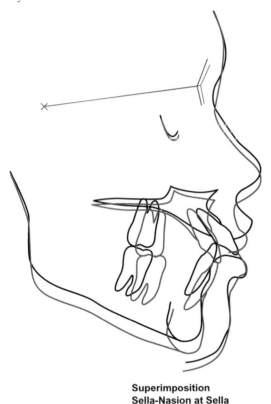

**Superimposition
Sella-Nasion at Sella**

Figure 33.15 Profile cephalometric tracings before and after treatment. Reproduced with permission from Elsevier.

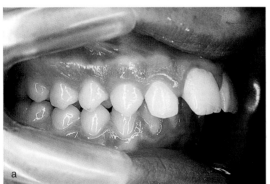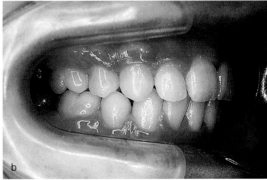

Figure 33.16a,b A 12 mm overjet treated in 17 months. Reproduced with permission from Elsevier.

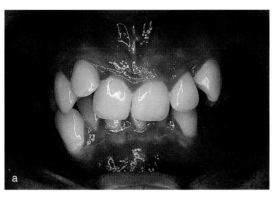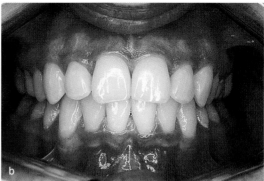

Figure 33.17a,b A severely crowded Class II division 2 case treated in 23 months. Reproduced with permission from Elsevier.

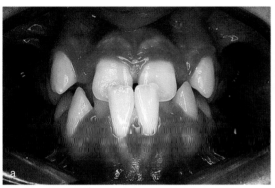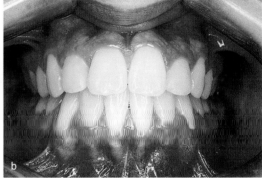

Figure 33.18a,b A crowded Class III case treated in 20 months. Reproduced with permission from Elsevier.

References

1. Begg PR. Light arch wire technique employing the principles of differential force. Am J Orthod 1961;47:30–48.
2. Kesling PC. Expanding the horizons of the edgewise arch wire slot. Am J Orthod 1988; 94:26–37.
3. Kesling PC. Dynamics of the Tip-Edge bracket. Am J Orthod 1989;96:16–28.
4. Parkhouse RC. Rectangular wire and third order torque: a new perspective. Am J Orthod 1998;113:421–30.
5. Parkhouse RC, Parkhouse PS. The 'Tip-Edge' torquing mechanism: a mathematical validation. Am J Orthod Dentofacial Orthop 2001;119:632–9.
6. Galicia-Ramos GA, Killiany DM, Kesling PC. A comparison of standard edgewise, preadjusted edgewise, and tip-edge in Class II extraction treatment. J Clin Orthod 2001;35:145–53.
7. Kesling CK. Differential anchorage and the edgewise appliance. J Clin Orthod 1994; 28:84–92.
8. Kesling CK. The Tip-Edge concept: eliminating unnecessary anchorage strain. J Clin Orthod 1992;26:165–78.
9. Kesling PC. Tip-Edge PLUS Guide and the Differential Straight-Arch Technique, 6th edn. TP Orthodontics, LaPlaza, IN.
10. Parkhouse RC. Tip-Edge Orthodontics and the Plus Bracket. Mosby, Edinburgh, 2003.

34
Clear aligners

INTRODUCTION

A number of clear aligner systems are on the market and a popular one in use today, which will be the focus of this chapter, is the Invisalign system. Although the concept of producing tooth movement using a removable tooth positioning device instead of conventional fixed appliances has been around since at least 1945,[1] it was not until Align Technology computerized the process in the late 1990s that it became practical to use the method for anything beyond minor tooth movement.[2] In order to accurately produce complex tooth movement with removable appliances, it is necessary to manufacture a series of patient casts with the teeth reset, each progressively incorporating a small amount of tooth movement until the teeth have been placed into their ideal position.[3] A series of tooth positioners, or aligners, are then fabricated from those casts.

PROCESS

As with any case requiring orthodontic treatment, the first step in the Invisalign process is to obtain diagnostic records. However, unlike treatment with conventional fixed appliances, impressions must be taken with poly-vinyl siloxane (PVS) due to its superior accuracy and stability.[4] The patient's impressions, PVS bite registration, photographs (both intraoral and extraoral) and radiographs are submitted to Align Technology in addition to the completed treatment form so that the fabrication process can begin. The PVS impressions and bite registration are scanned by computed tomography (CT) in order to create accurate three-dimensional digital models, registered in maximum intercuspation. The models are digitally processed by a technician using a software program that recognizes and removes artefacts. Technicians digitally separate the teeth and add gingiva around them.

Orthodontics: Principles and Practice, First Edition. Edited by Daljit S. Gill, Farhad B. Naini.
© 2011 Daljit S. Gill, Farhad B. Naini and Dental Update. Published 2011 by Blackwell Publishing Ltd.

A trained Invisalign computer technician then moves the teeth to their final positions in a series of stages according to the doctor's prescription. This preliminary plan is submitted to the doctor for approval in the form of a computerised movie that is downloaded from Invisalign's website and viewed via their ClinCheck software. Using the software, the doctor can communicate any additional instructions to the Align Technology technicians until they are satisfied with the progression of tooth movement and the final results.

Once the sequence and amount of tooth movement per stage are approved by the doctor, a series of casts are created using stereolithography, a three-dimensional printing process that makes a solid object from a computer image by using a computer-controlled laser to draw the shape of the object onto the surface of liquid plastic. The complete set of clear plastic aligners are made from these casts and sent directly to the doctor.[5] Each aligner is prescribed to be worn for 2 weeks and is only removed for eating, drinking, brushing and flossing.

INDICATIONS

Invisalign was developed when surveys showed that there was a huge potential adult market with unmet needs. Typically, adult orthodontic patients are apprehensive about the lack of aesthetics, difficult oral hygiene practices, pain and discomfort associated with conventional fixed appliances.[6] Some patients present with relapse from previous orthodontic treatment and do not want to undergo the same treatment again. The Invisalign appliance offers a removable, aesthetic alternative to patients with these concerns. Studies have demonstrated that patients treated with Invisalign have improved periodontal health[7] and experience less pain[8] than those treated with conventional fixed appliances. Composite attachments bonded to specific teeth may be required in order to accomplish certain tooth movements.

Invisalign has been used successfully to treat a variety of malocclusions, albeit some more successfully than others. In order to improve case selection for the expertise level of the practitioner, Align Technology has developed software that will evaluate the difficulty level of a case and will not allow a practitioner to treat beyond their capabilities without the proper experience and training. Specific clinical parameters are identified as being appropriate to be treated by practitioners with limited case experience (Table 34.1). Auxiliary appliances and advanced orthodontic techniques may be necessary if a case exceeds the beginner-level parameters listed.

Minor crowding can be alleviated by transverse expansion, interproximal reduction or by proclination of anterior teeth (Figure 34.1). As with most removable appliances, aligners are quite efficient at tipping movements. Space closure cases can be best managed with Invisalign if lingual tipping of incisors is acceptable as opposed to bodily retraction of these teeth (Figure 34.2). Lower incisor extraction cases are managed using vertical attachments on teeth adjacent to the extraction site to minimise tipping movements and aid in bodily movement (Figures 34.3, 34.4).[9] Deep bite correction can be achieved by absolute intrusion, using attachments on posterior teeth to aid in retention of the aligner whereas mild anterior open bite correction occurs by intrusion of the posterior teeth due to the thickness of the aligners. Posterior crossbite correction is facilitated by the slight disclusion of posterior teeth that occurs during aligner wear, eliminating any interference.[10] Invisalign can also be used in a multidisciplinary approach to prepare a patient with malaligned teeth to receive extensive fixed restorations (Figure 34.5).

Some types of case and/or tooth movement are difficult to achieve with Invisalign alone and are better treated in combination with sectional conventional fixed appliances before or

Table 34.1 Case complexity based on tooth movement and malocclusion type

	Individual tooth movements	Case types
Beginner	Canines/premolar rotations (<25°) Incisor rotations (25–40°) Posterior rotation (<20°) Relative extrusion Intrusion (1 mm per arch)	Mild crowding/spacing (0–3 mm) Narrow arches Mild to moderate deep bite (2–6 mm) Diastema closure (1–2 mm) Mild orthodontic relapse Individual anterior crossbite
Intermediate	Canine/premolar rotations (25–45°) Incisor rotations (40–55°) Posterior rotation (>20°) Pure extrusions (<1.5 mm) Translations (<3 mm) Intrusion (1–2 mm)	Moderate crowding/spacing (3–6 mm) Class II/III correction up to 3 mm Double tooth anterior crossbite Deep bite correction
Expert	Canine/premolar rotations (>45°) Incisor rotations (>55°) Pure extrusions (>1.5 mm) Translations (>3 mm) Intrusion (>2 mm)	Severe crowding/spacing (>6 mm) Extrusion of high canines Bicuspids extractions Posterior crossbite correction Class II/III correction >3 mm Surgical treatments Severe deep bite (>6 mm)

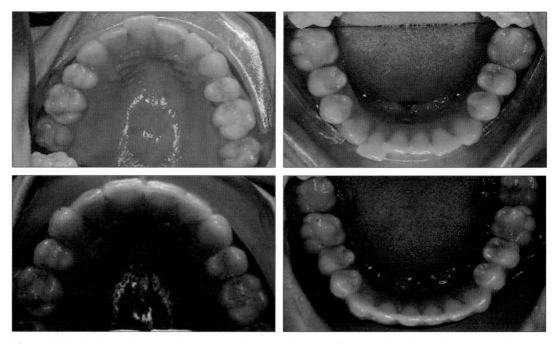

Figure 34.1 Patient presenting with minor crowding (top) alleviated after 6 months of Invisalign treatment (bottom).

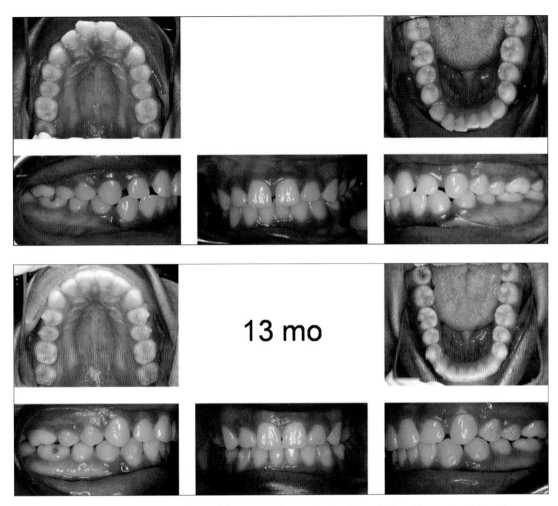

Figure 34.2 Patient presenting with need for space closure (top) achieved after 13 months of Invisalign treatment (bottom).

after aligner treatment. These include cases requiring root uprighting, as in premolar extraction cases, correction of severe rotations and extrusion.[9]

Invisalign Assist

Invisalign Assist was developed by Align Technology to provide product support for practitioners who want assistance making effective treatment choices that are consistent with their experience and comfort level (see www.aligntechinstitute.com). It helps the general practitioner select appropriate cases, keep the treatment on track and minimise failures. The first step in successful use of this product is selecting the right cases. A simplified prescription form is completed and the records

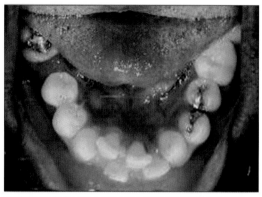

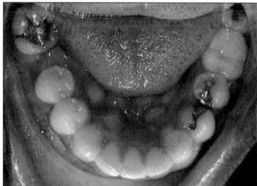

Figure 34.3 Alignment of lower incisor extraction case following 22 months of Invisalign treatment.

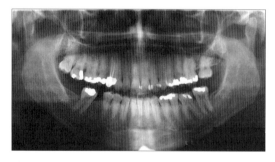

Figure 34.4 Panoramic radiograph showing good root alignment of lower incisors in a case treated with lower incisor extraction.

are submitted to Align Technology. Via a software tool, the case is reviewed to help determine if Invisalign Assist is the appropriate treatment option. The treatment plan should rely on the use of aligners only rather than utilising more complex orthodontics techniques and auxiliaries. If the chosen case does not fall within the product criteria, the practitioner has the option of treating the case with the standard Invisalign product, understanding that the use of auxiliaries and adjunctive therapy may be required. They also have the option of referring the case to a more experienced treatment provider or cancelling treatment.

A suggested task list for each patient appointment is included in this product, which provides additional resources to help the doctor prepare for each appointment, giving step-by-step instructions of what to do in each appointment (Figure 34.6). Invisalign Assist also has the benefit of helping treatment stay on track. About every eighteen weeks, the practitioner has the opportunity to send Align a new set of impressions to verify that the case is proceeding as expected via superimpositions of the patient's current impressions over the original approved treatment plan, verifying that the teeth are tracking with the aligners as planned. If necessary, adjustments are made to the next stage of the treatment and a new set of aligners are sent to the doctor.

CONCLUSION

Invisalign is an effective orthodontic treatment alternative which when used on the appropriate cases will result in excellent outcomes. Invisalign is *not* a product that simply runs through a computer which decides on patient treatment. Practitioners who decide to use Invisalign need to be knowledgeable in the basics of orthodontics for the best and consistent outcomes for their patients.

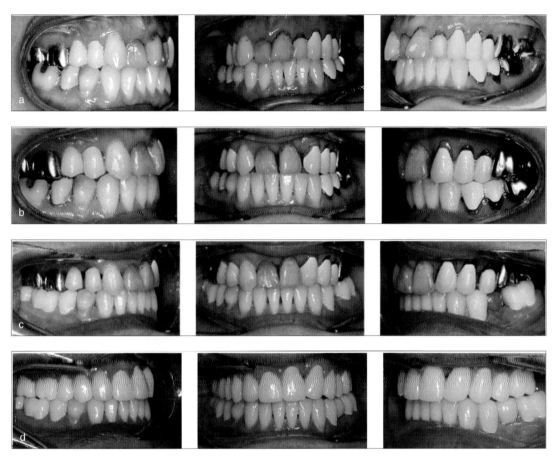

Figure 34.5 (a) Initial presentation. Treatment plan called for endodontic therapy, extraction of the upper left lateral incisor, orthodontic treatment with Invisalign initially followed by conventional fixed appliances for anterior alignment and referral to a general dentist for fixed restorations. (b) Presentation following 18 months of Invisalign. (c) Presentation following 6 months of fixed appliances. (d) Final presentation following delivery of fixed restorations.

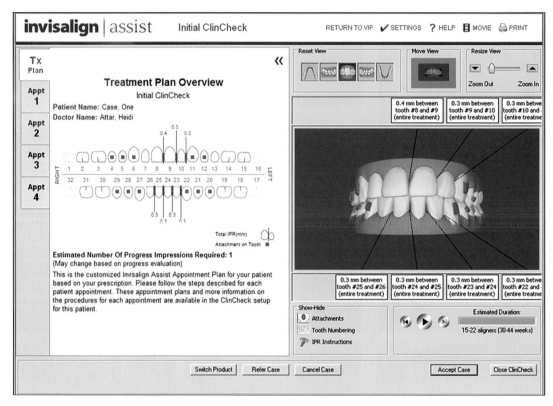

Figure 34.6 Example of the Invisalign Assist's ClinCheck and appointment plan.

References

1. Kesling HD. The philosophy of the tooth positioning appliance. Am J Orthod 1945;31:297–304.
2. Wong BH. Invisalign A to Z. Am J Orthod Dentofacial Orthop 2002;121:540–1.
3. Proffit WR, Fields HW. Contemporary Orthodontics. Mosby, St Louis, 2007.
4. Boyd RL, Miller RJ, Vlaskalic V. The Invisalign system in adult orthodontics: mild crowding and space closure cases. J Clin Orthod 2000;34:203–12.
5. Kuo E, Miller RJ. Automated custom-manufacturing technology in orthodontics. Am J Orthod Dentofacial Orthop 2003;123:578–81.
6. Womack WR, Ahn JH, Ammari Z, Castillo A. A new approach to correction of crowding. Am J Orthod Dentofacial Orthop 2002;122:310–16.
7. Taylor MG, McGorray SP, Durrett S, et al. Effect of Invisalign aligners on periodontal tissues. J Dent Res 2003;82:1483.
8. Miller KB, McGorray SP, Womack R, et al. A comparison of treatment impacts between Invisalign aligner and fixed appliance therapy during the first week of treatment. Am J Orthod Dentofacial Orthop 2007;131: 302.e1–9.
9. Boyd RL, Vlaskalic V. Three-dimensional diagnosis and orthodontic treatment of complex malocclusions with the Invisalign appliance. Semin Orthod 2001;7(4):274–93.
10. Boyd RL. Complex orthodontic treatment using a new protocol for the Invisalign appliance. J Clin Orthod 2007;41:525–47.

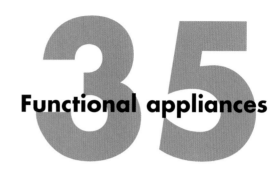

Functional appliances

WHAT ARE FUNCTIONAL APPLIANCES?

Functional appliances are removable or fixed orthodontic appliances that aim to utilise, eliminate or guide the forces arising from muscle function, tooth eruption and growth in order to alter skeletal and dental relationships. This chapter will be limited to the use of functional appliances in the treatment of Class II malocclusions. Without such treatment, most Class II cases remain unchanged or deteriorate. For example, among untreated pre-pubertal children with Class II malocclusion taking part in a randomised controlled clinical trial, only about one-third showed an improved sagittal jaw base relationship, as assessed by annual change in ANB angle; the relationship was unchanged in about half and worsened in one out of six children.[1]

The term 'functional appliance' is so named, because it was initially believed that altering muscle function can cause a change in growth response. Devices such as the fixed inclined anterior bite plane, posterior inclined planes attached to bands cemented onto posterior teeth and the original fixed functional appliance (Herbst appliance, Figure 35.1)[2] were described in a textbook 100 years ago.[1] In 1902, the monobloc appliance was devised to posture the mandible forward in babies born with severely retrognathic mandibles that compromised their airway. In the 1920s, Andresen used the same principle of posturing the mandible forward to treat malocclusions with his activator appliance.[3]

INDICATIONS AND DESIGNS OF FUNCTIONAL APPLIANCES

There are various indications and designs of functional appliances. The most common indication is to correct Class II malocclusion by posturing the mandible forward in growing patients in an attempt to utilise the individual's growth potential. The goal of this 'growth modification' is to change the anteroposterior occlusion between the upper and lower arches, and the procedure is often named the first-phase

Orthodontics: Principles and Practice, First Edition. Edited by Daljit S. Gill, Farhad B. Naini.
© 2011 Daljit S. Gill, Farhad B. Naini and Dental Update. Published 2011 by Blackwell Publishing Ltd.

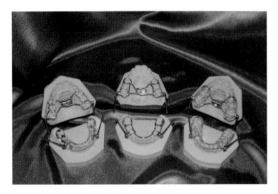

Figure 35.1 Herbst appliance, different designs. Reproduced with permission from Mr Wayne Robinson.

treatment. Because functional appliances cause some tilting of the teeth, part of the correction mediated by a functional appliance is actually attributable to this 'orthodontic camouflage', in addition to growth modification. If, after the first-phase treatment with a functional appliance, patients need further treatment to correct tooth irregularities and improve arch alignment, a second-phase treatment with a fixed appliance can be administered, with or without extractions. Some clinicians suggest that after the first phase of treatment there should be a period of retention with a functional appliance to consolidate the treatment results and stability. Finally, although functional appliances are primarily designed to treat Class II division 1 malocclusions, they can also be used to treat Class II division 2 malocclusions. Such treatment requires converting Class II division 2 incisor relationships to Class II division 1 relationships, to allow forward positioning of the mandible.

TIMING OF TREATMENT

Functional appliances should generally be used when patients are still growing so as to enhance the growth of the mandible. It has been suggested that treatment response is optimal during the pubertal growth spurt.[4] Accordingly,

standing height measurements, hand wrist radiographs, cervical vertebral maturation status and secondary sex characteristics have been advocated as tools to assess patients' maturity status and if the pubertal growth spurt has happened yet or is in progress. Studies have also shown that favourable treatment outcomes can be achieved before and after the pubertal growth spurt. However, very early treatment may be followed by relapse, and treatment that starts too late may decrease the skeletal treatment response.

In general, it is considered better to start functional appliance therapy in the late mixed dentition or early permanent dentition, as doing so will allow patients to progress to the second-phase treatment with a fixed appliance. This approach will also require less adjustment of the removable functional appliance so as to allow tooth exfoliation and eruption of the permanent teeth. In contrast, fixed functional appliances, such as the Herbst appliance, are usually used in the permanent dentition because the splint is cemented to the teeth. The Herbst appliance is primarily used during adolescence, but it can also be used in adults and has been demonstrated to be a valid alternative to surgical advancement of the mandible in adults with moderate mandibular retrognathism.[4] Nevertheless, early treatment with functional appliances to improve self-esteem is particularly important for patients who are being teased because their teeth are 'sticking out'.

TYPES OF FUNCTIONAL APPLIANCE

There are multiple classification systems of functional appliances. Functional appliances can be tissue-borne (e.g. the functional regulator),[5] or tooth-borne and active (twin block appliance; Figure 35.2)[6] or passive (Andresen appliance), and they may be removable or fixed.[4,7] They can also be myotonic with a wide mandibular opening (8–10 mm) and work by passive muscle stretching (e.g. Harvold activa-

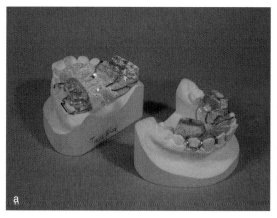
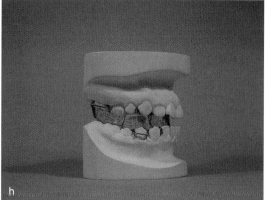

Figure 35.2a,b The twin block appliance. Reproduced with permission from Mr Wayne Robinson.

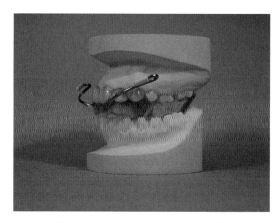

Figure 35.3 Headgear activator, van Beek style. Reproduced with permission from Mr Wayne Robinson.

tor),[8] or they can be myodynamic with moderate mandibular opening (<5mm) and work by stimulating muscle activity (e.g. Andresen activator).[3] The combined high-pull headgear activator attempts to enhance Class II correction by controlling both downward and forward maxillary growth (Figure 35.3).[9]

EFFECTS OF FUNCTIONAL APPLIANCES

When the mandible is postured, pressures are created by stretching of the muscles and soft tissues. These pressures are then transmitted to the dental arches and skeletal structures to produce dental effects (e.g. posterior movement of the upper teeth and anterior movement of the lower teeth) and skeletal effects (e.g. restriction of maxillary growth and enhancement of mandibular growth). Results of animal experiments seem to support that substantial changes in the skeletal structure, including condylar growth, remodelling of the glenoid fossa, mandibular growth and maxillary restraint, may be achieved with functional appliances.[10]

Clinically, the treatment effect is the treatment change after the natural growth change has been deducted. Most functional appliances have a statistically significant treatment effect on jaw base relationships, but the effects on prognathism of the maxilla and mandible are usually of small magnitude. After 12 months of treatment, the Andresen activator was found to have a restraining effect on the maxilla but no effect on the mandible,[11] whereas the bionator device had no effect on the maxilla and only a modest enhancement effect on the mandible.[1] In studies involving 18 months of treatment with the Harvold activator and the FRIII appliance,[12,13] and 12 months of treatment with the headgear-activator[9] with maximum mandibular advancement,[14] there were no significant treatment effects on the maxilla or mandible. By comparison, 12 months of treatment with the twin block appliance[15] and conventional Herbst appliance[16] had modest treatment effects on both jaws.

Effects of Stepwise Advancement of the Mandible

A noticeable effect on the mandible can be achieved after stepwise advancement of the mandible using the headgear activator, and an even more pronounced effect can result from 12 months of use of the headgear-Herbst appliance.[17] However, a study showed no difference in effect between gradual advancement and maximum advancement after 7 months of treatment with twin block appliances.[18]

DURATION OF TREATMENT

It has been suggested that the treatment time should not be less than 12 months, followed by a retention period of the same length, before the commencement of the second-phase treatment with a fixed appliance. Animal experiments have demonstrated that early removal of the bite-jumping device (brief treatment) leads to a period of sub-normal growth, whereas late removal (longer treatment) has a favourable outcome.

Choice of Retention Device

The choice of retention device after Herbst treatment has been shown to be critical. According to findings of clinical trials, the headgear-activator, which allows vertical control, maintains the new forward position of the mandible, whereas the Andresen activator's treatment effect vanishes within 6 months owing to the lack of vertical control.[19,20] High-pull headgear efficiently prevents downward growth of the maxilla and mandible, both

during active treatment and the immediate retention period.[20]

Long-term Effects

A follow-up study of 6 months of active treatment with the Herbst appliance revealed that mandibular growth was not normalised on a long-term basis despite immediate favourable growth changes.[4]

SUGGESTED TREATMENT PROTOCOL

There is a diverse range of opinion as to the best treatment approach with functional appliances. In this author's opinion the most predictable outcome in the treatment of Class II malocclusion is achieved with the following protocol.

1. Use of a non-compliant device, with stepwise advancement of the mandible over not less than 12 months when the patient's mandibular growth rate is high.
2. A retention period of a similar length using a device that maintains the new positioning of the mandible while mandibular growth rate is slowing down
3. Eventual treatment of the dental arches with a fixed appliance.

Vertical control of the first permanent molars is critical, and the use of miniscrews should be considered to avoid lengthening of the lower face. A preferred functional appliance is the splinted Herbst appliance with an expansion screw in the upper arch; tubes and brackets are attached to the splint to allow use of sectional archwires and brackets on the anterior teeth. Moreover, if extractions are needed to normalise the dental arch relationship, one should consider extracting the upper second molars during the functional appliance phase (especially if third molars are present), rather than commencing the second-phase treatment and extracting premolars. The use of the high-pull headgear is an efficient way of preventing enhanced downward positioning of the maxilla and mandible, both during active treatment and the immediate retention period.

References

1. Tulloch JF, Proffit WR, Phillips C. Influences on the outcome of early treatment for Class II malocclusion. Am J Orthod Dentofacial Orthop 1997;111:533–42.
2. Herbst E. Atlas und Grundriss der Zahnärztlichen Orthopädie. JF Lehmann's Verlag, München, 1910.
3. Andresen V, Haupl K. Funktionskieferorthopadie. Die Grundfagendes' norwegischen Systems. Herman Meusser Verlag, Leipzig, 1936.
4. Pancherz H, Ruf S. The Herbst appliance. Research-based clinical management. Quintessence Publishing, Berlin, 2000.
5. Frankel R. A functional approach to orotacial orthopaedics. Br J Orthod 1980;7:41–51.
6. Clark WJ. The twin block technique: A functional orthopedic appliance system, Am J Orthod Dentofacial Orthop 1988;93:1–18.
7. Proffit WR, Fields HW. Contemporary Orthodontics, 4th edn. Mosby, St. Louis, 2007.
8. Harvold EP. The Activator in Interceptive Orthodontics. Mosby, St. Louis, 1974.
9. van Beek H. Overjet correction by combined headgear and activator. Eur J Orthod 1982;4:279–90.
10. Peterson JE, McNamara JA. Temporomandibular joint adaptations associated with Herbst appliance treatment in juvenile rhesus monkeys (Macaca mulatta). Semin Orthod 2003;9:26–40.
11. Jacobsson SO, Paulin G. The influence of activator treatment on skeletal growth in Angle Class II: 1 cases. A roentgenocephlometric study. Eur J Orthod 1990;12:174–84.
12. Nelson C, Harkness M, Herbinson P. Mandibular changes during functional appliance treatment. Am J Orthod Dentofacial Orthop 1993;134:525–36.
13. Courtney M, Harkness M, Herbison P. Maxillary and cranial base changes during treatment with functional appliances. Am J Orthod Dentofacial Orthop 1996;109:616–24.
14. Wey MC, Bendeus M, Peng L, Hägg U, Rabie ABM, Robinson W. Stepwise advancement versus maximum jumping with headgear activator. Eur J Orthod 2008;29:283–93.
15. O'Brien K, Wright J, Conboy F, et al. Effectiveness of early orthodontic treatment with the twin-block appliance: a multicenter, randomized controlled trial. Part I: dental and skeletal effects. Am J Orthod Dentofacial Orthop 2003;124:128–37.
16. Du X, Hägg U, Rabike ABM. Effects of headgear Herbst and mandibular step-by-step advancement versus conventional Herbst appliance and maximal jumping of the mandible. Eur J Orthod 2002;24:167–74.
17. Hägg U, Rabie ABM, Bendeus M, et al. Condylar growth and mandibular positioning with stepwise versus maximum advancement. Am J Orthod Dentofacial Orthop 2008;134:525–36.
18. Banks P, Wright J, O'Brien K. Incremental versus maximum bite advancement during twin-block therapy: a randomized controlled clinical trial. Am J Orthod Dentofacial Orthop 2004;126:583–8.
19. Hägg U, Du X, Rabie ABM. Initial and late treatment effects of headgear-Herbst appliance with mandibular step-by-step advancement. Am J Orthod Dentofacial Orthop 2002;122:477–85.
20. Hägg U, Du X, Rabie ABM, Bendeus M. What does headgear add to Herbst treatment and retention? Sem Orthod 2003;9:57–66.

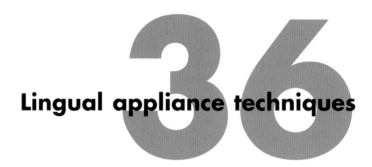

Lingual appliance techniques

INTRODUCTION

Lingual orthodontics was first introduced by K. Fujita in 1979[1] and C. Kurz in 1982.[2] J.C. Muir in 1991 reported that 'the technique is difficult to manage and should be used only by experienced orthodontists'.[3] Nowadays, this statement is not valid anymore, as state-of-the-art computer-assisted design/manufacture (CAD/CAM) technology, sophisticated laboratory procedures and detailed treatment protocols have transformed lingual orthodontics into a fully competitive treatment option. Now every orthodontist may treat as efficiently and successfully lingually as they do labially.

Lingual appliances considered sufficient for reliable orthodontic treatment consist of a bracket, wire and a laboratory process. By fully individualising all three components with the help of advanced computer and manufacturing technology, several major obstacles could be resolved, which in the past prevented lingual orthodontics from being regarded as a good treatment option. These were:

- Patient discomfort[4,5]
- Speech difficulties[6]
- Finishing and torque control (Figure 36.1a, b)
- Bonding and rebonding protocols were not easily implemented.

Much research has been carried out with respect to past problems: bonding and rebonding techniques,[7] laboratory[8] and clinical procedures,[9] patient comfort (Figure 36.1c)[10] and compliance,[11,12] through to comparing the forces and moments between labial and lingual orthodontics.[13] This has enabled the revolution of lingual appliance techniques.

There are many different lingual appliance systems in use. They differ according to the brackets, wires and level of laboratory complexity used. Only one lingual appliance is completely custom-made and this is Incognito.[14] Features such as fully individual bracket bases and bodies, custom-bent wires to compensate the different tooth thicknesses, and a laboratory procedure that incorporates the individualisation process into the bracket design itself,

Orthodontics: Principles and Practice, First Edition. Edited by Daljit S. Gill, Farhad B. Naini.
© 2011 Daljit S. Gill, Farhad B. Naini and Dental Update. Published 2011 by Blackwell Publishing Ltd.

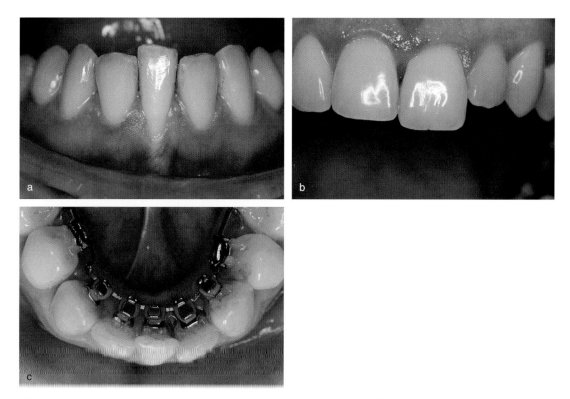

Figure 36.1 (a) Example of a torque control problem displaying itself as a vertical height discrepancy. (b) Torque control problem with upper incisors. (c) Non-customised lingual appliance, not flush to the tooth surface, adding to patient discomfort.

render Incognito extremely flat while maintaining the highest possible functionality This bespoke appliance enables every aspect of the patient's treatment to be taken into consideration and incorporated into the appliance while maximising speech adaptation and comfort.[15,16] Due to the computer-aided design and rapid prototyping manufacture, the appliance is capable of constantly evolving at unprecedented speed, being tailored therefore to both the patient and orthodontist.

A key component of successful lingual treatment is the precise calculation and manufacture of individual lingual archwires. The wire geometry is calculated in a CAD/CAM application and then sent to bending robots. Each wire in the sequence is fabricated to match the final set up of the teeth. Individual first order bends are

placed in all archwires necessary for treatment, from initial round superelastic, Nitinol (SE NiTi) arch wires, to stainless steel (SS) and full-size beta-titanium (TMA) archwires. In certain cases further three-dimensional correction values (e.g. extra torque or angulation) for specified teeth can be programmed into a separate TMA wire to facilitate finishing if necessary (Figure 36.2).

The precise individualisation of SE NiTi shape-memory materials reduces the number of archwires used in lingual treatment.[17] In contrast to the edgewise orientation of archwires known from fixed labial appliances, Incognito arch wires are used in a ribbon-wise configuration. A vertical slot insertion in the anterior region from canine to canine and a horizontal slot insertion in the lateral segments

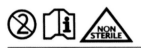

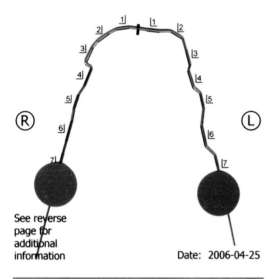

Customized **Upper** Archwire
0.0182" x 0.0182" TMA

See reverse page for additional information

Date: 2006-04-25

Figure 36.2 Three-dimensional correction values can be added to the TMA finishing wire, if needed, to simplify treatment.

is considered the optimum solution. A common archwire sequence for a non-extraction case is as follows: the wires have individual first-order bends in the lateral segments, the geometry is determined by the bracket configuration selected.

1. Initial wire: 0.014 inch SE NiTi
2. 0.016 × 0.022 inch SE NiTi
3. 0.0182 × 0.0182 inch TMA for finishing.

Elastics can be used with the TMA wire for a short time period; if elastic wear is more prolonged then a 0.016 × 0.024 inch SS is necessary before the finishing wire.

For an extraction case, the wires are straight in the lateral segment to allow for sliding during space closure in the posterior region:

1. Initial wire: 0.016 × 0.022 inch SE NiTi.
2. 0.016 × 0.024 inch SS for space closure and use of elastics if necessary.
3. In the upper arch a 0.016 × 0.024 inch SS with extra torque of 13° added to the wire in the anterior segment. This compensates for slot play when using an undersized wire during *en masse* retraction, elastic wear for long periods of time or when torque control is critical.
4. Finishing wire: 0.0182 × 0.0182 inch TMA, with individual first order bends in the lateral segment.

Another key factor for lingual orthodontics is optimal bracket positioning and slot precision.[18] Optimal bracket positioning has been developed using a laboratory procedure for indirect bonding. The Incognito system is a digitised system.[19] It uses a target set-up technique to facilitate the three-dimensional individualised positioning of brackets whilst allowing the brackets to be placed on the malocclusion model. A high resolution optical three-dimensional scanner permits non-contact scanning of the therapeutic set-up. It scans the set-up to generate a complete three-dimensional representation. This results is a three-dimensional digital representation of the teeth consisting of many thousands of minute triangles that can be observed and processed in the computer. Using CAD/CAM technology the model is aligned to ensure all the brackets slots are in the same plane. Each tooth is three-dimensionally assessed in order to create individualised bases to fit the lingual surfaces of the patient's teeth. Due to the high accuracy of the optical scan (minimum resolution: 20 μm) the bases mould precisely to the according lingual tooth surfaces. Large pad bases provide greater bond strength and allow for a direct rebonding procedure without the need of transfer trays or jigs in case of debonding. Once the bracket bases have been designed, the bracket bodies are selected and arranged using the software. The vertical height, angulation and torque are pre-set into each bracket so the need for maximum individuality is met and the patient's individual prescription is designed into the brackets. Only the first-order information is delivered via the archwire.

After bracket manufacture with the help of rapid prototyping technology, quality control steps in and ensures a slot tolerance of 0.0180–0.0183 inch (Incognito slot size is 0.018 × 0.025 inch). This is very important as variations in slot size affect torque control, which in turn affects the quality of the finish (Figure 36.1).

One of the outstanding features of Incognito is the ability to design and manufacture specific brackets to overcome anatomical limitations or to fulfil special requirements. For example, occlusal pads (Figure 36.3) can be used in deep bite cases to instantly improve the vertical dimension. With Incognito, vertical control, as in levelling the curve of Spee or controlling the overbite, is clinically more efficient than in edgewise labial or conventional lingual appliances because with a ribbon-wise configuration the big dimension of the archwire corrects the vertical plane.

Occlusal pads are essential in cases where a patient may have short clinical crown height, e.g. partially erupted teeth; this allows:

- Greater bonding surface area
- All teeth to be bonded at the same time rather than wait for full eruption of all teeth
- Treatment to commence immediately.

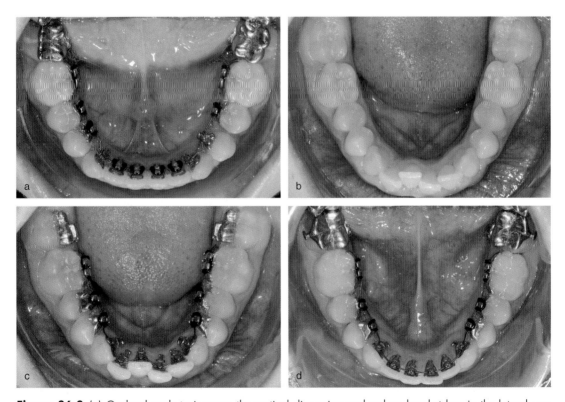

Figure 36.3 (a) Occlusal pads to improve the vertical dimension and reduce bracket loss in the lateral segments. (b) Patients with short clinical crown heights need a custom-made appliance so treatment can be commenced. (c, d) Half occlusal pads on the second molars, and occlusal pads on the first premolars and second right premolar, provide a greater bonding surface and all teeth can be bonded from the start.

Figure 36.3b displays a lower arch where a conventional lingual appliance could not be bonded due to partially erupted lower second molars and short clinical crown heights on the lower first premolars. As shown in Figure 36.3c this frequently observed limitation can easily be overcome with Incognito by using occlusal pads which are bonded to the second molars as well as the lower first premolars and second right premolar. The pads also help to prevent any premature contacts in the lateral segments, hence reducing bracket loss.

IMPACTED CANINES

Where a canine is impacted but the contralateral canine has erupted, a bracket for the unerupted canine can be made from the beginning of treatment by mirroring the image of the erupted canine. This avoids the need for having to take a mid-treatment impression and then ordering a new bracket (Figure 36.4).

Brackets in the lateral segments are designed with occlusal guides for direct rebonding. This 'positive lock' ensures that the brackets can only be seated into their correct position. In Figure 36.4b the left canine has been bonded directly and it can be seen that the bracket is easily placed as it can only fit in one position.

The same is true for all brackets as they curve to fit the shape of the respective lingual tooth surface so precisely, eliminating the problem associated with rebonding from the past.

To improve anchorage, control splints can be made to lock teeth together. Figure 36.5 shows two splints bonded on bridges extending from the first premolar to the first molar. Only the first premolars have bracket bodies and are incorporated on to the wire. Using the appropriate preparatory protocol for the respective artificial tooth surface, ceramic, gold, metal or composite, allows for a same time one step bond-up approach with a single tray.

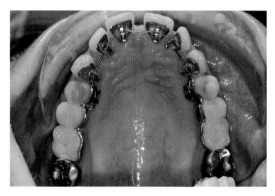

Figure 36.5 Splints from the first premolars to the first molars to improve anchorage control.

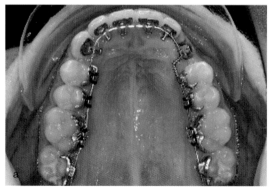 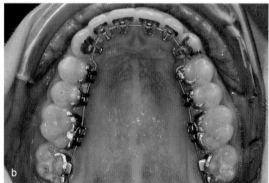

Figure 36.4 (a) Unerupted upper left canine. The bracket for it can be mirrored from the erupted upper right canine. (b) No need for mid-treatment impressions and delays in treatment time as the bracket can be bonded immediately. Fingers are placed on the bracket to help achieve the perfect bonding position.

SELF-LIGATION

Self-ligating slots have been designed to allow ease of placement of the first archwire and enable incorporation of all the teeth in crowded cases to maximise levelling and aligning in the initial stages of treatment. Self-ligating slots create a larger inter-bracket distance, thereby increasing the usable wire length and flexibility, hence all the teeth can be ligated. In combination with thin NiTi wires reduced friction forces of the self-ligation feature add another advantage as in more efficient initial alignment (Figure 36.6).

To aid clinical technique and reduce chairside time, for placement of power ties, grooves have been placed in the middle of the tie-wing of the upper and lower anterior segments (Figure 36.7a). A power tie is used to correct torque and angulation problems on both an under-sized and a full size archwire. It can be applied to anterior teeth when using a ribbonwise archwire in a slot with vertical insertion (Figure 36.7b).

Implementing today's state-of-the-art technology such as computer-aided design and rapid prototyping manufacture has achieved the creation of a new generation of lingual orthodontic appliances which overcome the core problems of conventional lingual appliances,

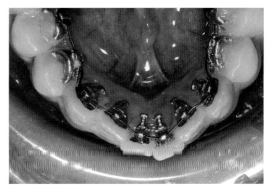

Figure 36.6 Self-ligating slots ease placement of the wire, reduce friction and create efficient initial alignment.

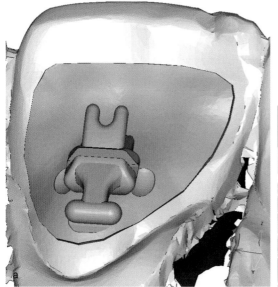

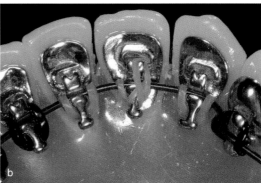

Figure 36.7 (a) To enable ease of placement of a power tie, a simple modification to the tie-wing creating a groove can be achieved with a custom-made appliance. (b) An example of a power tie to correct torque and angulation problems.

e.g. debonding and rebonding issues, patient discomfort and difficulties in finishing. Incognito provides maximum comfort for both the patient and the orthodontist by combining fully customised, intelligent design with high precision and maximum flatness, with exceptional clinical performance.

Lingual appliances can be used in combination with other devices, e.g. the Herbst appliance.[20] This is a fixed functional appliance for treatment of Class II malocclusions. It consists of a bilateral telescopic slide-out which is made up of a tube and plunger connecting the maxillary and mandibular dental arches with the mandible protruded. As the tubes are attached to the upper first molars and the plungers to the lower canines, custom-made upper first molar bands and lower canine bands with Herbst attachments are required.

CASE PRESENTATIONS

Case 1

An adolescent female presented with a Class II division 2 incisor relationship and Class II canine relationship a Class II skeletal base and a deep bite (Figure 36.8a–d). Figure 36.8e shows the Herbst attachments in place. Before the upper arch is bonded the upper first molar bands with Herbst attachments are tried in to ensure they fit well. They are not seated in the transfer tray but are bonded separately after the upper arch has been bonded. In the lower arch, standard brackets for the canines are used initially until the patient is nearly ready for the Herbst appliance to be fitted. The archwire sequence in a Herbst case differs from traditional lingual treatment as full size 0.018 × 0.025 inch SE NiTi and SS archwires are used. When the 0.018 × 0.025 inch SE NiTi is placed in the lower arch the canine brackets are removed and then replaced by bands with Herbst attachments. The wires are individual

in the lateral segments. The full size SE NiTi archwires prepare the arches for the insertion of the full size 0.018 × 0.025 inch SS archwires, which are the working wires during the whole bite correction phase. Therefore, the Herbst appliance is only fixed after the SS archwires have been placed in the upper and lower jaw.

Figure 36.8f and 36.8g show the SS archwires in place. Power chain is placed to ensure all spaces are closed and that spaces do not open up during the Herbst correction phase. It is possible that spaces occur distal to the lower canines and mesial to the upper first molars due to the forces from the Herbst appliance. The wires are turned back vertically instead of horizontally, distal to the second molars to prevent space opening. The patient postures up to an edge-to-edge relationship, (Figure 36.8h, i). Depending on the severity of the mandibular retrusion, further advancement is established later in treatment by adding activation rings in different millimetre sizes.

In children and adolescents the usual length of treatment time for the Herbst phase is 9 months and it is 12 months for adults. Once the Herbst appliance has been removed the lower canine attachments can be modified back to a normal bracket by removing the buccal aspect of the attachment. Class II elastics should be worn at night to maintain the Class II correction.

Figure 36.9a shows the patient's profile with the Herbst appliance *in situ*. Comparing with Figure 36.9b at the end of fixed appliance treatment, it can be noted that there has been a successful change in the patient's profile and occlusion (Figure 36.9c–e).

This case study shows the superior performance of a custom-made lingual appliance. It should be noted that only a small selection of different treatment stages are displayed for the case. Clinical appointments have occurred in between each treatment stage shown.

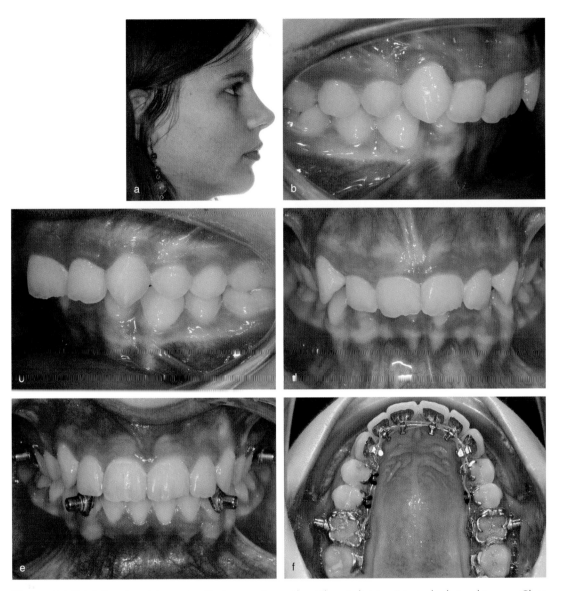

Figure 36.8 (a) Female adolescent patient presenting with a Class II division II incisal relationship on a Class II skeletal base; treatment with Herbst appliance was planned. (b–d) Pretreatment lateral and frontal views. (e) Herbst attachments on the upper first molars and lower canines. (f–g) Occlusal views of Herbst attachments on custom-made bands. (h) After levelling and aligning, in a full-size stainless steel wire, ready for Herbst appliance placement. (i) The Herbst appliance placed on attachments on the upper first molars and lower canines.

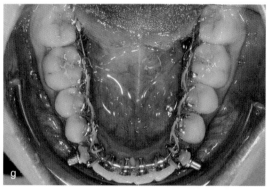

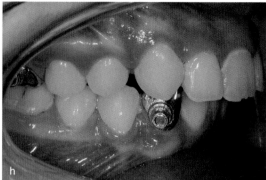

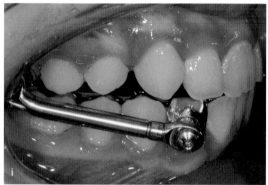

Figure 36.8 (Continued)

Case 2

An adolescent female presenting with a Class III skeletal base and increased lower anterior face height (Figure 36.10a–c). The malocclusion is Class III, complicated by an anterior crossbite involving the upper lateral and central incisors, which are retroclined (Figure 36.10d–h). The panoramic radiograph revealed heavily restored and decayed lower first molars with a radiolucent apical area in relation to the lower left first molar. The upper left second premolar was impacted. The lateral cephalogram confirmed the clinical findings (Figure 36.11a,b).

The treatment plan included extraction of the lower first molars, upper right first premolar and upper left second premolar. These teeth were extracted before treatment commenced. With the Incognito system, an indirect bonding protocol is used for the initial bond-up, extractions are usually only carried out after the appliance has been bonded. Any change in position of the teeth either side of the extraction site could prevent the tray from seating correctly. In this patient, the teeth had been extracted more than 1 year prior to treatment commencing so the occlusion was stable.

When looking at the bonded upper arch in Figure 36.12a, partial occlusal pads can be seen on the upper second molars with tubes. A 0.012 inch SE NiTi archwire was used in the upper arch to incorporate all the teeth. In the lower arch (Figure 36.12b), the initial archwire was a 0.014 inch SE NiTi. Tubing was placed between the second premolars and the second molars as the inter-bracket distance was large and the wire would have been uncomfortable for the patient.

The lower anterior region was relatively well aligned, so the archwire could be placed in the usual slots, but the lower second molars were bonded with brackets instead of tubes in place

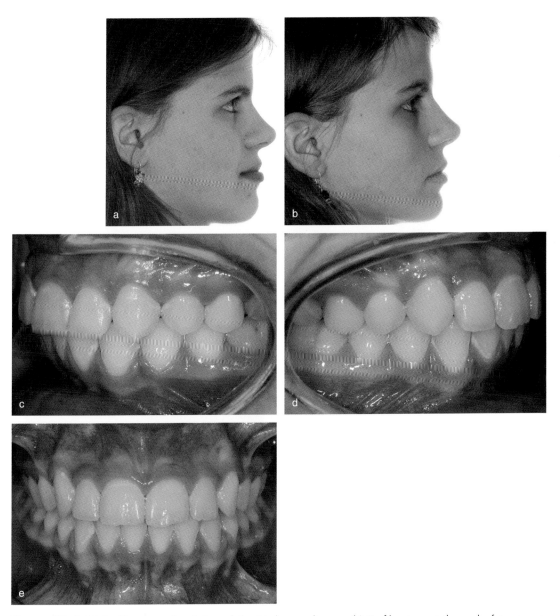

Figure 36.9 (a) Profile view after fitting of the Herbst appliance. (b) Profile view at the end of treatment. (c–e) The intraoral treatment result.

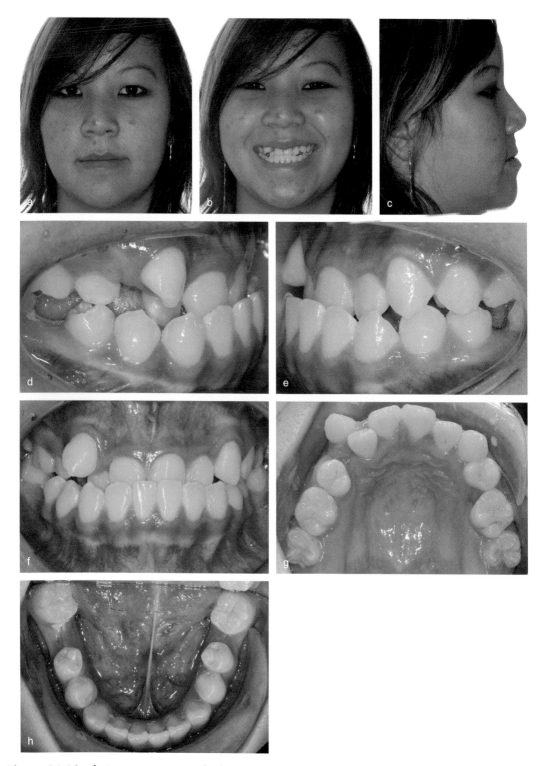

Figure 36.10a–h Pretreatment views of a female adolescent patient with a Class III skeletal base and a Class III malocclusion.

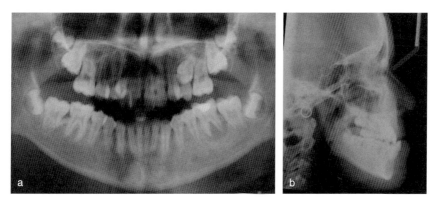

Figure 36.11a,b Pretreatment radiographs of the same patient as in Figure 36.10.

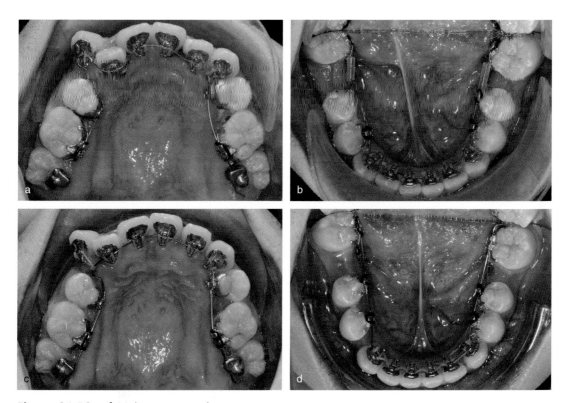

Figure 36.12a–d Mid-treatment mechanics.

(Figure 36.12d). This is because mesialisation of the second molar would have reduced the inter-bracket distance between this tooth and the second premolar, making it difficult to insert the wire into a tube. This would be further complicated if there was also a large first-order bend in the archwire to compensate for the difference in tooth thickness between the premolar and molar.

Usually in an extraction case, the initial archwire is a 0.016 × 0.022 inch NiTi and only the teeth that can be easily ligated on to the wire are incorporated, so as to prevent unwanted expansion and proclination. In Case 2, a round archwire incorporating all the teeth was used as proclination was required in the upper arch. In the lower arch the anterior segment was not crowded and the extractions were very distal, so unwanted tooth movement would not have occurred.

The first archwire change was to a 0.016 × 0.022 inch SE NiTi. In lingual orthodontics the majority of the mechanics required are carried out with this archwire in place. In extraction or non-extraction cases, usually three archwires are used for each arch. In the present case, in the upper arch (Figure 36.12c) the upper right canine was attached to the wire by a power chain to enable further alignment. The upper second premolar was ligated with a metal ligature to prevent the wire from slipping out. In the lower arch, a power chain was placed to gather the lower anterior segment. As the space to be closed between the lower left canine and lateral was small, a single module of power chain was used on the two teeth (Figure 36.12d).

Once the upper labial segment was aligned, power ties were placed from canine to canine to improve the torque control on an under-sized wire (Figure 36.13). With conventional orthodontics third-order problems unless severe are often undetected. With lingual appliances minor torque problems are apparent immediately and mainly appear as a vertical discrepancy. For example 10° of incorrect torque

will create about 1.2 mm of vertical height difference, which is already taking into consideration that this is with an extremely flat lingual appliance which is flush to the tooth surface. This will be noticed by both the patient and the orthodontist (Figure 36.1a,b).

For space closure, 0.016 × 0.024 inch SS archwires were used. In the upper arch the 0.016 × 0.024 inch SS archwire had extra torque of 13° from the upper canine to canine. Space closure was achieved using power chain running from the canines to the molars (Figure 36.14a, b). During space closure it may be necessary to use double cable mechanics. Double cable mechanics consist of two power chains, a transparent one running on the buccal side of the teeth and a grey one running on the lingual side. In this case, double cable mechanics were used in the lower right molar area as space closure was difficult and prolonged (Figure 36.14c).

The finishing archwires were 0.0182 × 0.0182 inch TMA. No finishing bends were required in this case (Figure 36.15a, b). Comparing Figure 36.15 with Figure 36.16, which shows the target set-up, it can be seen that the full Incognito prescription was achieved.

End of treatment records showed improved facial aesthetics (Figure 36.17), with a Class I canine and incisor relationship (Figure 36.18). To ensure excellent stability, in the upper arch a thermoplastic removable retainer was pro-

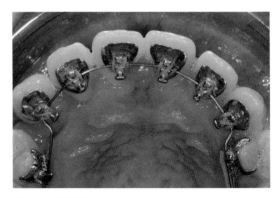

Figure 36.13 Power ties in place.

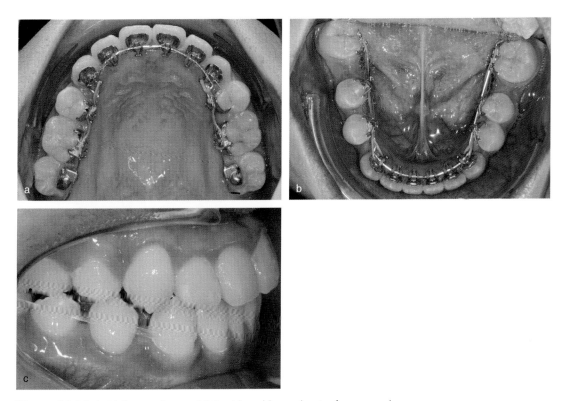

Figure 36.14 (a,b) Space closure. (c) Double cable mechanics for space closure.

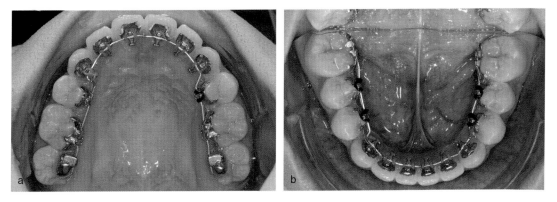

Figure 36.15a,b Finishing TMA wires with no finishing bends. Compare with Figure 36.16, the target set-up.

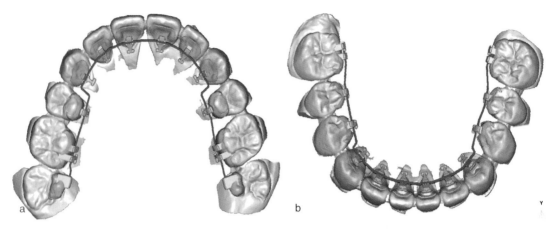

Figure 36.16 Planned set-up of (a) the upper arch and (b) the lower arch.

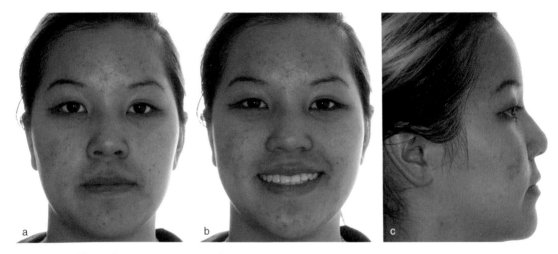

Figure 36.17a–c Post-treatment extraoral views.

vided because of the expansion achieved during treatment (Figure 36.19a). In the lower arch a bonded retainer was placed for life-long retention (Figure 36.19b). The post-treatment lateral cephalogram showed compensation of a Class III occlusion with maximum torque control of the lower incisors. The panoramic radiograph showed all spaces closed, parallel roots and sufficient space for the third molars to erupt (Figure 36.20).

The treatment time was 18 months.

CONCLUSION

No difference in treatment times have been observed with the use of labial and lingual orthodontic treatment techniques. Treatment goals and treatment planning are also identical. Lingual orthodontics may differ from labial orthodontics in certain areas of treatment mechanics or mechano-therapeutic aspects but the treatment results are the same. To be a good lingual orthodontist, time is required to learn

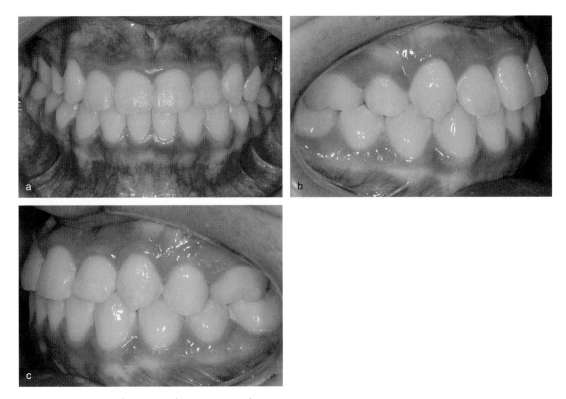

Figure 36.18a–c The intraoral treatment result.

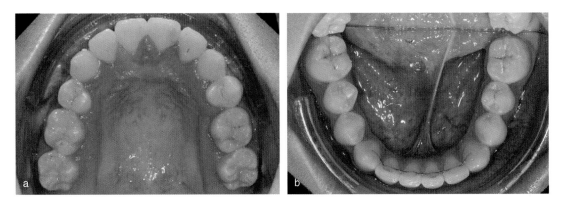

Figure 36.19 (a) Post-treatment upper occlusal view; no bonded retainer was used and a thermoplastic retainer was provided because of expansion during treatment. (b) The lower bonded retainer.

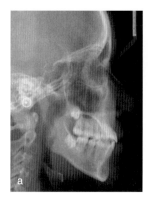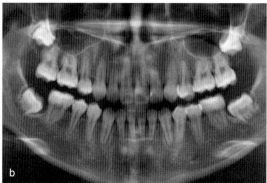

Figure 36.20a,b Post-treatment radiographs.

how to clinically treat patients. It is also important to appreciate the advantage of a custom-made lingual appliance that is extremely precise. Appliance customisation opens up the option for incorporation of special features to help achieve the best clinical results and eliminate many of the clinical problems associated with traditional lingual treatment. Not only does this improve clinical efficiency but it also maximises patient comfort. Advances in technology have allowed the refinement of lingual orthodontics and it is now a common treatment technique option for adults, adolescents and children.

References

1. Fujita K. New orthodontic treatment with lingual bracket mushroom arch wire appliance. Am J Orthod 1979;76(6):657–75.
2. Alexander CM, Alexander RG, Gorman JC, et al. Lingual orthodontics. A status report. J Clin Orthod 1982;16(4):255–62.
3. Muir JC. Lingual orthodontic appliances: invisible braces. N Z Dent J 1991;87(388): 57–9.
4. Hohoff A, Stamm T, Ehmer U. Comparison of the effect on oral discomfort of two positioning techniques with lingual brackets. Angle Orthod 2004;74(2):226–33.
5. Hohoff A, Fillion D, Stamm T, Goder G, Sauerland C, Ehmer U. Oral comfort, function and hygiene in patients with lingual brackets. A prospective longitudinal study. J Orofac Orthop 2003;64(5):359–71.
6. Hohoff A, Seifert E, Fillion D, Stamm T, Heinecke A, Ehmer U. Speech performance in lingual orthodontic patients measured by sonography and auditive analysis. Am J Orthod Dentofacial Orthop 2003;123(2): 146–5.
7. Wiechmann D. Lingual orthodontics (Part 3): Intraoral sandblasting and indirect bonding. J Orofac Orthop 2000;61(4): 280–91.
8. Wiechmann D. Lingual orthodontics (part 1): laboratory procedure. J Orofac Orthop 1999;60(5):371–9.
9. Wiechmann D. A new bracket system for lingual orthodontic treatment. Part 2: First clinical experiences and further development. J Orofac Orthop 2003;64(5):372–88.
10. Wiechmann D, Gerss J, Stamm T, Hohoff A. Prediction of oral discomfort and dysfunction in lingual orthodontics: a preliminary report. Am J Orthod Dentofacial Orthop 2008;133(3):359–64.
11. Hohoff A, Wiechmann D, Fillion D, Stamm T, Lippold C, Ehmer U. (2003). Evaluation of the parameters underlying the decision

by adult patients to opt for lingual therapy: an international comparison. J Orofac Orthop 2003;64(2):135–44.

12. Fritz U, Diedrich P, Wiechmann D. Lingual technique – patients' characteristics, motivation and acceptance. Interpretation of a retrospective survey. J Orofac Orthop 2002; 63(3):227–33.

13. Fuck LM, Wiechmann D, Drescher D. Comparison of the initial orthodontic force systems produced by a new lingual bracket system and a straight-wire appliance. J Orofac Orthop 2005;66(5):363–76.

14. Wiechmann D, Rummel V, Thalheim A, Simon JS, Wiechmann L. Customized brackets and archwires for lingual orthodontic treatment. Am J Orthod Dentofacial Orthop 2003;124(5):593–9.

15. Hohoff A, Stamm T, Goder G, Sauerland C, Ehmer U, Seifert E. Comparison of 3 bonded lingual appliances by auditive analysis and subjective assessment. Am J Orthod Dentofacial Orthop 2003;124(6):737–45.

16. Stamm T, Hohoff A, Ehmer U. A subjective comparison of two lingual bracket systems. Eur J Orthod 2005;27(4):420–6.

17. Wiechmann D. Lingual orthodontics (Part 4): Economic lingual treatment (ECO-lingual therapy). J Orofac Orthop 2000;61(5): 359–70.

18. Wiechmann D. A new bracket system for lingual orthodontic treatment. Part 1: Theoretical background and development. J Orofac Orthop 2002;63(3):234–45.

19. Mujagic M, Fauquet C, Galletti C, Palot C, Wiechmann D, Mah J. Digital design and manufacturing of the Lingualcare bracket system. J Clin Orthod 2005;39(6):375–82.

20. Wiechmann D, Schwestka-Polly R, Hohoff A. Herbst appliance in lingual orthodontics. Am J Orthod Dentofacial Orthop 2008;134(3):439–46.

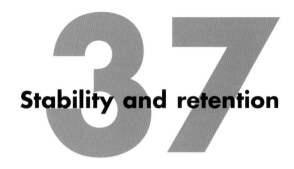

Stability and retention

INTRODUCTION

Relapse is perhaps the commonest risk of orthodontic treatment. Planning for post-treatment stability should be undertaken as part of the initial treatment plan and discussed with the patient as part of the consent process.

DEFINITION OF RELAPSE

Relapse has been officially defined by the British Standards Institute as the return, following correction, of the features of the original malocclusion.[1] However, post-treatment changes may not simply be a return towards the original malocclusion, but may also be movement caused by age changes and unrelated to the orthodontic treatment.

HOW STABLE IS ORTHODONTIC TREATMENT?

Relapse has always been recognised as a risk of orthodontic treatment, but the problem was highlighted in the 1980s with the publication of research following up cases 10 years after debond.[2] These were fixed appliance cases treated with extractions and retained with Hawley-type retainers for 1–2 years. After 10 years over 70% of cases had a severe need for re-treatment. The amount of observed relapse has differed between researchers,[3] which may be a reflection of different treatment techniques, different initial malocclusions and different retention regimens. However, the common finding in all these studies is the difficulty in identifying which cases will relapse and which will be stable. Indicators for stability have been particularly difficult to identify, with most cases having the potential for long-term relapse.

WHY DO ORTHODONTIC CASES RELAPSE?

There are a number of factors that can lead to relapse.[4]

Gingival and Periodontal Factors

Following tooth movement periodontal fibres need time to reorganise into the new position.

Orthodontics: Principles and Practice, First Edition. Edited by Daljit S. Gill, Farhad B. Naini.
© 2011 Daljit S. Gill, Farhad B. Naini and Dental Update. Published 2011 by Blackwell Publishing Ltd.

If orthodontic appliances are removed immediately and no retention used, then the fibres will tend to pull the tooth back towards its initial position. The collagen fibres within the periodontal ligament will take 3–4 months to remodel, but the elastic fibres – particularly those around the neck of the tooth, can take 8 months or more to remodel.[5] This is particularly a problem with rotated teeth. The orthodontist can reduce relapse caused by periodontal factors by ensuring teeth are maintained in their position long enough for the fibres to remodel. In rotated teeth the troublesome fibres around the neck of the teeth, the dentogingival and transseptal fibres, can be deliberately cut using a technique called 'pericision' (see Adjunctive Techniques to Enhance Retention).

Occlusal Factors

It has been suggested that the way teeth occlude may affect their stability. For example, after reducing an overbite it has been shown that the result will be more stable if the lower incisal edge lies anterior to the centre of the upper incisor root, known as the centroid.[6] Although it has been difficult to prove, it has been suggested that occlusions showing good interdigitation and vertically loaded teeth are more likely to be stable at the end of treatment. The orthodontist, with control of tooth positions, should be able to minimise relapse by controlling occlusal factors.

Soft Tissue Changes

The teeth lie in a zone of balance between the tongue lingually and the lips and cheeks buccally. Although the pressure from the tongue outweighs the pressure from the lips and cheeks, the teeth are maintained in a balance of equilibrium by the active metabolism of a healthy periodontal ligament. This equilibrium can be disturbed either by the teeth being moved out of this zone of stability, or by changes in the soft tissue pressures on the teeth. It is possible that with age the soft tissue pressures may change, which may lead to relapse.

Growth

Although the majority of growth is complete by the end of the late teens, there is potential for minor growth changes in the face and jaws throughout life. These changes are often unpredictable, but these subtle changes may be sufficient to affect the position of the teeth and the occlusion.

The orthodontist can influence the periodontal and occlusal factors. However, soft tissue and growth changes are unpredictable, and age changes are out of the control of the orthodontist. It is these latter factors that often account for the unpredictable long-term relapse that is sometimes observed after orthodontics.

RISK FACTORS FOR RELAPSE

There are certain features at the end of treatment, which are thought to be more prone to relapse (see Box 37.1). In these situations permanent fixed retainers are often required.

Third molars do not influence long-term stability. Prophylactic extraction of third molars as a means of preventing relapse of the lower labial segment is no longer recommended. Research

---

Box 37.1 Factors suggesting an increased risk of relapse

- Correction of severely rotated teeth
- Closure of diastema (or generalised spacing)
- Alteration of pretreatment lower arch form, particularly the intercanine width
- Excessive anteroposterior movement of the lower labial segment
- Correction of spacing secondary to adult periodontal disease
- Closure of anterior open bite
- Cleft lip and palate

has shown that their effect on the crowding of the lower labial segment is so small as to be clinically insignificant.[7]

CONSENT FOR ORTHODONTIC RETENTION

Clinicians must inform their patients of the risk of relapse and the unpredictable age changes that can occur in the long term. Patients can then choose to accept these late changes or be offered advice on the long-term wear of retainers to minimise the relapse. Patients should be advised to continue wearing retainers for as long as they wish to maintain straight teeth.

METHODS OF REDUCING RELAPSE AFTER TREATMENT

There is no agreed approach to reducing relapse after treatment[8] but this tends to involve:

* Retainers (removable or fixed)
* Adjunctive techniques to increase stability.

Removable retainers can be removed for cleaning and worn on a part-time basis. The long-term responsibility for reducing relapse is passed onto the patient who has to choose whether to wear the retainers or not. In contrast, fixed retainers will need long-term monitoring by a professional, but they have the advantage that the patient does not need to remember to wear them. They can also be useful when the result is very unstable (see Box 37.1) and for patients who cannot accept any relapse at all.

Removable Retainers

Except in cases with a high risk of relapse (Box 37.1), there is increasing evidence that removable retainers only need to be worn on a night-only basis. There are many different types, but

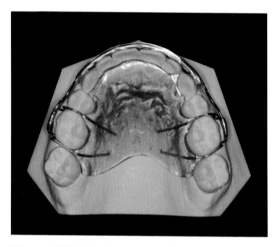

Figure 37.1 Hawley retainer. This Hawley retainer has been adapted – with acrylic facing over the labial bow – to improve stability. The patient had the upper first premolars extracted as part of their treatment, so the labial bow was soldered to the clasps on the first molars. This avoids wire work passing over the contact points between the canines and premolars, which could lead to relapse with the extraction space reopening after treatment.

the most popular are the Hawley and vacuum-formed retainers.

Hawley Retainer

The Hawley retainer was initially developed as an active removable appliance, but it was soon recognised that it makes an effective retainer (Figure 37.1). It is robust, with the capacity to maintain expansion and easily incorporate the addition of prosthetic teeth if required. It also allows greater 'settling' of teeth than vacuum-formed retainers.[9]

Vacuum-formed Retainers

The popularity of vacuum-formed retainers has increased in recent years (Figure 37.2). In comparison to Hawley retainers, at least in the short term, they are more cost-effective, preferred by patients and reduce relapse more effectively.[10,11]

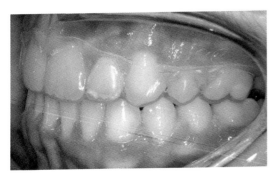

Figure 37.2 Vacuum-formed retainer. This vacuum-formed retainer is covering all the upper teeth. An area has been cut away over the gingival third of the upper canine teeth to allow the patient to more easily insert/remove the retainer.

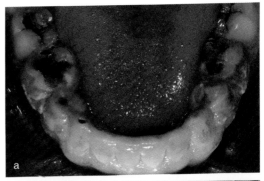

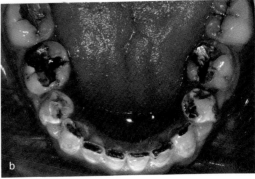

Vacuum-formed retainers are contraindicated in patients with poor oral hygiene. This is because this these retainers are retained by the plastic engaging the undercut gingival to the contact point. If the oral hygiene is poor, then hyperplastic gingivae can obliterate these areas of undercut.

Clear instructions are required to ensure the retainers are used safely and are effective. In particular it is important that patients do not eat or drink with the retainers in place, as they can act as a reservoir for the food and drink, which if cariogenic can severely damage the teeth (Figure 37.3).

Figure 37.3 Effects of a cariogenic diet when wearing a vacuum-formed retainer. It is vital that patients are instructed not to wear these retainers when eating or drinking. This patient wore a vacuum-formed retainer full-time (a), while regularly drinking fizzy drinks, leading to substantial tooth surface loss and caries (b). Photos courtesy of Jo Birdsall.

Fixed Retainers

Fixed or bonded retainers are usually attached to the palatal aspect of the upper or lower labial segment, using the usual acid-etch composite bonding technique. There are different types of bonded retainer:

- Multistrand stainless steel retainers bonded to each tooth (Figure 37.4)
- Special designed retainer chain (Figure 37.5)
- Rigid canine and canine retainers, which are only bonded to the canine teeth
- Reinforced fibres.

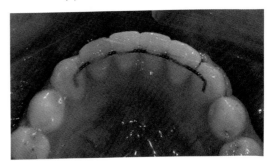

Figure 37.4 Multistrand bonded retainer.

The wires bonded to each tooth in the labial segment are the bonded retainer of choice. Retainers bonded only to the canines are associated with relapse of the incisors, and reinforced fibre retainers tend to fracture more frequently.[12]

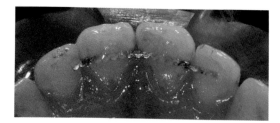

Figure 37.5 Ortho Flextech bonded retainer.

Bonding retainers is technique sensitive. The tooth surface should be thoroughly cleaned before bonding. A dry field must be maintained, and the wire held passively in position while bonding. Any active forces remaining in the wire can lead to unwanted tooth movement in the future.

Bonded retainers can be worn without causing long-term dental health problems;[13] however, the patient must maintain meticulous oral hygiene around the fixed retainer. This may involve threading floss under the wire below the contact points, or using small interdental brushes below the contact point (Figures 37.6, 37.7). The patient should be encouraged to regularly check that the retainer is in place – a disposable dental mirror can be useful for this.

Adjunctive Techniques to Enhance Retention

Adjunctive techniques include soft and hard tissue procedures to help enhance stability:

- Pericision
- Interdental stripping.

Pericision is also known as circumferential supracrestal fibrotomy. The principle is to cut the interdental and dento-gingival fibres above the level of the alveolar bone. It has been shown to be most effective in the maxilla, where it can reduce relapse by up to 30%.[14,15] There are no adverse effects on the periodontal health, provided there is no evidence of inflammation or

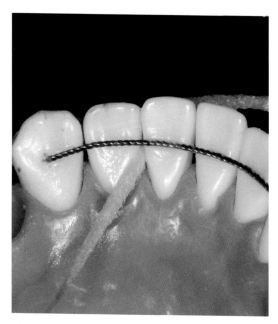

Figure 37.6 Superfloss used to maintain oral health around bonded retainer.

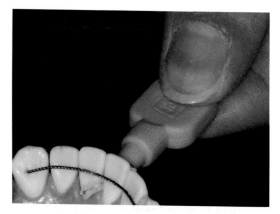

Figure 37.7 Interdental brush to maintain oral health around bonded retainer.

periodontal disease before the pericision. Undertaken under local anaesthesia, the fibres are cut around the neck of the tooth, without allowing the scalpel to touch the alveolar bone (Figure 37.8).

Enamel interproximal stripping, or reshaping of the interdental contacts is also known as

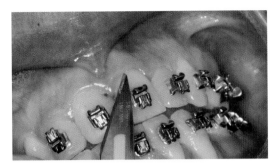

Figure 37.8 Pericision. The blade of the scalpel is placed vertically into the gingival sulcus, to cut the interdental and dento-gingival fibres around the neck of the tooth, just above the level of the alveolar bone.

reproximation. The theory is that flattening these contacts will increase the stability between adjacent teeth, although there is a lack of evidence to prove this.

LONG-TERM MAINTENANCE OF RETAINERS

It is the orthodontist's responsibility to ensure that the patient and their general dental practitioner are fully aware of how to look after the retainers in the long term, not only to ensure their effectiveness but also to reduce the risk of damage to the teeth and periodontium. Once a patient is discharged from the orthodontist, the general dental practitioner can keep the retainers under regular review. If problems arise the retainers can either be repaired, or the patient referred back to the orthodontist. It is therefore important to stress to patients that if they have problems with their retainer they should seek advice as soon as possible.

CONCLUSIONS

- Relapse after orthodontic treatment is unpredictable. It may be secondary to the treatment or due to age changes.
- Before treatment begins patients need to be informed about relapse and the need for

retention as part of the informed consent process.
- The patient must recognise their responsibilities in the retention phase of treatment.
- Fixed or removable retainers, in addition to adjunctive techniques, can be used to reduce relapse.

References

1. British Standards Institute. Glossary of Dental Terms (BS4492). BSI, London, 1983.
2. Little RM, Wallen TR, Reidel, RA. Stability and relapse of mandibular anterior alignment – first premolar extraction cases treated by traditional edgewise orthodontics. Am J Orthod 1981;80:349–65.
3. Littlewood SJ, Russell JR, Spencer RJ. Why do orthodontic cases relapse? Dent Update. In press.
4. Melrose C, Millet DT. Toward a perspective on orthodontic retention? Am J Orthod Dentofacial Orthop 1998;113:507–14.
5. Reitan K. Clinical and histologic observations on tooth movement during and after orthodontic treatment. Am J Orthod 1967;53:721–45.
6. Houston WJB. Incisor edge-centroid relationships and overbite depth. Eur J Orthod 1989;11:139–43.
7. Harradine NW, Pearson MH, Toth B. The effect of extraction of third molars on late lower incisor crowding: A randomised controlled trial. Br J Orthod 1998;25: 117–22.
8. Littlewood SJ, Millett DT, Doubleday B, Bearn DR, Worthington HV. Retention procedures for stabilising tooth position after treatment with orthodontic braces. Cochrane Database Syst Rev 2006;1: CD002283.
9. Sauget E, Covell DA Jr, Boero RP, Lieber WS. Comparison of occlusal contacts with use of Hawley and clear overlay retainers. Angle Orthod 1997;67:223–30.

10. Hichens L, Rowland H, Williams A, et al. Cost-effectiveness and patient satisfaction: Hawley and vacuum-formed retainers. Eur J Orthod 2007;29:372–8.

11. Rowland H, Hichens L, Williams A, et al. The effectiveness of Hawley and vacuum-formed retainers: A single-center randomized controlled trial. Am J Orthod Dentofacial Orthop 2007;132:730–7.

12. Rose E, Frucht S, Jonas IE. Clinical comparison of a multistranded wire and a direct-bonded polyethylene ribbon-reinforced resin composite used for lingual retention. Quintessence Int 2002;33:579–83.

13. Årtun J, Spadafora AT, Shapiro PA. A 3-year follow-up study of various types of orthodontic canine-to-canine retainers. Eur J Orthod 1997;19:501–9.

14. Edwards JG. A long-term prospective evaluation of the circumferential supracrestal fiberotomy in alleviating orthodontic relapse. Am J Orthod Dentofacial Orthop 1988;93:380–7.

15. Taner T, Haydar B, Kavuklu I, Korkmaz A. Short-term effects of fiberotomy on relapse of anterior crowding. Am J Orthod Dentofacial Orthop 2000;118:617–23.

Index

Orthodontics: Principles and Practice, First Edition. Edited by Daljit S. Gill, Farhad B. Naini.
© 2011 Daljit S. Gill, Farhad B. Naini and Dental Update. Published 2011 by Blackwell Publishing Ltd.